Clean Eating Made Simple

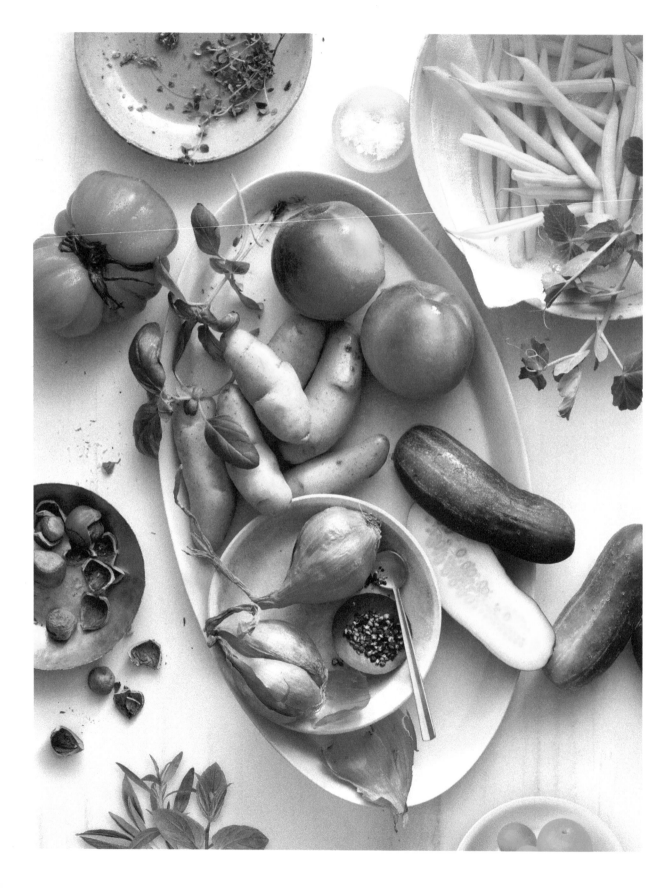

Clean Eating
Made Simple

A HEALTHY COOKBOOK WITH DELICIOUS
WHOLE-FOOD RECIPES FOR EATING CLEAN

ROCKRIDGE
PRESS

clean are key contributors to obesity. All the foods you eat—clean, healthy food—will fill you up and stop food cravings without adding empty calories to your body.

Decreased Risk of Cancer, Heart Disease, and Diabetes

Cancer, heart disease, and diabetes are the major causes of death around the world. These diseases can be prevented by diminishing their common risk factors, which include obesity, high blood pressure, high blood sugar, high cholesterol, and a sedentary lifestyle. All these risk factors are decreased when eating clean.

Improved Mood

Depression and mood disorders can have their roots in vitamin and nutrient deficiencies. Increased availability of vitamins and minerals through healthy eating can improve mood. Some whole foods also contain vitamins that help produce mood-elevating chemicals in the body, such as dopamine from vitamin B_6 contained in sunflower seeds and cooked tuna. Also, when you are energized and maintain a healthy weight, you will feel attractive and confident.

Prevention of Age-Related Ailments and Conditions

Many debilitating diseases associated with old age are preventable with healthy clean eating. No matter when you start eating clean (in your twenties, fifties, or even seventies), your body will respond by becoming the efficient machine it is meant to be. Providing the right fuel can keep joints lubricated and pain free, improve mobility, and help create a positive outlook well into the golden years.

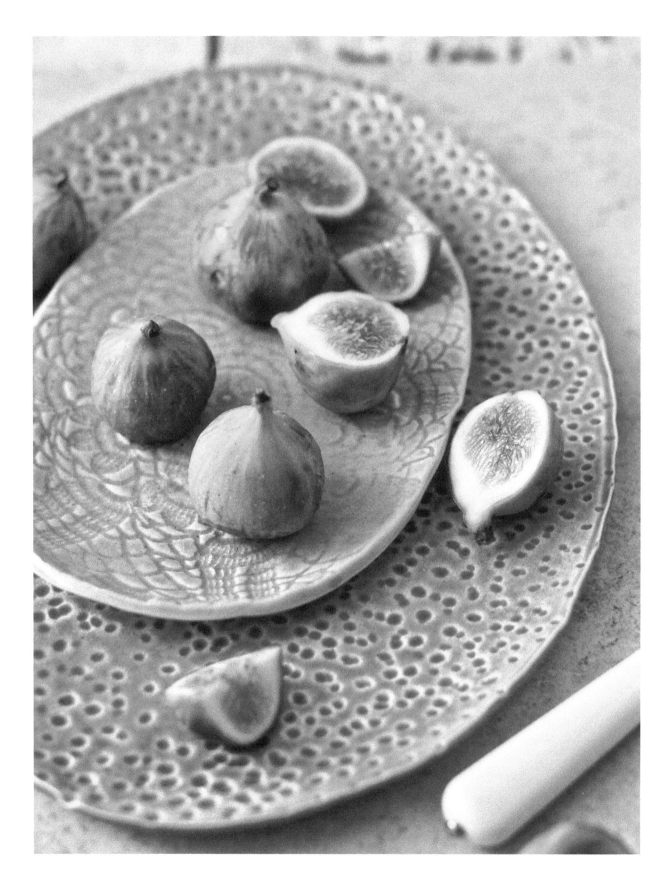

CHAPTER TWO

Clean Eating Foods

Many diets are all about what you can't eat in the interest of losing weight, but clean eating is about the abundance you *can* eat with vibrant good health as a goal and weight loss as a nice bonus. The foods included in this lifestyle are as close to their natural form as possible, with no additives, refining, or processing. You will be eating from every food group, even healthy fats, and not counting each calorie you put in your mouth.

Every food has a unique and valuable complement of nutrients that serve important functions in the body. This means variety is the key when meal planning and shopping. You will be reading labels and sourcing the best products possible from butchers, fishmongers, and farmers' markets. This might sound like a big commitment, but you will soon be making clean eating choices easily as they become a habit. The goal is to gravitate toward craving fresh blueberries rather than blueberry muffins and a handful of tasty almonds rather than salty potato chips. The supplements and nutrients your body needs already exist in food in their most natural form.

Don't worry if you do have an occasional clean eating lapse, such as eating a slice of your mother's famous pecan pie. Clean eating is a long-term lifestyle, which means perfection is not practical. Simply enjoy the moment and then go back to the numerous natural food choices that nurture your body.

What's On the Clean Eating Diet?

You will be delighted to see how many delicious foods are on the clean eating list. This is not a comprehensive list, but a guideline to give you an idea of the choices available. The bulk of your diet should be fruits, vegetables, whole grains, lean proteins, and healthy fats.

Foods to Include in Your Diet

- All fruits, fresh and frozen
- All vegetables, fresh and frozen
- Almond milk
- Applesauce, unsweetened
- Baking powder
- Baking soda
- Brown rice cakes
- Canned tomatoes (sodium-free)
- Canned tuna and salmon (packed in water)
- Chicken breast (skinless, boneless)
- Cocoa powder
- Coffee
- Cooking spray, fat-free
- Cream cheese
- Dried fruit
- Edamame
- Eggs, organic free-range, if possible
- Feta cheese, low-sodium
- Fish (except the ones considered to be high in mercury)
- Game meats (elk, venison, bison, buffalo, rabbit)
- Granola (homemade or unsweetened store-bought)
- Grass-fed beef, trimmed
- Greek yogurt, plain
- Green tea
- Ground beef, extra lean
- Ground chicken, lean
- Ground lamb, lean
- Ground pork, lean
- Ground turkey, extra lean
- Herbal teas
- Herbs and spices
- Hot sauce
- Hummus
- Lamb rack
- Legumes (black beans, black eyed peas, chickpeas, lentils, kidney beans)
- Kefir
- Ketchup (organic, low-sugar)
- Mustard
- Nuts (in smaller amounts)
- Nut butters (in moderation)
- Nut flours
- Nut milks
- Nutritional yeast

- Olives

- Pickles

- Pork chops or roast, trimmed

- Pork tenderloin

- Protein powder (all-natural)

- Pure vanilla extract

- Salsa

- Sauerkraut

- Seafood (lobster, crab, scallops, clams, mussels, shrimp)

- Sea salt

- Seeds (chia, sunflower, flax, pumpkin, sesame)

- Skim milk

- Soba noodles

- Stock, low-sodium, fat-free (vegetable, beef, chicken)

- Tahini

- Tofu and tempeh

- Turkey breast (skinless, boneless)

- Veal

- Vinegars (apple cider, rice, balsamic)

- Whole grains

- Whole-grain breads, pitas, tortillas

- Whole-grain flours (whole-wheat, oat, quinoa, amaranth, spelt)

- Whole-grain pasta

- Whole-wheat bread crumbs

- Yogurt, plain

Foods to Cut Down on or Use Sparingly

These are foods that are still considered to be clean, but due to their fat, sodium, or sugar content (naturally occurring), they should be used in small amounts in the cooking process or as an ingredient.

- Avocado oil

- Coconut oil

- Fruit juices

- Grapeseed oil

- Honey

- Maple syrup

- Olive oil

- Pumpkin seed oil

- Sea salt

- Stevia

- Sunflower oil

- Tamari or low-sodium soy sauce

- Unsalted butter

- Walnut oil

Foods to Eliminate

This list contains refined or processed items that you need to stay away from to reap the benefits of clean eating. Eliminate any food that contains these items as ingredients. Also eliminate any food that has ingredients you don't recognize.

- Alcohol
- Artificial sweeteners
- Chocolate spreads
- Foods high in saturated fats or trans fats
- Frozen dinners
- Fruit drinks and cocktails (not labeled as juice or 100 percent juice)
- Hydrogenated oils
- Junk foods
- Marshmallow spreads
- Processed meats
- Preservatives
- Soda
- Sugar
- White flour
- White pasta

What's the Problem with Processed Foods?

People eat much more processed food than they realize. Many would be horrified if they added it all up for a typical day. Processed foods are convenient, designed to taste good, and difficult to avoid. One of the problems with processed foods is the lack of information about what happens to the food before it hits the grocery shelf—and worse, what it does to your body. Since processed foods have become the bulk of most people's diets, the prevalence of diseases such as obesity, heart disease, diabetes, and cancer have skyrocketed.

Food processing sounds like it should be relatively simple: Take raw ingredients and turn them into food products that are safe to eat. Unfortunately, processed foods are changed to the point where they are almost unrecognizable—all in the interest of a longer shelf life, approved food safety, and supposed enhancement of the natural product. Some processed foods still make the clean eating list, particularly if you "process" them yourself. Freezing and dehydrating are great preservation methods that do not change the nutritional makeup of the original food very much. Look for frozen foods that are flash frozen with no additives and for dehydrated foods that have no preservatives or sugar added.

Unfortunately, most commercial processing techniques affect the raw natural ingredients catastrophically. Processing strips food of nutrients, phytonutrients, flavor, moisture, and texture. Some processing techniques are designed to add these lost components back into the food, along with preservatives, dyes, synthetic flavors, stabilizers, anti-caking agents, emulsifiers, humectants, fats, and sugars. When you consider these extra ingredients, processed food suddenly does not look as appetizing. These many changes to the food turn it into something unnatural to the body, and that can create major health issues.

Some of the reasons to avoid eating processed foods include:

- **Chronic illness and general poor health.** Many diseases are caused by chronic inflammation in the body. Inflammation is a natural response of the body to something that is damaging. Unfortunately, this inflammation cycle can become destructive to the body itself when the damaging agent is constantly reintroduced or the immune system starts to attack healthy tissue. Heart disease, cancer, asthma, Crohn's disease, arteriosclerosis, dementia, neurological problems, and rheumatoid arthritis have all been linked to chronic inflammation. Many studies (a host of them published in the *American Journal of Clinical Nutrition*) have shown that refined flour and sugar, vegetable oils, and other additives in processed foods cause chronic inflammation.

- **Addiction to processed foods.** This is a huge bonus for food manufacturers, because you start craving processed foods and purchase more. This addiction is caused by the fact that ingredients in processed foods increase your body's production of a pleasure neurotransmitter called dopamine.

- **Genetically modified ingredients.** Many processed foods are made up of genetically modified ingredients. They are not usually included on clean eating plans because they are not considered to be completely natural. How delicious does your corn cereal taste when you know it was initially created in a laboratory?

- **Weight gain.** Common ingredients in processed foods, such as high-fructose corn syrup and hydrogenated vegetable oil, are conclusively linked with obesity.

- **Negative effects on mental health.** Spiking blood sugar from sugary processed foods and nutritionally substandard ingredients can create mental fog, mood swings, an inability to concentrate, fatigue, depression, and headaches.

- **Increased aging.** Phosphate additives in processed foods can contribute to loss of bone density, kidney disease, and accelerated aging of the cells in the body.

Clean Eating Food Groups

Clean eating is not about eliminating any one food group. You will see carbohydrates, proteins, and fats in the meal plans and recipes in this book. In most cases you will not have to go out of your way to get enough fat in your diet, because healthy oils such as olive oil, as well as the oils that occur naturally in products like peanut butter, are used in recipes in recommended quantities. There is a great deal of flexibility in the clean eating food groups, so you will never feel deprived or hungry.

Complex Carbohydrates

How many servings should you eat?

Six to ten servings a day (55 percent of your diet; made up of 35 percent dietary fiber and 20 percent starchy carbs)

What are complex carbohydrates?

The carbohydrates you eat are found in two forms: simple and complex. Complex carbohydrates are the type that is consumed on the clean eating plan, except for a few simple carbs in the form of some fruit. Complex carbohydrates consist of at least three sugars held together to form a chain. These chains don't create a quick rise in blood sugar because they take longer to digest. There are two types of complex carbohydrates: starches and dietary fiber. They are found mainly in fruits, vegetables, nuts, seeds, and grains.

What do they do in the body?

Complex carbohydrates are used for fuel in the body. When you eat carbohydrates, either simple or complex, the body breaks them down into sugar to use as fuel. When the sugar levels in the blood rise, the pancreas produces insulin, which stimulates the cells to absorb the sugar, causing blood sugar levels to fall again. If blood sugar levels fall too low, the pancreas produces a hormone called glucagon that prompts the liver to release stored sugar into the blood. This delicate balancing act ensures that the cells of the body have a constant supply of energy. The glycemic index is a tool used to rank carbohydrates based on how much and how fast the blood sugar levels rise after eating a food. This scale ranks food from 0 to 100, with foods scoring between 0 and 55 considered to be low on the glycemic index. This is the range where most complex carbohydrates fall.

Benefits

Complex carbohydrates are required primarily in the body as fuel, powering all the body's functions. If you don't eat enough of them, you will experience fatigue, mental fogginess, mood swings, and irritability.

They also have other benefits. The fiber in these foods improves digestion. Fiber is the part of the complex carbohydrate that is not digested. It acts as a broom sweeping through your digestive system. This fiber pushes the food through the system, along with other undigested substances and toxins. Complex carbs also contain important vitamins, minerals, phytonutrients, and antioxidants. These nutrients are crucial to help prevent most diseases and keep the body as healthy as possible.

Dangers

Some people experience problems when eating certain complex carbohydrates if they are sensitive to gluten, a protein found in cereal grains. This sensitivity manifests as celiac disease or gluten intolerance. Gluten causes an atypical immune response that can cause damage in the lining of the small intestine, creating unpleasant symptoms and malabsorption of nutrients.

Shopping guide

When you are eating clean, most of your shopping cart should be filled with complex carbohydrates, because this group includes fresh produce, nuts, whole grains, and multigrain pastas and breads. Try to buy your fruit and vegetables locally and in season, paying particular attention to their freshness and ripeness. Also consider buying organic whenever possible, especially for the items on the Dirty Dozen list created every year by the Environmental Working Group, which ranks the amount of pesticide contamination in commercially grown produce. Produce on this list contains the most pesticide residue. (Since the list does change a bit from year to year, it's worth checking it out yourself at www.ewg.org/foodnews/summary.php. They also put out a Clean Fifteen list (page 205) that shows the least contaminated produce.) Local co-ops, farmers' markets, and even your own garden are the best places to find great clean eating fruits and vegetables.

Whole grains can be purchased year round and can be found in the bulk section of most supermarkets. When you get your grains home, you will need to store them more carefully because they have healthy oils in them. Store your whole grains in airtight containers in a cool, dry place or in the freezer for up to six months.

Lean Proteins

How many servings should you eat?

Five to six servings a day (27 percent of your diet)

What are lean proteins?

Protein molecules are made up of amino acids held together by peptide bonds. Proteins perform a wide variety of functions within the body and are also the building blocks of cells. Twenty amino acids are required to synthesize protein, and each type of protein is made of an exact combination of amino acids in a certain order. Nine of these amino acids cannot be synthesized in the body, so they must come from the food we eat. Amino acids cannot be stored, which means you need to consume them in your diet to meet the daily needs of the body.

What do lean proteins do in the body?

A better question might be, what doesn't protein do in the body? Protein plays a part in almost every function in the body. Some of the roles protein plays include:

- Carrying oxygen in the blood
- Making antibodies
- Helping muscle contract and move
- Making enzymes
- Making hormones
- Acting as neurotransmitters
- Storing iron in the liver
- Building, repairing, and strengthening cells, protective coverings, and connective tissue

Benefits

Since protein is essential to so many functions in the body, it is obvious that eating it has many benefits. Beyond supporting all the bodily functions and general good health, including lean protein in your diet can help build muscle after a hard workout by repairing and rebuilding the muscle. Eating protein supports weight loss by helping you feel full longer. Eating lean protein instead of proteins that are loaded with saturated fats can cut the risk of heart disease by lowering cholesterol and blood pressure levels. And protein helps boost the immune system.

Dangers

There are problems with both too little and too much protein, as well as eating proteins that contain too much fat. Too little or poor-quality protein in your diet can create a deficiency that may cause poor digestion, water retention, repressed immunity, slow wound healing, hair loss, and, in severe cases, liver damage. Diets that are too high in protein can increase the risk of osteoporosis and cancer, put a strain on the kidneys, and create a nutritional deficiency. The reason *lean* proteins are the clean eating choice is because the saturated fat in fattier protein sources can contribute to cancer, heart disease, diabetes, and other health problems.

Shopping guide

Clean eating proteins include a broad range of foods. The most common protein sources are meats, poultry, fish, seafood, and eggs. Protein can also be found in dairy foods, grains, nuts, seeds, and vegetables, although most vegetables need to be combined with other types of food to create a complete protein that contains all nine essential amino acids.

When shopping for meats, get the freshest, leanest cuts possible. Look for meat with little fat marbling and trim off any excess fat before using it in your recipes. Go for skinless chicken, or take the skin off yourself and trim any visible fat. When buying fish or seafood, do your homework on what types are caught locally or in season and make sure it is fresh. Your fish should never have a strong scent or be slimy.

Grains, nuts, and seeds are an important part of the clean eating diet, so try to buy your staples in bulk whenever possible to save money. Store these products in sealed containers in the refrigerator or freezer to keep them fresh longer.

Healthy Fats

How many servings should you eat?

Two to three servings a day (18 percent of your diet)

What are healthy fats?

Fat is an essential nutrient that provides energy, helps the body function, and helps other nutrients do their jobs. There are four kinds of fat—two associated with eating clean and two to be avoided. The two healthy fats allowed in moderation on the clean eating plan are monounsaturated fats and polyunsaturated fats, which include omega-3 and omega-6 fatty acids. The two unhealthy fats to be avoided are saturated fats and trans fats.

What do healthy fats do in the body?

The healthy fats allowed on the clean eating diet have many functions in the body. These include:

- Providing a source of immediate and stored energy
- Helping the body absorb fat-soluble vitamins, such as vitamins A, D, E, and K
- Insulating the body
- Providing essential nutrients cell function and repair
- Helping regulate blood sugar
- Promoting mental clarity and memory retention
- Playing a crucial part in hormone production

Benefits

Healthy fats have a great many benefits in the body. Despite the bad reputation fat has in general with the healthy eating community, healthy fat can:

- Decrease your risk of heart disease and type 2 diabetes
- Help prevent belly fat
- Protect against irregular heartbeat
- Improve good cholesterol levels
- Improve blood pressure
- Help prevent plaque build-up in the arteries
- Strengthen the immune system
- Support healthy skin

Dangers

Many people don't realize that the danger associated with fat is specific to the type of fat and amount consumed. You will be eliminating saturated fat and trans fat from your diet, so health issues associated with those fats will be minimal. Healthy fats still represent a danger if you eat too much of them. Consuming more monounsaturated fat than is recommended can lead to weight gain, although it will not increase your risk of heart disease. Too much polyunsaturated fat can lower good (HDL) cholesterol and increase your cancer risk.

Shopping guide

Healthy fats are found in many types of foods, including vegetable oils, nuts, seeds, some fruit (such as avocado), and fish. Buying fresh is the key to great fish. Research the varieties that are local or in season in your area, or find a knowledgeable fishmonger who can point you in the right direction. Fish with high mercury levels, such as fresh tuna, shark, swordfish, and orange roughy, should be eaten infrequently to limit your exposure to the metal. (To learn more about which fish have the highest and lowest mercury levels, check out the Natural Resources Defense Council's guide at www.nrdc.org/health/effects/mercury/guide.asp.)

Take a careful look at the bottles of oil on your grocery shelf. Make sure the seals are tight and there isn't any dust on them. The oils should also be stored out of direct sunlight and away from heat sources. Nuts and seeds can be purchased in bulk and stored for several months in sealed containers either in a cool, dry place or the refrigerator.

As for oils, clean eating oils include:

- Almond oil
- Avocado oil
- Coconut oil
- Extra virgin olive oil

- Unrefined safflower oil
- Unrefined sunflower oil
- Unrefined walnut oil

Clean eating oils *do not* include:

- Canola oil
- Corn oil
- Hydrogenated oil

- Palm or palm kernel oil
- Vegetable oil

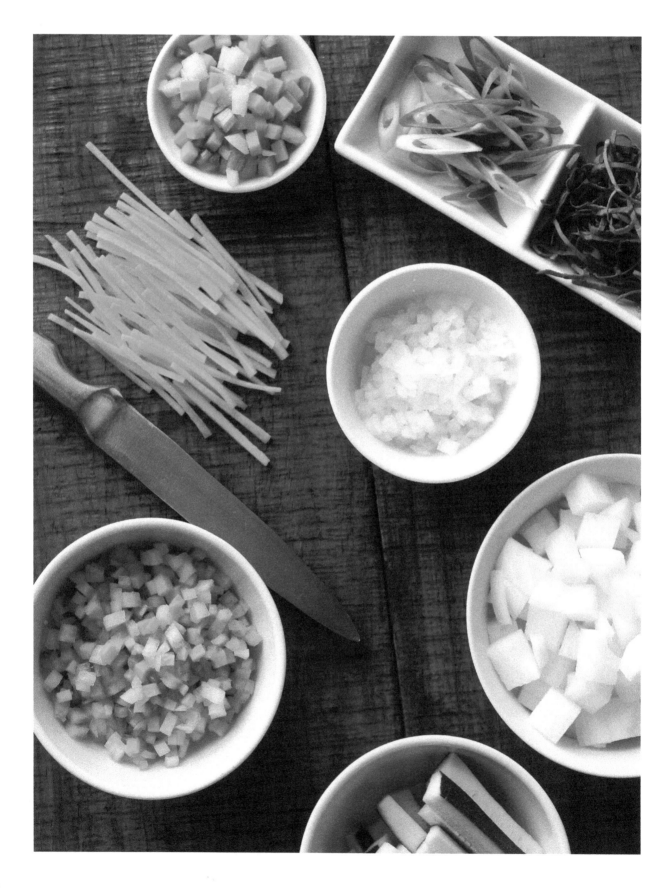

CHAPTER THREE

Everyday Clean Eating Plan

You will have well over a thousand opportunities a year to choose clean eating and support your healthy lifestyle. If you eat five small meals a day, every day that's 1,825 meals each year! That's a lot of meals to organize, so it is clear that meal plans are crucial for success. Fortunately, with so many delicious natural ingredients to choose from in the pantry and the refrigerator, clean eating meal plans are flexible. This means your meal plans can take your lifestyle and diet into consideration.

Meals consisting of nutritious, unprocessed food are only part of a successful clean eating strategy. You also have to consider exercise. A healthy body requires regular exercise to function effectively, and clean eating includes exercise, both cardio and weight training, as an integral component. Plan for a minimum of thirty minutes of exercise a day, four days a week, in your daily clean eating routine.

Make a Weekly Plan

An important part of eating clean is having a meal plan in place each and every week. This is key to ensure that you have clean eating choices on hand at home and when you go to work or school. The plan's flexibility allows for leftovers or eating out on occasion, as long as you follow the general parameters as outlined in chapter one. A typical clean eating day, whether omnivore or vegetarian, should include the following:

- Five to six small meals, spaced out every few hours (no skipping meals) to guarantee stable blood sugar levels; these meals are breakfast, lunch, and dinner, with two or three snacks in between

- Appropriate portion sizes

- A minimum of eight glasses of water, with water as the main drink in your plan

- A combination of complex carbohydrates and protein in each meal, including snacks

- Healthy fats, because fat is not the enemy as long as it makes up no more than 18 percent of your calories

- A focus on eating fresh, natural, high-quality food; everything else will fall into place

People have different palates, health conditions, and schedules. This means the typical clean eating meal plan will be slightly different for each person, even when following the basic guidelines listed here. Remember, there is no set food per meal, beyond combining complex carbs and protein.

A Day in the Life of a Clean Eater

Wake Up

Always start your day with a mug of hot water and freshly squeezed lemon juice to detoxify the liver and hydrate the body. This morning routine will be the same for the omnivore and vegetarian meal plans.

Breakfast

Many people skip breakfast in the interest of losing weight or because they are in too much of a hurry to eat anything in the morning. Breakfast is crucial to a healthy body. After sleeping all night, you need to replenish your fuel stores. Also, people who skip breakfast usually crave high-sugar foods later in the day, creating a destructive cycle of blood sugar spikes and deficits. There is no excuse for missing this important meal, especially when you have a clean eating plan in place.

Ten Clean Eating Breakfast Ideas

1. Oatmeal with fresh fruit, chopped nuts, dried fruit, applesauce, or Greek yogurt

2. Breakfast sandwiches with vegetables, eggs, lean meats, or nut spreads

3. Omelets, frittatas, poached eggs, hardboiled eggs (either vegetarian or made with lean meats, fish, or seafood)

4. Low-fat whole-grain quick breads or muffins (made with added protein powder or another protein source, such as almond milk or nut flour)

5. Whole-grain toast with nut butter and fresh fruit

6. Whole-wheat pancakes, waffles, or crêpes (made with added protein powder or another protein source, such as almond milk or nut flour)

7. Greek yogurt with grains, granola, or fresh fruit

8. Smoothies

9. Homemade protein cookies or bars

10. Fresh vegetables with hummus or peanut butter dip

Breakfast Tips

■ Eat leftovers from the night before

■ Whip up a breakfast casserole the night before and bake it in the morning

■ Put oats or grains in your slow cooker overnight for a nutritious, quick breakfast

■ Make a tray of frittatas and freeze individual portions; simply thaw and make a handy breakfast wrap

■ Layer pretty Greek yogurt fruit parfaits for a special meal

■ Make pancakes or clean eating waffles and freeze them for future meals; pop them into the toaster and serve with fresh fruit or Greek yogurt

Lunch

Lunch is often as rushed as breakfast, because people are at work or school, and time is limited. This is why taking a packed clean eating cooler is essential to make sure your food choices are healthy and natural. You should have a nutritious snack about two hours before lunch, so that you're not super hungry or craving sugar. Lunch should recharge you as well as help boost flagging energy and concentration to take you through the afternoon. As with every other clean eating meal, lunch should be a balance of complex carbohydrates, lean protein, and healthy fats.

Ten Clean Eating Lunch Ideas

1. Whole-grain wraps or sandwiches stuffed with lean meat, eggs, vegetables, fruit, whole grains, or nut butters

2. Clean eating soup or stew (combining protein and complex carbs)

3. Vegetable or whole-grain salads topped with lean meats, nuts or seeds, avocado or fruit

4. Whole-grain pastas with a variety of toppings and combinations

5. Leftovers from dinner the night before

6. Cut-up vegetables or fruit with nut butters, Greek yogurt, or hummus

7. Your favorite grilled or broiled protein (chicken breast or salmon) with steamed vegetables

8. Clean eating casserole or baked egg dish

9. A smoothie with some substance, such as added protein powder, Greek yogurt, oatmeal, or avocado

10. Homemade protein cookies or bars with fresh fruit

Lunch Tips

- Bring your favorite salad and stuff it into a pita or wrap

- Make sure your dressings and juicy sandwich toppings are packed separately, or the bread will be soggy

- Cook chicken breasts in bulk and store them in individual bags or containers until you need them for a meal

- Try adding cooked whole grains to your favorite soups and stews instead of noodles

Dinner

Dinner is a meal that should be light but satisfying. Many people consider dinner the biggest meal of the day because the entire family is at the table and it is a time to socialize. But dinner should be no larger than any other main clean eating meal. You can still have a substantial meal, but try to have smaller portions of protein and limited fat.

Ten Clean Eating Dinner Ideas

1. Salad topped with fruit and grains, lean meats, fish, or low-fat dairy products

2. Clean eating casserole or stew

3. Soup topped with Greek yogurt, served with a crusty multigrain roll

4. Whole-grain pasta with tomato sauce or pesto, fresh vegetables, and lean meat, fish, or seafood

5. Stir-fry with tofu or lean meat and vegetables, served over brown rice or cooked whole grains

6. Grilled, broiled, or baked meat, poultry, or fish with whole grains and salad or steamed vegetables

7. Sandwich or wrap stuffed with fish, lean meat, tofu, or low-fat dairy, with whole grains and vegetables

8. Egg dishes

9. Curries and stews

10. Protein- and carb-packed smoothie with a fresh green salad

Dinner Tips

- Make double batches of all your soups, stews, and casseroles and freeze the extra for quick and easy meals the following week

- Invest in a slow cooker and set up your dinner in the morning so it cooks all day

- Have breakfast for dinner

- Try to include vegetarian meals regularly, even if you are an omnivore

Snacks

The importance of snacking is underestimated. If you have ever experienced a mid-morning or midafternoon energy crash, you will appreciate how much your body needs stable blood sugar. Clean eating snacks provide wholesome fuel to keep the body on an even keel. These snacks should be eaten about two hours after break-fast and two hours after lunch. You can also include a snack a few hours after dinner, especially if you tend to eat early, are doing something active, or are staying up later. Snacks should still include lean protein and complex carbs. Carry them in a cooler when you leave home, so you always have them on hand. And you don't have to wait until *exactly* two hours after breakfast or lunch to snack. Listen to your body and have a snack when you are hungry, or your energy and concentration start to lag.

Ten Clean Eating Snack Ideas

1. Cut-up fresh fruit or vegetables with a protein-packed dip (such as hummus or tzatziki)

2. A handful of nuts and dried fruit or trail mix

3. A hardboiled egg and fresh sliced tomatoes or radishes

4. Roasted chickpeas

5. Homemade fruit leathers (see the recipe in chapter six)

6. Whole-wheat pinwheels with vegetables and lean meat

7. Cut-up apple with nut butter

8. Greek yogurt topped with fruit

9. Whole-wheat pita "pizzas" with hummus and cut-up fruit or vegetable toppings

10. Clean eating chia pudding with Greek yogurt and fruit

Snack Tips

- Pack your dips at the beginning of the week in handy two-ounce or four-ounce sealed containers

- Cut up an assortment of fresh vegetables to keep in containers in your refrigerator for quick grab-and-go snacks

- Pop ripe grapes in the freezer in a resealable plastic bag to preserve them as a chilly snack

- Save a bit of lunch or breakfast for a quick snack later in the day

Choose Protein and Carbohydrate Combos

When you're planning meals, the recipes in part two of this book are a great place to start. If you are still not sure about what to eat, try using the table below to pair proteins with complex carbohydrates in your own clean eating meals. Many of the standard clean eating meal plan ideas are also vegetarian options. Consider your specific diet needs when looking at the ideas and tips in this book. This list is not comprehensive, but it should give you a good idea of what you can mix and match.

Complex Carbohydrates

Clean eating granola

Fresh fruit

Fresh vegetables

Hot or cold whole-grain cereals

Legumes

Oatmeal

Seeds

Sweet potatoes, yams

Whole-grain bread, wraps, and pita

Whole grains and grasses (brown rice, buckwheat, bulgur, chickpeas, lentils, quinoa)

Proteins

Cheeses and dairy

Chickpeas, lentils, quinoa, split peas

Edamame

Eggs or egg whites

Fish and seafood

Greek yogurt

Lean meats (beef, pork, game meats, veal)

Legumes

Nuts

Nut milks

Natural nut butters

Poultry (skinless and trimmed)

Seeds

Some vegetables and fruits, such as avocadoes, peas, corn, broccoli, dark leafy greens, artichokes, asparagus, Brussels sprouts, and beets

Tofu and tempeh

Don't Forget About Exercise

Eating clean, wholesome foods is just the start of your healthy living plan. The other component is exercise. Start exercising at least three times a week for thirty minutes per session, and build up to five or six times a week for forty-five to sixty minutes a day. This might sound like a big commitment if you're not exercising now, but your energy levels will be considerably higher when you're fueling your body with clean food, and exercise will be a pleasure. You will not reach optimum health without doing at least the minimum amount of exercise recommended by the plan.

Some benefits of regular exercise include:

- Increased energy
- Improved immune system
- Reduced body fat
- Increased muscle mass
- Better sleep
- Improved libido
- Reduced risk of diseases such as diabetes and heart disease
- Faster metabolism
- Fewer food cravings

It is also important to combine cardio and strength training as part of a balanced exercise approach. The benefits of weight training are incredible, and you will actually be able to sculpt your body, depending on the areas you concentrate on in your workout. Pay particular attention to your core—your abdominal, lower-back, and mid-back muscles—because a strong core will support the rest of your body.

The nice part about building more muscle is that muscle burns more calories, even when you're at rest. Your body will also burn calories faster and more efficiently, facilitating weight loss and maintenance. The cardio component of your exercise routine can be anything that gets your heart rate up and your body moving. You can jog, swim, bike, walk, play with your dog, play a sport, or even dance.

As with any life choice, it is essential to keep the exercise component of clean eating in perspective and at a healthy level. Don't get caught up and overtrain, or you will set yourself back physically and actually jeopardize your health. Remember to rest between your workouts, or at least rest certain body parts so they can recover and get stronger. For example, if you do a back workout on Monday, do not work the same muscle group on Tuesday—work on your legs or chest instead. Balance is the key to getting the most benefits from your exercise regime. It is also important to consult with your health provider before starting any exercise routine.

Clean Eating Tips to Kick-Start Your Diet

1. **Clean out your refrigerator, freezer, and cupboards.** This process might not be too drastic if your eating habits were relatively healthy to begin with, but if you are a junk food addict prepare yourself for a very empty kitchen. Removing all the temptations from your personal space will give you the best chance of starting off right and not falling off the wagon a couple of days later when you stumble upon the old Halloween candy in the back of a drawer.

2. **Make a weekly clean eating meal plan.** Clean eating is about making a mindful, informed choice about the food you are putting into your body. Starting each week with a balanced, prepared meal plan is the best tool for success. You will know what you are eating each day and cooking for each meal. This will eliminate those drive-through fast food meals you grab when you have no idea what you're having for dinner. Meal plans will also make shopping a breeze and cut down on midweek stops at the store.

3. **Make a shopping plan.** Never shop without a plan, because stores are designed to entice you to make impulse purchases. Why do you think sugary cereals are at kids' eye level, and snack foods are found next to the cash registers? A shopping list, with sections for each food group (produce, meat, dairy, and pantry items) will get you through the store quickly and efficiently with no surplus purchases. Never plan to shop right after a workout or a long day at work when you will be hungry and everything will look yummy.

4. **Plan for leftovers.** One of the most efficient cooking strategies to save money and time is to make double batches of all your favorite recipes and freeze the extra portions in sealed containers or plastic bags. Some recipes obviously don't transfer well from the pot to the freezer, but you certainly can double up on most soups, stews, casseroles, and chilies, as well as cooked grains and beans. This will ensure you have clean eating meals available even when you are in a schedule crunch. Simply take a container out of the freezer in the morning and thaw it in the refrigerator all day.

5. **Invest in a food processor.** You can certainly prepare lovely clean eating meals with just a few pots, a knife, and a cutting board, but why not make your life easier? Your processor does not need to be an outrageously expensive model with grinding attachments and twelve speeds. You can find effective midrange machines for a reasonable price and cut your kitchen prep time in half.

6. **Learn to read labels and then pay attention to them.** You might as well accept the fact that your grocery shopping trips are going to be a little longer, because if you pick up a can or package, you will be reading the label. Some clean eating foods will be prepackaged because there are some great items on the market made with clean eating in mind. The majority of your cart will be single-ingredient items such as chicken breasts, vegetables, and whole grains, but you also might want to pick up some dried gluten-free pasta or prepared beans. When reading the label, pay the most attention to the ingredient list—unless you are on a strict diet that limits ingredients such as sodium. Then by all means scan the sodium content first to see if the product passes. On the ingredient list, look to make sure that every item is recognizable and on your clean eating list. If not, put it back and keep looking until you find what you need.

7. **Buy locally grown, in-season produce whenever possible.** Organic produce is also a wonderful idea if you can afford it and live in an area that supports that buying choice. If 100 percent organic is not possible, try to at least buy organic for the foods found on the "dirty dozen" list of pesticide-contaminated produce, to reduce your exposure to toxins. Pick up produce that is in season and grown locally to ensure freshness and optimum nutrition. Produce that sits in trucks on the long haul to various supermarkets loses nutrients in transit. Fresh-picked fruit and vegetables also taste better, which means you will want to eat them! Whenever possible, get your produce at local farmers' markets to save money and be informed about where your food is grown.

8. **Throw out preconceived notions about your meals.** When following the clean eating diet, you will often find yourself eating something for one meal that you usually would reserve for another. There is nothing wrong with having a lovely mixed bean and vegetable salad for breakfast or a plate of oatmeal pancakes for dinner. Food is meant to nourish and delight. Use the entire day as your culinary palette and enjoy unique healthy food creations when you want them.

9. **Learn about clean eating ingredients.** You might already know a great deal about many of the foods found on the clean eating shopping list, such as apples, carrots, or chicken. However, there are also going to be new choices and clean eating substitutions for familiar products that might require a bit of research. For example, cooking clean foods might require using an oil that's different from the one you are used to using. Obviously, you will only be using a little oil, but healthy fats are desirable. It is best to be acquainted with the clean eating choices before shopping, so you know what to look for in the aisles.

10. **Cook your meals from scratch.** If you are one of those people who would rather watch a cooking show on television than wield the knife yourself, plan to spend more time in the kitchen. You might never become an avid cook, but making each clean eating meal from scratch allows you to control and choose the ingredients that end up on your plate. You also might think you don't have time to putter around in the kitchen every day. This is where precise planning will be invaluable. Spend one of your days off cooking the food for the week. Prepare cooked chicken breasts and hardboiled eggs, cut up vegetables that hold well, and freeze portions of your favorite meals for later in the week.

11. **Don't drink your calories.** You might not even realize how many calories you consume as beverages until you add it up. Depending on your beverage choices, you can be adding as much as 500 to 600 extra calories per day. Fruit juices, drinking your coffee with cream or sugar, and enjoying full-fat milk are all habits you should change immediately when eating clean. Always pick water first, then herbal teas, either cold or hot, when you are thirsty.

12. **Consider your unique needs.** Clean Eating is not a one-size-fits-all plan. It is flexible enough to include any diet factor or health concern, so you should also consider your unique circumstances when planning your Clean Eating journey. If you don't look at you own needs, the whole diet strategy will fail because you will not be able to stick with it. For example, if you are an athlete, your carbohydrate intake might need to be higher than someone who is just starting to exercise.

13. **Keep track of your goals and successes.** Every diet plan encourages keeping a food journal, and this is a very good plan to keep on track. You don't have to write pages and pages of food descriptions, physical reactions, and inspirational quotes, unless you want to record these thoughts. Try keeping a small book or even a phone app where you can write your weight or health goals. This written record keeps you accountable to the reason you are eating clean, and it focuses you on long-term changes rather than just fitting into your jeans by the weekend.

14. **Add meatless Mondays to your week.** The actual meatless day doesn't matter as much as that you start incorporating vegetarian meals into your weekly routine because they are healthy and usually embody the Clean Eating priorities. If you are a hardcore carnivore, it might be a good idea to make a favorite dish such as chili with vegetarian ingredients or a simple stir-fry. Eventually a couple vegetarian meals a week is a wonderful way to get all the benefits of wholesome foods, such as produce and grains.

15. **Start cooking clean.** One of the easiest methods of getting the benefit of Clean Eating is to make sure your food preparation and cooking techniques aren't sabotaging your efforts. Watch the amount of oil you use when sautéing or use nonstick pans with water or stock instead of butter and tablespoons of vegetable oil. Make sure you lighten up on breading, bake instead of fry, and use half the dressing you usually use on salads or sandwiches. Cooking clean will allow you to taste the unique flavors of fresh foods as well, so you can gain a new appreciation for your ingredients and the combinations of herbs, spices, and other seasonings.

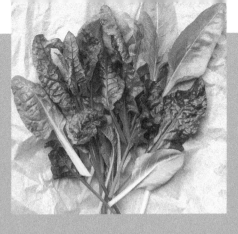

Recipe Key

Selecting Recipes for Your Clean Eating Plan

The recipes in part 2 come with a great deal of additional information to help you pick and choose what foods you wish to include in your clean eating plan. Each recipe contains labels indicating what special diets it is suitable for, plus nutritional information and handy tips.

Special Diet Labels

The recipes in this book clearly indicate when they are appropriate for certain diets. You can quickly glance at a recipe and get this information right in the beginning without having to search through all the ingredients. We use the following special diet labels:

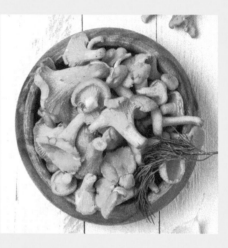

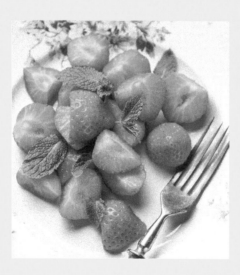

FODMAP-free: This may be a diet you are unfamiliar with if you do not suffer from Crohn's disease, irritable bowel syndrome, or colitis. It is designed to provide relief from the unpleasant symptoms associated with these conditions, such as abdominal pain, bloating, bowel changes, and gas. This diet came about when studies showed that some types of carbohydrates caused irritation in the bowels, which creates these symptoms. The carbohydrates that affect the bowels are called fermentable oligosaccharides, disaccharides, monosaccharides, and polyols, known by the acronym FODMAP. The range of foods that are not allowed on this diet include:

- Some fruits
- Some vegetables, including all alliums (such as onions, garlic, and chives)
- Grains and cereals
- Some nuts
- Sugars and other sweeteners
- Prebiotic foods
- Some alcohols
- Dairy foods

Gluten-free: This diet is often prescribed to treat celiac disease. Celiac disease affects the digestive system and can damage the small intestine, which hinders the absorption of nutrients from food. Those who suffer from this condition cannot eat gluten, a protein in wheat, barley, and rye. Avoiding gluten in all its forms can help people with celiac disease control and minimize their uncomfortable symptoms. Foods that are allowed on a gluten-free diet include:

- Some grains, such as corn, rice, and soy
- Nuts
- Seeds such as quinoa, sesame, and sunflower
- Beans
- Most dairy products
- Fresh meats, fish, eggs, and poultry
- Fruits and vegetables
- Any product specifically labeled as gluten-free

Low-fat: A great deal of research in the past few decades has pinpointed high fat consumption to an increased risk of diseases such as cardiovascular disease, obesity, and cancer. A low-fat diet decreases the likelihood of developing these conditions and many others, while supporting weight loss. Simply stated, a low-fat diet is any diet that includes no more than 30

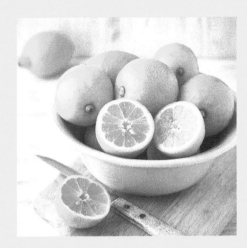

percent of total calories as fat, and saturated fat should be no more than 10 percent. Most attention is paid to saturated fats and trans fats, which are not healthy, as opposed to monounsaturated and polyunsaturated fats, which are healthy. Foods to be avoided include red meat and whole-fat dairy products. Allowed foods include fruits, vegetables, healthy whole grains, low-fat dairy products, and lean poultry.

Low-sodium: A low-sodium diet includes no more than 1,500 mg to 2,400 mg of sodium per day. Your body needs some sodium to function efficiently, but an excess of sodium can lead to health problems such as high blood pressure, heart disease, and kidney disease. Sodium is found naturally in many foods, especially meats and fish, but it is also added through processing, cooking, and at the table via the saltshaker. If you are a healthy young adult, you can eat up to 2,300 mg of salt a day with no problems, but you should consume no more than 1,500 mg a day if:

- are fifty-one or older
- have high blood pressure, kidney disease, heart disease, or diabetes
- are African-American

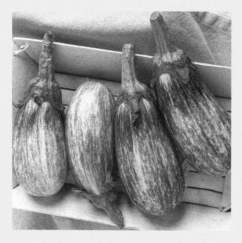

Nightshade-free: Some people have a genetic intolerance to a group of vegetables in the Solanaceae family of plants, known collectively as nightshades. These vegetables naturally produce alkaloids and saponins to protect themselves from the ravages of insects, and these substances are poisonous in large amounts. People who are sensitive to nightshade vegetables can experience gastrointestinal problems (leaky gut, bloating, nausea, and diarrhea), aching or arthritic joints, headaches, and absorption issues in the digestive tract leading to anemia and osteoporosis. Although cooking nightshade vegetables can lower the alkaloid levels by about 40 percent to 50 percent, a nightshade-free diet simply eliminates the vegetables themselves. Nightshade vegetables include:

- Capsicum family (bell peppers, jalapeño peppers, chili peppers, cayenne pepper)
- Tomato
- Potato
- Eggplant (aubergine)
- Tamarillo
- Goji berry
- Ground cherry
- Tomatillo

Vegan: A vegan diet excludes all animal products. This is why it is difficult to state definitively what a vegan diet contains, because fat-laden processed foods can be as vegan as organic fresh produce. There are many reasons why people might choose to follow a vegan diet, including health, environmental, and ethical concerns. There is a great deal of research pointing to the fact that a healthy, clean eating vegan diet reduces the risk of many diseases, including diabetes, obesity, heart disease, and cancer. The China Study by T. Colin Campbell and Thomas M. Campbell is a great resource outlining the research linking vegetable-based diets to improved health. A healthy, clean eating vegan diet includes vegetables, fruit, grains, healthy oils, nuts, legumes, and seeds. The vegan recipes in this book exclude:

- Animal or animal by-products (including meat, fish, shellfish, poultry, gelatin, rennet)
- Dairy (including milk, cheese, yogurt)
- Eggs
- Honey

Vegetarian: There are many types of vegetarian diets, depending on what you want to restrict and the reason you follow the diet. Plant-based diets can be a healthy lifestyle choice if a broad range of wholesome foods are consumed and unhealthy foods containing saturated fats and sugar are limited. A standard vegetarian diet excludes animal foods and animal by-products. However, many vegetarians still eat eggs and dairy products, and some eat fish and seafood. The recipes in this book that have the vegetarian (but not the vegan) label assume a lacto-ovo approach to diet. This means they include dairy products, eggs, and honey but do not include meat, fish, or seafood.

Nutritional Value per Serving

Calories: This is the fuel found in food that powers your body. Calories are essential for providing energy. The amount required by the body varies from person to person, depending on the individual's metabolism and activity level. If you are not an athlete or following a vigorous exercise routine, you will need between 1,600 and 2,200 calories a day to function effectively. Clean eating is not about calorie counting, but if you are trying to lose weight, you will need to eat fewer calories than you burn. If you eat an assortment of high-quality, nutritious foods and avoid processed foods, saturated fat, and sugar, you should naturally take in the right amount

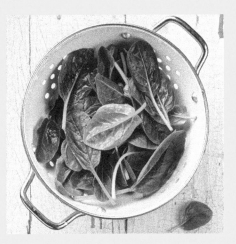

of calories. The recipes in this book assume you are following a 2,000-calorie-per-day meal plan.

Calories from fat: All calories are not created equal. This number simply reflects the calories from the fat in the dish. Do not get hung up on this piece of information unless you are on a low-fat diet, because many nutrient-packed clean eating ingredients contain a fair amount of fat. Keep in mind that this number reflects the total fat in the dish, including healthy fats that the body needs to produce hormones and absorb vitamins.

Total fat: In a healthy diet, such as a clean eating diet, you should be getting about 20 percent to 35 percent of your calories from fat. This total fat number includes all types of fat in the recipe—saturated fat, trans fat, monounsaturated fats, and polyunsaturated fats (which include omega-3 and omega-6 fatty acids). A high total-fat number can be a cause for concern, but only if it is accompanied by high saturated-fat and trans-fat percentages as well.

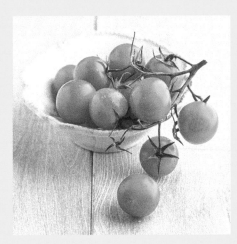

Saturated fat: Generally speaking, saturated fats are unhealthy fats—although coconut oil is an exception and can be part of a healthy diet in moderation. Saturated fats are usually animal fats. They are solid at room temperature (imagine a big, greasy brick of lard). Consuming too much saturated fat has been linked to cancer, obesity, heart disease, and other diseases. The clean eating diet recommends getting less than 10 percent of your daily calories from saturated fat.

Trans fat: This may be the most unhealthy type of fat found in food because it rarely occurs naturally—only in small amounts in some red meats and dairy products. Most trans fats are created in food production when hydrogen is added to liquid vegetable oil to make it solid. Trans fat should be almost nonexistent in a clean eating diet because it is mostly found in processed foods that are avoided on this diet. Trans fats increase the risk of heart disease, diabetes, and stroke and raise cholesterol levels. This fat should be consumed as little as possible, which is why there is no maximum

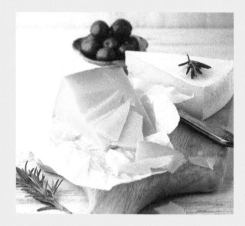

percentage of daily calories from trans fat on a clean eating list.

Sodium: When following a clean eating diet, you should try to stay under 2,300 mg of sodium a day. This basically means following a low-sodium diet. Too much sodium can create serious health problems, but clean eating plans recognize that sea salt can be a healthy part of the diet if consumed in moderation. Also remember that the sodium information in a recipe reflects one meal in a daily total. If, for example, you want to have crab for lunch, which is naturally high in sodium, balance it out with a sodium-free salad for dinner. When it comes to salt, it is the daily total that is important.

Carbs: This number shows the amount of total carbohydrates in the recipe, including fiber, starch, and sugar. The fiber in food is the indigestible part of complex carbohydrates that is found in plant foods. It is very beneficial for the digestive system and can help reduce your risk of heart disease and type 2 diabetes. Fiber does not increase blood sugar or provide energy.

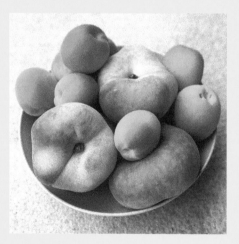

Sugar: This number shows both naturally occurring sugars and added sugars in the recipe. Refined white sugar is on the list of foods to avoid when eating clean, and you will not find that ingredient in any recipe in this book. Honey, maple syrup, and molasses, along with fruits and some vegetables, make up the majority of sugar grams in the recipes. Natural sweeteners are allowed in moderation when eating clean, but there is no set guideline for recommended grams of sugar per day.

Protein: This macronutrient is present in every cell and organ in the body and needs to be replenished daily from the food you eat. It is recommended that 10 to 35 percent of your daily calories come from protein; the amount will vary depending on your age and gender. The clean eating diet does not have a threshold number of protein grams per day, but rather advises a varied whole-food diet to ensure you don't get too much or too little protein.

Recipe Tips

These tips and insights are designed to give you more information about each recipe. You might learn an interesting preparation technique, handy shopping advice, or even how to convert a recipe to another type of diet, such as vegan or gluten-free.

- **Cooking tip:** These hints and tips will help you effectively prepare your recipes, provide advice about storage, or suggest interesting cooking techniques or shortcuts.

- **Diet tip:** The information found here will help you change the ingredients or technique in the recipe to create a dish that follows one of the special diets listed previously in this section.

- **Leftovers tip:** What happens if you use only half of an ingredient in a recipe or have leftovers from your meal? This tip will give you ideas about how to use up the ingredient or create a new dish the next day using the leftovers.

- **Nutrition tip:** You will find specific health benefits and unique characteristics of certain ingredients in the recipe here.

- **Shopping tip:** These are tips about the best seasons to buy specific foods, what to look for to get the best ingredients, and ideas on how to save money on more expensive ingredients.

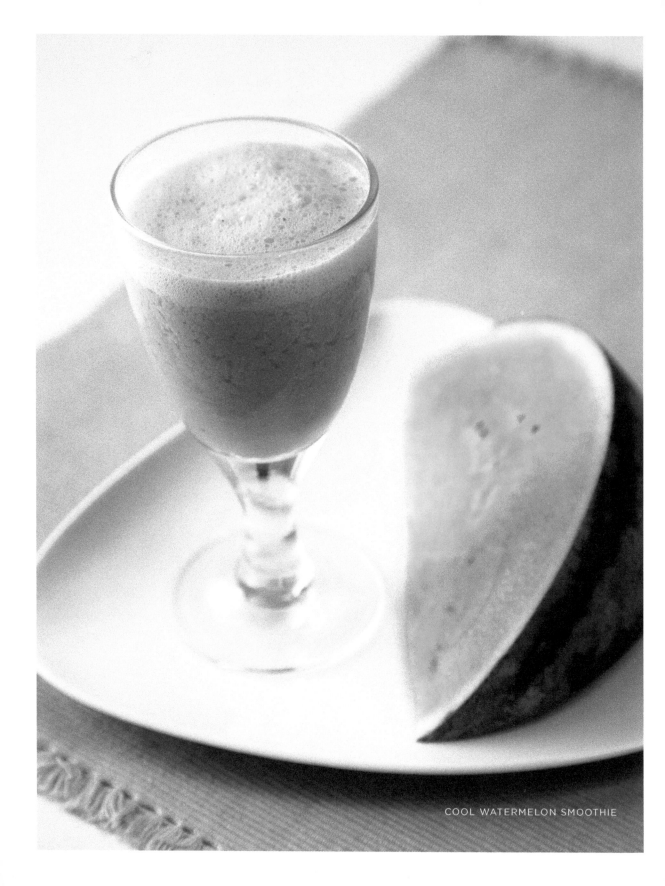

COOL WATERMELON SMOOTHIE

Smoothies

Gluten-free
Low-fat
Low-sodium
Nightshade-free
Vegetarian

CHAPTER FOUR

SMOOTHIES

Green Tea, Blackberry, and Banana Smoothie

Green tea might not be the first ingredient you think of when making a smoothie, but it can be a delicious, healthy choice to combine with your favorite fruits or vegetables. Green tea has been used as a medicinal drink in Asia for centuries and is linked to improving or preventing many health problems, such as high blood pressure, diabetes, and cancer. Green tea is not processed, like black teas, so it contains powerful antioxidants.

Cooking tip If you want to make green tea a regular ingredient in your smoothies, you can steep a large batch of tea and keep it in your refrigerator in a sealed container for easy use.

⅓ cup hot water (not boiling)

1 green tea bag

2 tablespoons honey

3 cups fresh blackberries

1 medium banana

2 cups vanilla almond milk

3 cups ice cubes

1. In a small bowl, pour the water over the tea bag.
2. Steep the tea for about 4 minutes and then remove the tea bag.
3. Stir the honey into the tea and put the tea in the refrigerator until cool, about 20 minutes.
4. In a blender, combine the blackberries, banana, and vanilla almond milk and pulse until smooth.
5. Add the tea and the ice cubes and blend until the drink is smooth.
6. Pour into glasses and serve.

Serves 2. Prep time 7 minutes.

Calories **239** / Calories from fat **32** / Total fat **3.6g** / Saturated fat **0.0g** / Trans fat **0.0g** / Sodium **164mg** / Carbs **52.5g** / Sugars **34.8g** / Protein **4.6g**

Papaya Yogurt Smoothie

Gluten-free
Low-fat
Low-sodium
Nightshade-free
Vegetarian

SMOOTHIES

This smoothie is a lovely pastel pink and is packed with flavor and energy-boosting ingredients. If you are looking for relief from sports injuries or other aches and pains, the enzyme found in papaya—papain—and the enzyme in pineapple—bromelain—are effective treatments. Papaya is also heart-friendly and can help prevent atherosclerosis.

Shopping tip Ripe papayas are slightly soft to the touch and have orange skin. The antioxidant level of the fruit increases as the fruit ripens. Store ripe papayas in the refrigerator and eat them within two or three days.

2 medium papayas, peeled, seeded, and cut into chunks

2 cups Greek yogurt

1 cup fresh pineapple, peeled, cored, and cut into chunks

1 tablespoon pure vanilla extract

3 cups ice cubes

1. In a blender, combine all the ingredients except the ice and pulse until smooth.
2. Add the ice cubes and blend until smooth.
3. Pour into glasses and serve.

Serves 2. Prep time 6 minutes.

Calories **384** / Calories from fat **90** / Total fat **10.0g** / Saturated fat **6.2g** / Trans fat **0.0g** / Sodium **113mg** / Carbs **54.7g** / Sugars **42.5g** / Protein **22.0g**

Gluten-free
Low-fat
Low-sodium
Nightshade-free
Vegetarian

SMOOTHIES

Cool Watermelon Smoothie

Summer in a glass is the best description of this tasty treat. Watermelon is extremely high in antioxidants, especially lycopene, which is wonderful for the cardiovascular system. It can help improve blood flow, which can reduce blood pressure. Watermelon is also a good source of iron and zinc, which are minerals that support a healthy heart.

Nutrition tip Watermelon has the highest amount of antioxidants when ripe and juicy red. Once a watermelon is ripe, the antioxidant levels stay stable for about two days. Choose red watermelons rather than yellow if you want the greatest lycopene benefits.

4 cups chopped watermelon

½ cup unsweetened apple juice

4 cups ice cubes

1. In a blender, combine the watermelon and apple juice and pulse until blended, about 30 seconds.
2. Add the ice cubes and blend until smooth, about 30 seconds.
3. Pour into glasses and serve immediately.

Serves 2. Prep time 4 minutes.

Calories **112** / Calories from fat **5** / Total fat **0.5g** / Saturated fat **0.0g** / Trans fat: **0.0g** / Sodium **29mg** / Carbs **30.2g** / Sugars **22.0g** / Protein **3.9g**

Oatmeal–Peanut Butter Smoothie

If you have a busy day planned, peanut butter is the perfect food to boost your energy and help you feel full longer. Peanut butter has many nutrients such as protein, potassium, fiber, and healthy fat. It is also a good source of magnesium and vitamin E.

Shopping tip Try to buy natural peanut butter. The fat content of most peanut butters is the same regardless of whether it is processed, but natural products contain only healthy fats, while processed peanut butter can have other unhealthy fats added.

1 large banana

½ cup rolled oats

½ cup Greek yogurt

½ cup skim milk

2 tablespoons natural peanut butter

2 cups ice cubes

1. In a blender, combine the banana, oats, yogurt, milk, and peanut butter, and blend until smooth.
2. Add the ice cubes and blend until smooth.
3. Pour into glasses and serve.

Serves 2. Prep time 5 minutes.

Calories **336** / Calories from fat **102** / Total fat **11.3g** / Saturated fat **3.3g** / Trans fat: **0.0g** / Sodium **77mg** / Carbs **39.3g** / Sugars **16.3g** / Protein **20.4g**

Creamy Orange Smoothie

Oranges are one of the most popular fruits because they are so sweet and have a glorious, cheerful color. This smoothie, with the combination of mango and orange, is like sunshine in a glass. Oranges help prevent several types of cancer, improve heart health, and promote good vision.

Cooking tip If you want your drink to be smooth and silky, you can segment your orange before putting it in a blender rather than leaving all the membranes intact. Simply peel the orange using a sharp paring knife to cut away the pith as well as the peel. Then cut the segments out of the orange by following the membranes.

1 cup plain Greek yogurt

1 cup almond milk

1 large mango, peeled and cut into chunks

1 large orange, peeled and chopped into chunks

1 teaspoon pure vanilla extract

2 cups ice cubes

1. In a blender, combine the yogurt, almond milk, mango, orange, and vanilla and pulse until smooth.
2. Add the ice cubes and blend until smooth.
3. Pour into glasses and serve.

Serves 2. Prep time 5 minutes.

Calories **237** / Calories from fat **60** / Total fat **6.6g** / Saturated fat **3.2g** / Trans fat **0.0g** / Sodium **130mg** / Carbs **34.2g** / Sugars **28.9g** / Protein **11.9g**

Kiwi Mint Smoothie

Gluten-free
Low-fat
Low-sodium
Nightshade-free
Vegan
Vegetarian

SMOOTHIES

The cool, minty goodness of this smoothie might remind you of a breeze-kissed veranda in the South. Kiwi is one of the safest fruits to consume if you do not buy organic. For several years it has been on the list of produce that is least contaminated with pesticides. You can also use golden kiwi in this recipe, but the smoothie might not be as green.

Cooking tip If you have a nice big bunch of fresh mint and don't use it all in one recipe, try puréeing the mint and freezing the purée in ice cube trays. For this smoothie, add one frozen mint cube instead of using fresh leaves.

2 large kiwis, peeled and cut into slices
2 cups fresh pineapple, peeled, cored, and cut into chunks

1 cup almond milk
15 fresh mint leaves
1 cup ice cubes

1. In a blender, combine the kiwis, pineapple, almond milk, and mint, and pulse until smooth.
2. Add the ice and blend until the drink is well mixed and smooth.
3. Pour into glasses and serve.

Serves 2. Prep time 4 minutes.

Calories **172** / Calories from fat **18** / Total fat **2.0g** / Saturated fat **0.0g** / Trans fat **0.0g** / Sodium **78mg** / Carbs **40.4g** / Sugars **27.4g** / Protein **2.8g**

FODMAP-free
Gluten-free
Low-fat
Low-sodium
Nightshade-free
Vegan
Vegetarian

SMOOTHIES

Cucumber Ginger Smoothie

Several ingredients in this refreshing drink are beneficial to the digestive system. It is great for improving an upset stomach or even as part of a healthy detox plan. Ginger soothes the intestines, eliminates gas, and can relieve the symptoms of motion or morning sickness.

Nutrition tip Cucumbers have a high water and fiber content, which can assist the digestive process. They can help clear toxins from the body, and, as part of a daily meal plan, can improve heartburn, gastritis, and ulcers.

1 large English cucumber, washed and cut into chunks
1 teaspoon grated fresh ginger
1 cup water, plus more if necessary

Juice of ½ large lemon
¼ cup mint leaves
1 cup ice cubes

1. In a blender, combine the cucumber, ginger, water, lemon juice, and mint. Blend until smooth.
2. Add the ice and blend until smooth, adding more water if the smoothie is too thick.
3. Pour into glasses and serve.

Serves 2. Prep time 5 minutes.

Calories **35** / Calories from fat **5** / Total fat **0.5g** / Saturated fat **0.0g** / Trans fat **0.0g** / Sodium **10mg** / Carbs **7.1g** / Sugar **0.0g** / Protein **1.4g**

Green Strawberry Smoothie

Gluten-free
Low-fat
Low-sodium
Nightshade-free
Vegan
Vegetarian

SMOOTHIES

This refreshing smoothie has all the goodness of spinach, with a surprising strawberry taste. The texture is not completely smooth because of the strawberry seeds, but the seeds are a rich source of fiber so are a healthy addition to the smoothie.

Cooking tip You can use fresh strawberries for this smoothie for a more intense berry taste. If you use fresh berries, you have to add an extra cup of ice or use a frozen banana to get the right thick texture.

1½ cups unsweetened almond milk

2 cups packed baby spinach greens

1 cup frozen unsweetened strawberries

1 banana

1 cup ice

1. Place the almond milk, spinach, strawberries, and banana in a blender and purée until smooth.
2. Add the ice and blend until the smoothie is a milkshake consistency. Pour the smoothie into 2 glasses to serve.

Serves 2. Prep time 10 minutes.

Calories **107** / Calories from fat **18** / Total fat **2.0g** / Saturated fat **0.0g** / Sodium **159mg** / Carbs **21.8g** / Sugars **11.6g** / Protein **2.2g**

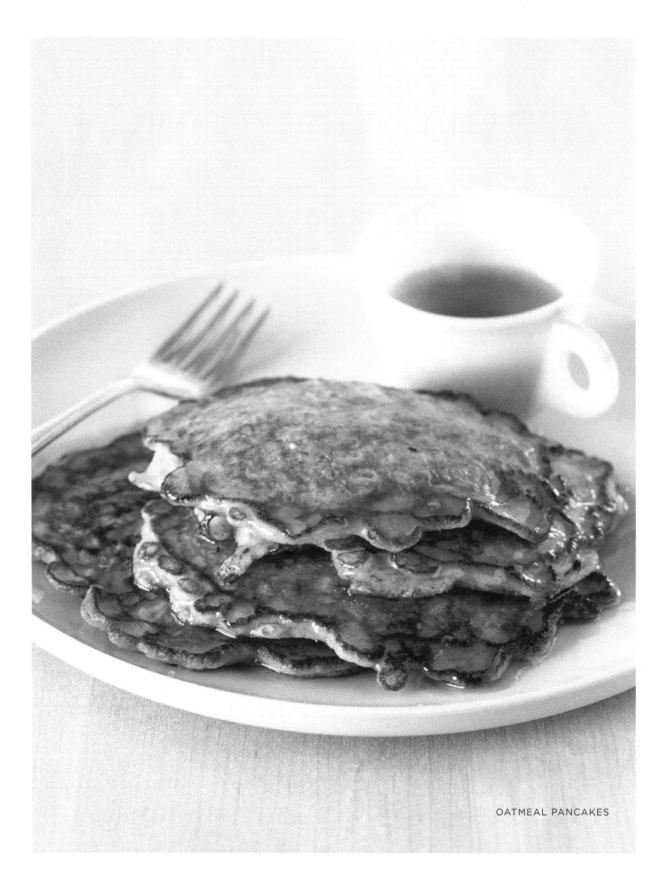

OATMEAL PANCAKES

CHAPTER FIVE

Breakfast

Oatmeal Chia Breakfast Pudding

You will love the convenience of this creamy porridge because there is no cooking involved, and it can be made the night before. Chia seeds can absorb about ten times their volume, so make sure you use enough liquid in your preparation. Chia supports healthy weight-loss goals, can help stabilize blood sugar, and promotes an efficient digestive system.

Diet tip If you want to create a gluten-free dish, buy gluten-free oats instead of regular ones. Chia seeds are already gluten-free.

1½ cups vanilla almond milk

¼ cup chia seeds

¼ cup rolled oats

¼ cup honey

1 teaspoon ground cinnamon

1 teaspoon pure vanilla extract

1 large banana, peeled and sliced

½ cup sliced strawberries

1. In a medium bowl, stir together the almond milk, chia seeds, oats, honey, cinnamon, and vanilla until very well combined.
2. Let the mixture sit for about 15 minutes in the refrigerator, until the liquid is absorbed.
3. Serve topped with sliced banana and strawberries.

Serves 2. Prep time 15 minutes.

Calories **395** / Calories from fat **119** / Total fat **13.3g** / Saturated fat **1.0g** / Trans fat **0.0g** / Sodium **138mg** / Carbs **67.4g** / Sugars **46.0g** / Protein **9.3g**

Coconut Quinoa Porridge

Quinoa is an ancient grain that fits right into the clean eating diet. Although cooked like a grain, this tasty food is actually a seed, making it gluten-free. Quinoa is a complete protein, which means it contains the nine essential amino acids that the body does not produce. There are more than one hundred varieties of quinoa, but you will probably find only the white, red, and black types in your local grocery store.

Cooking tip Always wash your quinoa thoroughly. It is coated with saponins, which have a slightly bitter, soapy taste. Some people are sensitive to this substance, which makes this step a must.

¼ teaspoon extra-virgin coconut oil

1 teaspoon ground cinnamon

½ cup quinoa, rinsed

½ cup almond milk

½ cup light coconut milk

1 teaspoon honey

1 tablespoon unsweetened shredded coconut

1 cup blueberries

1. In a medium saucepan over medium-high heat, heat the oil and cinnamon for about 1 minute.
2. Add the quinoa and stir until coated with the oil.
3. Stir in the almond milk and coconut milk and bring the mixture to a boil.
4. Reduce the heat to low so the mixture simmers and then cover the saucepan.
5. Continue to simmer until the quinoa has absorbed all the milk, about 10 minutes.
6. Stir in the honey.
7. Serve topped with coconut and blueberries.

Serves 2. Prep time 10 minutes. Cook time 15 minutes.

Calories **247** / Calories from fat **38** / Total fat **4.2g** / Saturated fat **1.1g** / Trans fat **0.0g** / Sodium **64mg** / Carbs **37.8g** / Sugars **14.9g** / Protein **8.7g**

Sunny Corn Cakes

They are less dense than traditional cornbread and are best if you use fresh corn taken right off the cob. You can leave out the maple syrup if you are watching your sweetener intake; these cakes will still be just as tasty without it.

Diet tip This recipe can be vegan if you exclude the yogurt. These cakes are delicious even without the creamy topping.

½ cup vanilla almond milk

½ teaspoon apple cider vinegar

¼ cup yellow cornmeal

¼ cup whole-wheat pastry flour

1 teaspoon baking powder

Pinch of sea salt

Pinch of ground nutmeg

2 tablespoons pure maple syrup

1 tablespoon olive oil

½ cup fresh or frozen corn kernels

Nonstick cooking spray

4 tablespoons Greek yogurt

1. In a medium bowl, whisk together the almond milk and vinegar and set aside for 5 minutes to thicken.
2. In a small bowl, combine the cornmeal, flour, baking powder, salt, and nutmeg and set aside.
3. Add the maple syrup and olive oil to the almond milk mixture and stir to combine.
4. Add the dry ingredients and the corn into the milk mixture and stir until just combined.
5. Put the batter in the refrigerator for about 10 minutes.
6. In a large skillet over medium-high heat, add a light coat of cooking spray.
7. Add the batter, 3 tablespoons per cake, and cook until bubbles form, about 2 minutes. Flip the cakes over and cook the other side until golden, about 1 minute.
8. Transfer to a plate and repeat with remaining batter.
9. Serve three cakes per portion, topped with 1 tablespoon of yogurt.

Serves 4. Prep time 15 minutes. Cook time 15 minutes.

Calories **155** / Calories from fat **46** / Total fat **5.1g** / Saturated fat **1.0g** / Trans fat **0.0g** / Sodium **94mg** / Carbs **24.4g** / Sugars **7.8g** / Protein **4.6g**

Apricot Cranberry Breakfast Bars

Once you try homemade granola bars, you will never buy the packaged, processed version again. You can use any dried fruit or nuts in these bars, such as raisins, dried blueberries or cherries, pecans, and cashews for interesting variations.

Cooking tip These bars freeze very well, so make a double batch and keep some stored for a quick grab-and-go breakfast or even a snack throughout the day.

Olive oil cooking spray

4 cups rolled oats

1 cup whole-wheat flour

½ teaspoon ground nutmeg

½ teaspoon ground cinnamon

4 egg whites

1 cup unsweetened applesauce

¼ cup honey

1 teaspoon pure vanilla extract

½ cup chopped dried apricots

½ cup dried cranberries

4 tablespoons slivered almonds

1. Preheat the oven to 350°F. Lightly coat a 12-by-8-inch baking dish with cooking spray and set aside.
2. In a medium bowl, stir together the oats, flour, nutmeg, and cinnamon. Mix well.
3. In a large bowl, whisk together the egg whites, applesauce, honey, and vanilla until well blended.
4. Add the oat mixture to the wet ingredients and stir to combine.
5. Stir in the apricots, cranberries, and almonds.
6. Spoon the mixture into the baking dish, smoothing out the top.
7. Bake for 20 to 25 minutes, or until a toothpick inserted in the center comes out clean.
8. Let the uncut bars cool on a wire rack until they reach room temperature. Cut into 16 bars and store in a sealed container in the refrigerator or freezer.

Makes 16 bars. Prep time 15 minutes. Cook time 25 minutes.

Calories **146** / Calories from fat **20** / Total fat **2.2g** / Saturated fat **0.0g** / Trans fat **0.0g** / Sodium **16mg** / Carbs **27.3g** / Sugars **6.8g** / Protein **4.8g**

Oatmeal Pancakes

You would never know these pretty golden pancakes have cottage cheese in them as a base. Although technically it's not clean, cottage cheese is an excellent source of protein, calcium, vitamin B_{12}, and phosphorus. The extra fiber from the oatmeal makes this an incredibly nutritious start to the day.

Tasty Tip The vanilla extract adds a lovely sweet taste to these pancakes, but you can substitute almond extract for a satisfying nutty taste. If you opt for almond extract, sprinkle some slivered almonds on the pancakes to double up on the flavor.

3 egg whites

½ cup low-fat cottage cheese

1 tablespoon pure maple syrup

½ teaspoon pure vanilla extract

½ teaspoon ground cinnamon

½ cup rolled oats

Nonstick cooking spray

1. In a food processor combine the egg whites, cottage cheese, maple syrup, vanilla, and cinnamon and pulse until very well blended, about 1 minute.
2. Add the oatmeal and pulse for an additional 30 seconds.
3. In a large skillet over medium heat, add a light coat of cooking spray.
4. Pour about ¼ cup of batter onto the skillet for each pancake; do not overcrowd.
5. Cook until the tops of the pancakes start to bubble and then flip the pancakes over.
6. Cook for an additional minute until the pancakes are cooked through and golden brown.
7. Repeat until all the batter is used up.
8. Serve 3 pancakes, warm or cold, per person.

Makes 2 servings. Prep time 2 minutes. Cook time 15 minutes.

Calories **185** / Calories from fat **26** / Total fat **2.9g** / Saturated fat **1.0g** / Trans fat **0.0g** / Sodium **314mg** / Carbs **23.5g** / Sugars **6.8g** / Protein **15.9g**

Simple Potato Frittata

Potatoes have a bad reputation with healthy eaters, but they are actually very nutritious. It is the deep frying of French fries and the fatty toppings on baked potatoes, such as sour cream and butter, that make them seem bad. Potatoes in their clean form are packed with fiber and low in calories.

Leftovers tip Frittatas are just as delicious cold. Cut your leftover frittata into portions and store them individually for a quick snack, light lunch, or a no-hassle breakfast the next day.

10 new potatoes, washed and cut
    into quarters

1 egg

6 egg whites

3 teaspoons skim milk

3 tablespoons finely chopped fresh parsley

1 tablespoon chopped fresh rosemary

Pinch of freshly ground black pepper

Pinch of sea salt

1 teaspoon olive oil

1 small sweet onion, peeled and diced

1 teaspoon minced garlic

1. In a medium saucepan, cover the potatoes with water by about 1 inch and bring to a boil over medium-high heat.
2. Reduce the heat to low, and simmer until the potatoes are tender, about 10 minutes.
3. Drain the potatoes and set aside.
4. In a medium bowl, whisk together the egg, egg whites, milk, parsley, rosemary, pepper, and salt.
5. In a medium skillet over medium-high heat, heat the oil and sauté the onion until it is tender and lightly browned, about 5 minutes.
6. Add the garlic and sauté for an additional minute.
7. Add the cooked potatoes to the skillet and stir to combine.
8. Pour the egg mixture into the skillet, shaking the pan gently to distribute the egg evenly.
9. Cover the skillet and cook until the eggs are just set, about 10 minutes.

continued ➤

Simple Potato Frittata *continued*

10. Remove the skillet from the heat and let the frittata sit for about 15 minutes.
11. Cut the finished frittata into 4 wedges and serve.

Serves 4. Prep time 10 minutes. Cook time 35 minutes.

Calories **271** / Calories from fat **26** / Total fat **2.9g** / Saturated fat **0.7g** / Trans fat **0.0g** / Sodium **121mg** / Carbs **36.7g** / Sugars **4.8g** / Protein **12.4g** /

Poached Eggs over Sweet Potatoes

This is a truly lovely dish that is simple to put together and makes a meal for a large gathering, if you double or triple the recipe. Don't worry if the yolks on the eggs break; they will simply run into the hash underneath and the dish will still taste delicious.

Diet tip The sunny, rich yolks of these poached eggs are an important part of a healthy diet because they contain essential fatty acids and vitamins. Yolks are beneficial to the heart because they can help reduce homocysteine in the liver, which is a compound that can increase the risk of heart disease.

1 teaspoon olive oil

2 medium sweet potatoes, peeled and diced into ½-inch pieces

½ small sweet onion, peeled and diced into ½-inch pieces

¼ teaspoon ground cumin

¼ teaspoon smoked paprika

Pinch of sea salt

Pinch of freshly ground black pepper

2 tablespoons finely chopped fresh parsley

1 teaspoon white vinegar

2 eggs

1. In a large skillet over medium heat, heat the olive oil and sauté the sweet potatoes and onions, stirring frequently, for about 15 minutes or until the potatoes are tender.
2. Add the cumin, paprika, salt, and pepper. Continue sautéing until the potatoes are browned, about 5 minutes.
3. Stir in the parsley and sauté for 1 minute more.
4. Set the skillet aside, covered.
5. Meanwhile, in a large saucepan over high heat, boil 4 to 5 inches of water.
6. Stir in the vinegar, and bring to a boil again.
7. Reduce the heat to low, so the water is gently simmering.
8. Crack one egg into a small bowl.

continued ➤

9. Gently slip the egg into the simmering water and repeat with the other egg.
10. Poach the eggs for about 3 minutes, or until the whites are firm.
11. Remove the poached eggs with a slotted spoon and drain them on paper towels.
12. Spoon the sweet potato hash onto two plates and top each portion with a poached egg.

Serves 2. Prep time 5 minutes. Cook time 25 minutes.

Calories **280** / Calories from fat **69** / Total fat **7.7g** / Saturated fat **2.0g** / Trans fat **0.0g** / Sodium **86mg** / Carbs **44.4g** / Sugars **2.0g** / Protein **8.9g** /

Vegetable Hash

Gluten-free
Low-fat
Low-sodium
Vegan
Vegetarian

BREAKFAST

The broccoli elevates this hash into super-food territory. This vegetable may help prevent many types of cancer and detoxify the body. Broccoli is an excellent source of vitamins K, C, and A, plus fiber and chromium. It is also very low on the glycemic index, which means eating plenty of this vegetable can decrease your risk of kidney disease, type 2 diabetes, and cardiovascular disease.

Cooking tip To save time, roast the squash and potatoes the day before and then sauté them along with the onion and broccoli to warm them up.

½ small butternut squash, peeled and cut into ½-inch chunks

10 small new potatoes, quartered

1 teaspoon chopped fresh thyme

¼ teaspoon sea salt

¼ teaspoon freshly ground black pepper

2 teaspoons olive oil, divided

½ small sweet onion, peeled and diced

1 head broccoli, cut into small florets

1 small red bell pepper, seeded and cut into thin strips

1 teaspoon fresh lemon juice

1 teaspoon chopped fresh parsley

1. Preheat the oven to 425°F. Line a baking sheet with foil and set aside.
2. In a large bowl, toss the squash and potatoes together with the thyme, salt, pepper, and 1 teaspoon of the oil until well combined.
3. Transfer the squash and potatoes to the baking sheet and bake, stirring occasionally, until the vegetables are tender, about 20 minutes.
4. Remove the squash and potatoes from the oven and set aside.
5. In a large skillet over medium-high heat, heat the remaining 1 teaspoon of olive oil and sauté the onion and broccoli until tender, about 5 minutes.
6. Add the red pepper and sauté for an additional minute.
7. Add the squash and potatoes to the skillet along with the lemon juice and parsley, and stir until heated through and well mixed, about 5 minutes.
8. Serve warm.

Serves 6. Prep time 5 minutes. Cook time 35 minutes.

Calories **194** / Calories from fat **17** / Total fat **1.9g** / Saturated fat **0.0g** / Trans fat **0.0g** / Sodium **98mg** / Carbs **21.3g** / Sugars **4.8g** / Protein **4.7g**

Turkey Sausage Patties

Sausage can be a lovely, lean addition to any breakfast if you make your own and use extra-lean turkey breast as a base. This sausage has a definite fiery kick to it, with lots of ginger and fresh jalapeño pepper. If you want to reduce the heat, simply decrease the quantities of these ingredients.

Diet tip If you are trying to avoid nightshade vegetables, omit the jalapeño pepper from your ingredients.

1 pound extra-lean ground turkey breast

1 small apple, peeled, cored, and
   diced small

2 large green onions, chopped finely

1 fresh jalapeño pepper, seeded and
   chopped finely

1 tablespoon grated fresh ginger

1 tablespoon chopped fresh cilantro

Pinch of sea salt

Pinch of freshly ground black pepper

1 tablespoon olive oil

1. In a medium bowl, combine all the ingredients except the oil until very well mixed.
2. Form the sausage mixture into 8 patties, each about 3 inches in diameter.
3. In a large skillet over medium heat, heat the oil and cook the patties until golden and completely cooked through, about 4 minutes per side.
4. Serve 2 patties per person with greens or a hardboiled egg.

Serves 4. Prep time 5 minutes. Cook time 10 minutes.

Calories **179** / Calories from fat **42** / Total fat **4.6g** / Saturated fat **0.5g** / Trans fat **0.0g** / Sodium **131mg** / Carbs **7.0g** / Sugars **4.3g** / Protein **26.4g**

Eggs Baked in Ratatouille

Gluten-free
Low-sodium
Vegetarian

BREAKFAST

Ratatouille is considered to be a rustic dish, but there is an elegance to the perfect combination of textures, tastes, and colors. It is even more perfectly balanced by the rich, almost buttery baked eggs. The mix of different colored vegetables ensures you will be eating a healthy range of nutrients as well.

Cooking tip The best eggs for baking are the freshest you can find, because the whites thin out after about a week in the refrigerator. Thin whites mean your eggs will not hold together as well. This is also true for poaching eggs.

1 teaspoon olive oil

1 medium red onion, peeled and chopped

1 tablespoon minced garlic

1 red bell pepper, seeded and diced

1 yellow bell pepper, seeded and diced

1 small eggplant, diced

2 small zucchini, diced

3 large tomatoes, diced

½ cup water

2 teaspoons balsamic vinegar

1 tablespoon chopped fresh oregano

Pinch of crushed red pepper flakes

4 eggs

1. In a large skillet over medium-high heat, heat the oil and sauté the onion until tender, about 3 minutes.
2. Add the garlic and sauté for 1 minute more.
3. Add the peppers, eggplant, and zucchini and sauté for 3 minutes.
4. Add the tomatoes, water, and vinegar and stir to combine.
5. Bring the vegetable mixture to a boil.
6. Reduce the heat to low and simmer the ratatouille, uncovered, for 20 minutes.
7. Stir in the oregano and the red pepper flakes.
8. With the back of a large spoon, make four deep indents in the vegetable mixture and carefully crack an egg into each indent.
9. Cover the skillet and cook for 4 more minutes, or until the egg whites are firm.
10. Serve immediately.

Serves 4. Prep time 15 minutes. Cook time 40 minutes.

Calories **162** / Calories from fat **62** / Total fat **6.9g** / Saturated fat **1.8g** / Trans fat **0.0g** /
Sodium **81mg** / Carbs **19.9g** / Sugars **9.1g** / Protein **9.4g**

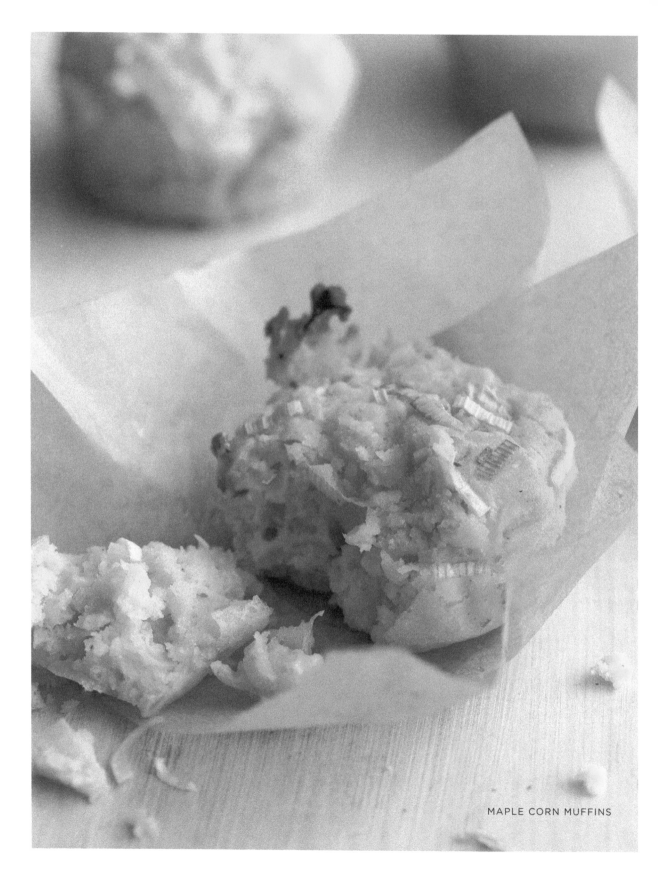

MAPLE CORN MUFFINS

Snacks

Gluten-free
Low-sodium
Nightshade-free
Vegan
Vegetarian

CHAPTER SIX

SNACKS

Garlic Roasted Chickpeas

Roasting chickpeas creates a crunchy, golden treat that makes a great grab-and-go snack for kids and adults alike. You can flavor these with any assortment of seasonings you feel will work, such as chili powder, thyme, and curry. You can also omit the savory ingredients and try cinnamon or nutmeg instead.

Cooking tip Do not skip the step of drying your chickpeas, because otherwise the oil will not coat evenly and your finished snack will not be crunchy.

3 cups canned sodium-free chickpeas,
    rinsed and drained
2 teaspoons olive oil

1 teaspoon minced garlic
Pinch of sea salt
Freshly ground black pepper

1. Lay out paper towels on a work surface and spread the chickpeas on the towels to dry for about 30 minutes.
2. Preheat the oven to 375°F.
3. In a large bowl, toss the dried chickpeas with the oil, garlic, salt, and pepper until well coated.
4. On a baking sheet, spread the chickpeas evenly and bake until golden and crisp, about 45 minutes.
5. Allow the chickpeas to cool completely. Store them in a sealed container at room temperature for up to 5 days.

Serves 5. Prep time 10 minutes. Cook time 45 minutes.

Calories **70** / Calories from fat **23** / Total fat **2.5g** / Saturated fat **0.0g** / Trans fat **0.0g** / Sodium **52mg** / Carbs **8.1g** / Sugar **0.0g** / Protein **3.7g**

Apple Pie Fruit Leathers

Fruit leathers sold in colorful packaging to kids are nothing like these flavorful apple-packed treats. The trick to great fruit leather is to spread the ingredients very thinly and evenly on the baking sheets. Try using a metal baker's spatula (also called an offset spatula) to achieve the perfect layer.

Nutrition tip Apples are one of the most nutritious foods on the planet, and eating one a day might really keep the doctor away! They are incredibly high in antioxidants that help repair the effects of free radicals and fight disease.

4 cups unsweetened applesauce

1 teaspoon ground cinnamon

½ teaspoon ground nutmeg

½ teaspoon ground ginger

Pinch of ground cloves

1. Preheat the oven to the lowest setting possible, or 140°F. Line two baking sheets with parchment paper and set aside.
2. In a medium bowl, combine all the ingredients until very well mixed.
3. Spread 2 cups of the apple mixture onto each baking sheet. Take your time, and make the layer even and thin.
4. Bake or dehydrate the mixture in the oven until it is completely dried and no longer tacky, about 6 hours.
5. Remove the baking sheets from the oven and cut the leathers into 20 pieces.
6. Store the leathers in a sealed container in the refrigerator for up to 1 week.

Makes 20 fruit leathers. Prep time 5 minutes. Cook time 6 hours.

Calories **22** / Calories from fat **0** / Total fat **0.0g** / Saturated fat **0.0g** / Trans fat **0.0g** / Sodium **1mg** / Carbs **5.7g** / Sugars **4.9g** / Protein **0.1g**

Low-fat
Low-sodium
Nightshade-free
Vegan
Vegetarian

SNACKS

Gingerbread Granola Bars

These bars have a complex, warm taste enhanced by the molasses. Gingerbread often contains molasses as a natural complement to the flavor, but molasses is also very healthy. It is a safe sweetener for diabetics because it is not high on the glycemic index. Molasses is also rich in iron, copper, calcium, and magnesium.

Cooking tip If you are a true ginger enthusiast, replace the ground ginger with 2 tablespoons of freshly grated ginger.

3 cups rolled oats

½ cup cranberries

½ cup slivered almonds

1 teaspoon ground ginger

1 teaspoon ground cinnamon

½ teaspoon ground nutmeg

¼ teaspoon baking soda

½ cup unsweetened applesauce

⅓ cup pure maple syrup

3 tablespoons molasses

1 teaspoon pure vanilla extract

1. Preheat the oven to 350°F. Line a 9-by-13-inch baking dish with parchment paper and set aside.
2. In a large bowl, combine the oats, cranberries, almonds, ginger, cinnamon, nutmeg, and baking soda.
3. In a small bowl, stir together the applesauce, maple syrup, molasses, and vanilla.
4. Add the wet ingredients to the dry ingredients and stir until mixed well.
5. Transfer the oat mixture to the baking dish, spread evenly, and press down firmly.
6. Bake for 20 minutes and then remove the dish from the oven.
7. Allow the mixture to cool for about 30 minutes and then score, but do not cut, into 16 bars.
8. Cool completely and slip the parchment paper with the scored-bars from the pan. Cut through the score marks.
9. Store the granola bars in a sealed container in the refrigerator for up to 1 week.

Makes 16 bars. Prep time 5 minutes. Cook time 20 minutes.

Calories **111** / Calories from fat **23** / Total fat **2.5g** / Saturated fat **0.7g** / Trans fat **0.0g** / Sodium **22mg** / Carbs **19.7g** / Sugars **7.2g** / Protein **2.7g**

Thai Chicken Endive Boats

Gluten-free
Low-sodium
Nightshade-free

SNACKS

Belgium endive leaves make perfect crunchy containers for all sorts of tasty fillings, and they don't add extra fat or calories to the finished dish. Endive is high in vitamin A, vitamin C, calcium, iron, potassium, and fiber. It can be slightly bitter, especially if the leaves are bigger. Try to pick the medium to small leaves for these filled boats.

Leftovers tip The endive leaves that are too big or small for this dish can be used in a salad or shredded for sandwiches and wraps.

One 6-ounce boneless, skinless cooked
    chicken breast, shredded

1 cup shredded carrots

1 cup bean sprouts

1 green onion, finely chopped

2 tablespoons chopped fresh cilantro

2 tablespoons fresh lime juice

2 teaspoons grated fresh ginger

1 tablespoon natural almond butter

1 teaspoon rice vinegar

1 teaspoon olive oil

2 large Belgium endive heads, separated
    into 12 medium leaves

1. In a medium bowl, combine the chicken, carrot, bean sprouts, green onion, cilantro, lime juice, and ginger until well mixed.
2. In a small bowl, whisk the almond butter, vinegar, and oil together to make the dressing and set aside.
3. Arrange the endive leaves on a serving plate and spoon the chicken mixture into the leaves.
4. Drizzle the stuffed endive leaves with the dressing and serve.

Makes 12 appetizers. Prep time 15 minutes.

Calories **64** / Calories from fat **22** / Total fat **2.4g** / Saturated fat **1.2g** / Trans fat **0.0g** / Sodium **35mg** / Carbs **5.5g** / Sugars **0.9g** / Protein **6.0g**

Spiced Chicken Meatballs

This is a perfect choice for a slightly exotic casual dish for a party, although it is a bit messy to eat if you use flatbread. It can even be placed in the center of the table for a family-style meal. You can substitute lean ground turkey or pork in this dish for a different taste and texture.

Diet tip If you want a gluten-free dish, omit the flatbreads and serve the curried meatballs over quinoa or brown rice.

1 pound lean ground chicken

2 green onions, finely chopped

Pinch of sea salt

1 teaspoon olive oil

2 teaspoons grated fresh ginger

1 teaspoon ground coriander

½ teaspoon ground cumin

4 cups fat-free, low-sodium chicken stock

1 bay leaf

3 cups cauliflower florets

1 teaspoon chopped fresh cilantro

2 whole-wheat flatbreads, cut in half

1. In a medium bowl, mix together the chicken, green onions, and salt until well combined.
2. Form the chicken mixture into 12 meatballs and set aside.
3. In a large skillet over medium-high heat, heat the oil and sauté the ginger, coriander, and cumin until fragrant, about 1 minute.
4. Add the stock and bay leaf to the skillet and bring to a boil.
5. Reduce the heat to low, so the stock is simmering, and add the meatballs and cauliflower.
6. Simmer until the meatballs are cooked through and the cauliflower is tender-crisp, about 10 minutes.
7. Remove the bay leaf.
8. Top with cilantro and serve with flatbreads.

Serves 4. Prep time 15 minutes. Cook time 25 minutes.

Calories **259** / Calories from fat **95** / Total fat **10.6g** / Saturated fat **2.5g** / Trans fat **0.0g** / Sodium **900mg** / Carbs **23.9g** / Sugars **2.9g** / Protein **29.6g**

Crab and Celery Root Lettuce Cups

Crab is usually a very high-sodium ingredient so you might be surprised that this recipe is low-sodium. This is because of the relatively small amount of crab in each portion. Crab is often a very good choice for a healthy meal, despite the sodium, because it is also low in fat and calories. Crab is also a great source of protein and vitamin B$_{12}$.

Shopping tip Crab can be expensive, but you need only 4 ounces for these tasty appetizers. If you don't have a great source for fresh seafood, you can also get good quality canned crabmeat packed in water.

½ small celery root, washed, peeled, and grated

1 green onion, finely chopped

½ cup (about 4 ounces) cooked lump crab-meat, drained, shell pieces removed

2 tablespoons plain Greek yogurt

1 teaspoon fresh lime juice

1 teaspoon Dijon mustard

½ teaspoon finely chopped fresh thyme

Pinch of sea salt

Pinch of freshly ground black pepper

Pinch of cayenne pepper

12 small Boston lettuce leaves

1. In a medium bowl, stir together the celery root, green onion, and crabmeat.
2. In a small bowl, whisk together the yogurt, lime juice, mustard, thyme, salt, pepper, and cayenne until very well blended.
3. Add the yogurt mixture to the crab mixture and stir to mix.
4. Spoon about 3 teaspoons of filling into each lettuce leaf and serve immediately.

Makes 12 appetizers. Prep time 10 minutes.

Calories **16** / Calories from fat **2** / Total fat **0.4g** / Saturated fat **0.0g** / Trans fat **0.0g** / Sodium **53mg** / Carbs **2.0g** / Sugars **0.5g** / Protein **1.5g**

Maple Corn Muffins

These tender muffins might seem to have a lot of saturated fat in them, but it comes entirely from coconut oil, which is a healthy fat alternative. Saturated vegetable fats such as coconut oil do not have the same destructive effect as saturated animal fats. Coconut oil is burned very quickly in the body because it is composed mostly of medium-chain triglycerides rather than the long-chain fats found in butter and bacon fat. This means coconut oil is heart-friendly and is less likely to be stored as fat in the body.

Diet tip Substitute almond flour or spelt flour for the whole-wheat flour if you want a gluten-free recipe.

1½ cups cornmeal

1½ cups whole-wheat flour

1 tablespoon baking soda

1 teaspoon baking powder

Pinch of sea salt

2 eggs

½ cup pure maple syrup

½ cup almond milk

3 tablespoons coconut oil, melted

1 tablespoon apple cider vinegar

1 tablespoon pure vanilla extract

1. Preheat the oven to 350°F. Line a muffin tin with paper liners and set aside.
2. In a large bowl, combine the cornmeal, flour, baking soda, baking powder, and salt.
3. In a medium bowl, mix together the eggs, maple syrup, almond milk, coconut oil, vinegar, and vanilla until well blended.
4. Add the wet ingredients to the dry ingredients and stir until just combined.
5. Spoon the batter into the muffin cups until they are two-thirds full. Bake until a toothpick inserted in the center of a muffin comes out clean, about 15 minutes.
6. Cool the muffins completely before serving.

Makes 12 muffins. Prep time 5 minutes. Cook time 15 minutes.

Calories **214** / Calories from fat **66** / Total fat **7.3g** / Saturated fat **5.4g** / Trans fat **0.0g** / Sodium **355mg** / Carbs **33.4g** / Sugars **8.5g** / Protein **4.1g**

Spinach Dip

This version of spinach dip is much lower in fat and calories than the traditional sour cream and mayonnaise recipe. Make sure you don't skip blanching the spinach in this recipe, because cooking your spinach makes the nutrients more available for the body. This means cooked spinach is healthier than raw!

Shopping tip To save time, you can buy a good-quality frozen chopped spinach instead of blanching your own. Make sure you thaw it completely and squeeze out all the liquid before adding the spinach to the rest of the ingredients, or your dip will be watery.

2 cups packed spinach leaves

1 cup cottage cheese

1 green onion, cut into 1-inch pieces

1 tablespoon chopped fresh parsley

1 teaspoon minced garlic

Freshly ground black pepper

1. Fill a medium saucepan with water and bring the water to a boil over medium-high heat.
2. Add the spinach and blanch until tender, about 2 minutes.
3. Drain the spinach and run it under cold water.
4. Squeeze as much water as possible out of the blanched spinach.
5. In a food processor, combine the spinach, cottage cheese, green onion, parsley, and garlic and pulse until blended but not smooth.
6. Transfer the spinach mixture to a medium bowl and season with pepper to taste.
7. Cover the dip, and put it in the refrigerator until you are ready to serve it.
8. Serve with vegetables or baked pita bread.

Serves 6. Prep time 5 minutes. Cook time 25 minutes.

Calories **40** / Calories from fat **8** / Total fat **0.8g** / Saturated fat **0.0g** / Trans fat **0.0g** / Sodium **162mg** / Carbs **2.1g** / Sugar **0.0g** / Protein **5.6g**

Gluten-free
Low-fat
Low-sodium
Vegan
Vegetarian

SNACKS

Sweet Potato Hummus

This very tasty, slightly sweet hummus is an absolutely glorious reddish orange color. The texture is very close to the traditional chickpea version, so try it as a spread on wraps and sandwiches as well as a veggie and pita dip. You can even toss it with whole-grain pasta for a delicious, simple meal.

Diet tip If you need to follow a FODMAP-free diet, remove the maple syrup and enjoy this dip with vegetables on the approved list, like cucumbers, carrots, and green beans.

2 large sweet potatoes
1 large red bell pepper
Olive oil
¼ cup fresh lemon juice
1 teaspoon cumin

1 teaspoon pure maple syrup
½ teaspoon minced garlic
Pinch of cayenne pepper
Sea salt

1. Preheat the oven to 350°F. Line a baking tray with foil.
2. Prick the sweet potatoes with a fork and lightly coat the red pepper with olive oil.
3. Place the potatoes and pepper on the baking tray and bake until they are soft.
4. After about 20 minutes, remove the pepper from the oven and put it in a small bowl. Cover the bowl tightly with plastic wrap and set aside while the potatoes continue to bake, about another 20 minutes.
5. Remove the potatoes from the oven and let them cool for about 10 minutes. Then scoop out the flesh into a food processor.
6. Carefully remove the pepper from the bowl, peel off the skin, remove the seeds, and place the flesh in the food processor with the sweet potatoes.
7. Add the remaining ingredients and pulse until the hummus is smooth.
8. Transfer the mixture to a serving bowl and refrigerate for at least an hour until cool.
9. Serve with cut-up vegetables.

Serves 6. Prep time 5 minutes. Cook time 45 minutes.

Calories **75** / Calories from fat **3** / Total fat **0.3g** / Saturated fat **0.0g** / Trans fats **0.0g** / Sodium **8mg** / Carbs **16.8g** / Sugars **2.3g** / Protein **1.2g**

Fresh Fruit Salsa

This salsa is not too sweet, despite the fruit, and has a definite kick from the jalapeño pepper and green onion. Peaches are consistently on the "dirty dozen" list of pesticide-contaminated produce. Make sure you buy organic whenever possible and thoroughly scrub your peaches before using them.

Cooking tip Your peaches and mango should be just ripe or even a little green, so that this salsa is not mushy. If they are too ripe, use them for another dish or eat them cut up as a snack.

2 large ripe peaches, peeled, pitted, and cut into chunks

½ mango, peeled, pitted, and cut into chunks

1 large tomato, cut into 8 wedges

1 green onion, coarsely chopped

1 jalapeño pepper, chopped with the seeds

½ cup fresh cilantro

1 tablespoon minced garlic

1 teaspoon fresh lime juice

Baked tortilla chips or pita bread

1. In a food processor, combine the peaches, mango, tomatoes, onion, jalapeño, cilantro, garlic, and lime juice and pulse until the salsa is coarsely chopped but not completely smooth. Scrape down the sides of the bowl at least once.
2. Transfer to a serving bowl and serve with tortilla chips or pita bread.

Serves 6. Prep time 15 minutes.

Calories **44** / Calories from fat **2** / Total fat **0.3g** / Saturated fat **0.0g** / Trans fats **0.0g** / Sodium **3mg** / Carbs **9.9g** / Sugars **8.0g** / Protein **1.1g**

Southwestern Bean Dip

Bean dips are usually fatty and ooze with cheese, which does not fit into your eating clean diet. But this healthy recipe is just as tasty as its calorie-laden counterpart. There is no cheese in this dip; instead, there's a touch of tahini for a nutty, rich taste. Tahini is made from ground-up sesame seeds and is a great source of calcium, magnesium, and vitamins B_1, B_2, and E.

Shopping tip You will come across two kinds of tahini in your local grocery store: hulled and unhulled. Whenever possible, try to get unhulled tahini because leaving the hull on the sesame seeds when grinding them up makes the finished paste more nutritious.

2 cups canned sodium-free navy beans, rinsed and drained

1 cup homemade salsa

¼ cup tahini

Juice of 1 lime

1 teaspoon ground cumin

¼ teaspoon ground coriander

Pinch of crushed red pepper flakes

Baked tortilla chips or pita bread

1. In a food processor, combine the navy beans, salsa, tahini, lime juice, cumin, coriander, and pepper flakes and pulse until mixed but not completely smooth.
2. Scrape down the sides of the food processor and pulse until smooth.
3. Transfer to a serving bowl and serve with baked tortillas.

Serves 6. Prep time 5 minutes.

Calories **181** / Calories from fat **49** / Total fat **5.5g** / Saturated fat **0.8g** / Trans fat **0.0g** / Sodium **232mg** / Carbs **18.3g** / Sugars **2.7g** / Protein **12.4g**

Spinach and Sun-Dried Tomato–Stuffed Mushrooms

Gluten-free
Low-sodium
Vegan
Vegetarian

SNACKS

This is an elegant hors d'oeuvre that takes very little time to put together. Instead of button mushrooms, you can also use small portobellos or cremini mushrooms to change the taste and texture a little. Mushrooms are the only fruit or vegetable that are rich in vitamin D, so make sure you eat them regularly in the winter months, especially in the northern climates that have less daily sunshine exposure.

Cooking tip Oil-packed sun-dried tomatoes are delicious, but some people want to avoid the extra fat and calories. If you get the dried version without oil, soak them in water for at least an hour to plump them up.

16 large button mushrooms

1 tablespoon olive oil

1 green onion, finely chopped

1 tablespoon minced garlic

½ red bell pepper, seeded and finely chopped

¼ cup sun-dried tomatoes, finely diced

1 cup finely shredded baby spinach

½ cup finely chopped pecans

Freshly ground black pepper

1. Preheat the oven to 375°F. Line a baking sheet with foil.
2. Remove the stems from the mushrooms, creating a hollow, and set the stems aside. Place the mushrooms on the baking sheet, hollow side up.
3. Bake the mushroom caps for about 5 minutes until softened. Remove the caps from the oven and pour off any liquid that has purged from the mushrooms. Set aside.
4. Finely chop half the mushroom stems and set aside. Reserve the remaining half in a sealed bag to use in a stew or frittata.
5. In a skillet over medium-high heat, heat the oil and sauté the chopped mushroom caps, green onion, garlic, and red pepper until the vegetables are softened, about 3 minutes.

continued ➤

Spinach and Sun-Dried Tomato–Stuffed Mushrooms *continued*

6. Add the sun-dried tomatoes and sauté for an additional minute.
7. Add the spinach and pecans to the skillet and stir until the spinach is wilted, about 3 minutes.
8. Remove the mixture from the heat and season with pepper to taste; stir to combine.
9. Spoon the filling into the mushroom caps and put them back in the oven for 5 minutes.
10. Serve warm, four per person.

Serves 4. Prep time 10 minutes. Cook time 20 minutes.

Calories **162** / Calories from fat **123** / Total fat **13.7g** / Saturated fat **1.3g** / Trans fat **0.0g** / Sodium **84mg** / Carbs **8.9g** / Sugars **4.2g** / Protein **5.2g**

Sesame-Crusted Chicken Tenders

FODMAP-free
Gluten-free
Low-sodium
Nightshade-free

SNACKS

You can eat these tempting golden strips as a filling snack with a dip, or as a light meal with a nice mixed green salad. They would be perfect after a workout because the chicken and sesame seeds are rich in the protein needed for muscle recovery. Protein is essential for building muscle tissue, and these tenders have over 40 grams per portion.

Leftovers tip If you have chicken tenders left over, simply store them in the refrigerator in a sealed plastic bag and use them in a pita or wrap the next day for lunch.

Nonstick olive oil cooking spray

1 egg white

1 tablespoon water

1 cup sesame seeds

12 chicken tenders, about 1 pound

1. Preheat the oven to 350°F. Line a baking sheet with foil and lightly coat it with the cooking spray; set aside.
2. In a small bowl, whisk the egg white and water together and set aside.
3. Put the sesame seeds on a small plate and set up next to the egg white mixture.
4. Pat the chicken dry with paper towels.
5. Dip a tender in the egg white mixture and allow the excess to drip off. Then dredge the chicken in the sesame seeds to coat completely.
6. Place the coated tender on the baking sheet.
7. Repeat with the remaining tenders.
8. Lightly spray the tenders with the cooking spray and bake until the chicken is cooked through and the tenders are light golden brown, turning once, about 15 minutes.
9. Serve three per person with a salad or your favorite clean eating dip.

Serves 4. Prep time 5 minutes. Cook time 15 minutes.

Calories **397** / Calories from fat **197** / Total fat **21.9g** / Saturated fat **2.5g** / Trans fat **0.0g** / Sodium **149mg** / Carbs **8.5g** / Sugar **0.0g** / Protein **43.7g**

Avocado Stuffed with Chicken Salad

The pastel green of the avocado, white chicken, and flecks of orange carrot and red pepper combine to create visual and culinary appeal. If your avocado halves do not have very deep cavities when you remove the pits, carefully scoop out a bit more flesh so there is room for the chicken salad. Use the scooped-out avocado in a smoothie or dip.

Cooking tip Chicken breast is a popular ingredient in clean eating. To save time, bake four or five breasts at the beginning of the week and store them in the refrigerator in a sealed container for when you need them.

1 cup finely chopped cooked
    chicken breast
½ cup shredded carrot
1 red bell pepper, seeded and chopped
2 green onions, finely chopped
2 tablespoons chopped fresh cilantro

1 tablespoon fresh lemon juice
2 tablespoons Greek yogurt
Freshly ground black pepper, to taste
2 avocados, sliced in half lengthwise
    and pitted

1. In a medium bowl, mix together the chicken, carrot, red pepper, green onion, cilantro, lemon juice, yogurt, and pepper until well combined.
2. Spoon the chicken mixture into each avocado half and serve one avocado half per person.

Serves 4. Prep time 10 minutes.

Calories **291** / Calories from fat **192** / Total fat **21.4g** / Saturated fat **4.4g** / Trans fat **0.0g** / Sodium **64mg** / Carbs **12.7g** / Sugars **3.0g** / Protein **15.2g**

Cucumber Feta Dip

Gluten-free
Low-fat
Nightshade-free
Vegetarian

The flavor of this dish is so delicious you might want to eat it as a dip, spread, salad dressing, and maybe even on its own with just a spoon! The cucumber adds nice texture and a refreshing taste, along with the lemon juice. Lemon juice is packed with antioxidants and vitamin C, so it can help detoxify the body, boost the immune system, and improve digestion.

Nutrition tip Greek yogurt seems to be a healthy eating trend that is here to stay. It has twice the protein and less lactose than regular yogurt, because the whey is strained out.

2 cups plain Greek yogurt

¼ large English cucumber, grated, liquid squeezed out

¼ cup feta cheese

1 teaspoon minced garlic

3 teaspoons fresh lemon juice

3 teaspoons chopped fresh oregano

Freshly ground black pepper, to taste

1. In a large bowl, mix together all the ingredients until very well combined.
2. Cover the bowl and put it in the refrigerator until you are ready to serve.
3. Serve with pita bread or fresh cut vegetables.

Serves 4. Prep time 10 minutes.

Calories **128** / Calories from fat **60** / Total fat **6.7g** / Saturated fat **4.5g** / Trans fat **0.0g** / Sodium **144mg** / Carbs **6.6g** / Sugars **5.0g** / Protein **11.6g**

Clean Eating Made Simple   83

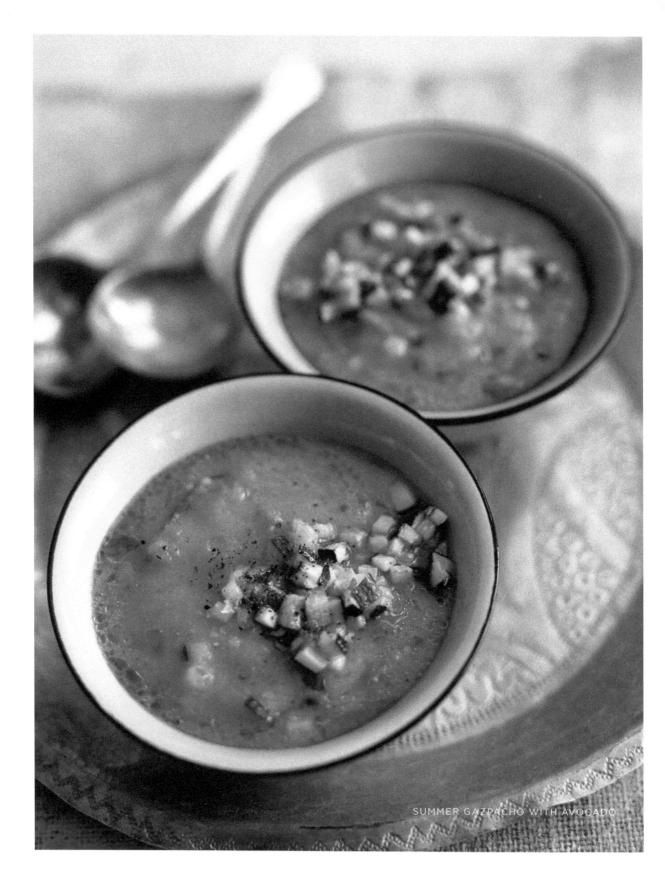

SUMMER GAZPACHO WITH AVOCADO

Soups and Salads

Gluten-free
Low-fat
Nightshade-free
Vegetarian

CHAPTER SEVEN

SOUPS AND
SALADS

Carrot Soup with Yogurt

Carrots are the superstars of this pretty soup, with very good reason. They are delicious, versatile, and packed with vitamins and other nutrients. Carrots contain a great deal of vitamin A (more than 200 percent of the daily recommended requirement), as well as vitamin C, iron, and calcium. Carrots promote healthy vision and can help prevent cancer.

1 teaspoon olive oil

½ small sweet onion, peeled and chopped

1½ pounds carrots, peeled and cut into
    1-inch chunks

3 cups fat-free, low-sodium
    vegetable stock

1 teaspoon grated fresh ginger

½ teaspoon ground nutmeg

Freshly ground black pepper

½ cup plain Greek yogurt

1. In a large saucepan over medium heat, heat the oil and sauté the onion until tender, about 3 minutes.
2. Add the carrots and stock and bring the mixture to a boil.
3. Reduce the heat to low and simmer until the carrots are tender, about 20 minutes.
4. Add the ginger and nutmeg and simmer for an additional 2 minutes.
5. Remove the mixture from the heat and purée the soup with an immersion blender or in a food processor until very smooth.
6. Season with pepper.
7. Serve topped with yogurt.

Serves 4. Prep time 10 minutes. Cook time 30 minutes.

Calories **114** / Calories from fat **22** / Total fat **2.4g** / Saturated fat **1.0g** / Trans fat **0.0g** / Sodium **464mg** / Carbs **19.1g** / Sugars **10.0g** / Protein **4.8g**

Rustic Tomato Soup

Gluten-free
Low-fat
Vegan
Vegetarian

SOUPS AND
SALADS

Homemade tomato soup rarely resembles the thin, flavorless, processed version most people are familiar with from childhood. This soup is rich with chunks of tomato, celery, and carrot, as well as an abundance of fresh herbs. Commercially produced hothouse tomatoes are often pale and flavorless. The best tomatoes for this soup are organic locally grown tomatoes—or better yet, grow your own!

Nutrition tip Did you know that tomatoes are actually healthier for you when cooked? Your body can absorb more of the lycopene in tomatoes after they are cooked.

1 teaspoon olive oil

1 sweet onion, peeled and diced

3 teaspoons minced garlic

2 celery stalks, diced

10 large ripe tomatoes, chopped

3 medium carrots, peeled and diced

4 cups fat-free, low-sodium
    vegetable stock

2 tablespoons chopped fresh basil

2 tablespoons chopped fresh parsley

1 teaspoon chopped fresh oregano

Freshly ground black pepper

1. In a large pot on medium heat, heat the olive oil and sauté the onion, garlic, and celery until softened, about 5 minutes.
2. Add the tomatoes, carrots, and stock and bring to a boil.
3. Reduce the heat to low and simmer the soup until the carrots are tender, about 25 minutes.
4. Remove the soup from the heat and purée with an immersion blender or in a food processor until the soup reaches the desired consistency. It is better a little chunky.
5. Stir in the basil, parsley, and oregano; season with pepper and serve warm.

Serves 4. Prep time 10 minutes. Cook time 30 minutes.

Calories **134** / Calories from fat **21** / Total fat **2.4g** / Saturated fat **0.0g** / Trans fat **0.0g** / Sodium **112mg** / Carbs **30.0g** / Sugars **16.1g** / Protein **5.4g**

Gluten-free
Nightshade-free
Vegan
Vegetarian

SOUPS AND
SALADS

Roasted Beet Soup

Beets are an underused vegetable, mostly because many people have no idea what to do with them and beets can be very messy to prepare. Beets are a smart clean eating choice because they contain no saturated fat and no trans fat. They are also high in iron, fiber, and vitamins A and C. Beets can help fight cancer and protect you from heart disease.

Shopping tip Beets are available all year round in most areas, so try this soup in every season. When buying beets, try to get ones with the greens still attached so you can use the greens for a healthy, delicious salad. Detach the greens immediately and try to use them as soon as possible. The roots will keep for weeks in your refrigerator.

8 medium beets

½ small sweet onion, peeled and cut into chunks

2 garlic cloves, peeled

1 tablespoon olive oil

2 tablespoons apple cider vinegar

2 cups almond milk

¼ cup chopped fresh parsley

1. Preheat the oven to 350°F. Line a baking sheet with foil.
2. Peel the beets and cut them into quarters.
3. On the baking sheet, arrange the beets, onion, and garlic and drizzle the vegetables with the oil.
4. Bake until the beets are fork tender, about 35 minutes.
5. In a food processor, combine the vegetables, including any juices on the baking sheet, with the vinegar and almond milk, and process into a very smooth soup.
6. Serve warm, topped with parsley.

Serves 4. Prep time 10 minutes. Cook time 35 minutes.

Calories **152** / Calories from fat **55** / Total fat **6.1g** / Saturated fat **2.6g** / Trans fat **0.0g** / Sodium **159mg** / Carbs **25.5g** / Sugars **16.4g** / Protein **3.6g**

Cream of Vegetable Soup

Gluten-free
Nightshade-free
Vegan
Vegetarian

SOUPS AND
SALADS

Don't let the ingredient list of this recipe limit the vegetables you want to use. Pretty much any combination would taste fabulous, so try about seven or eight cups of chopped vegetables of any type. If you add potatoes, eggplant, or peppers to the mix, you can no longer consider the finished dish nightshade-free.

Nutrition tip Tofu is a great, inexpensive food that can make your sauces, soups, and smoothies lovely and creamy. It is high in protein, low in saturated fat, and low in calories.

1 teaspoon olive oil

¼ cup chopped sweet onion

2 celery stalks, diced

1 teaspoon minced garlic

4 cups fat-free, low-sodium
   vegetable stock

2 cups chopped cauliflower florets

1 cup chopped broccoli florets

1 cup shredded spinach

8 ounces silken tofu

1 teaspoon white wine vinegar

½ teaspoon ground nutmeg

Freshly ground black pepper

1. In a large pot over medium heat, heat the oil and sauté the onion, celery, and garlic until softened, about 3 minutes. Add the stock and bring the liquid to a boil.
2. Add the cauliflower and broccoli and reduce the heat to low so the soup simmers.
3. Cover the pot and cook until the vegetables are tender, about 25 minutes.
4. Add the spinach and simmer an additional 3 minutes.
5. Transfer the soup to a food processor and purée until it is smooth.
6. Add the tofu and vinegar and purée until the soup is very silky and smooth.
7. Season with the nutmeg and pepper to taste.
8. Serve warm.

Serves 6. Prep time 15 minutes. Cook time 40 minutes.

Calories **89** / Calories from fat **27** / Total fat **3.0g** / Saturated fat **0.0g** / Trans fat **0.0g** / Sodium **126mg** / Carbs **8.1g** / Sugars **2.9g** / Protein **7.9g**

Summer Gazpacho with Avocado

Cold soups can be an acquired taste for those who have never tried them, but the fresh, unadulterated taste of vegetables and fruits can be addictive. The flavor of this soup is sharpened and brightened by a splash of fresh lemon juice and chopped cilantro. Try to use fresh vegetable juice whenever possible, and good, organic canned products if not, for the best taste.

Cooking tip Gazpacho is usually a chunky soup because the texture is part of the whole cold soup experience. If you enjoy a smoother soup, simply purée all the ingredients until you get the desired texture.

8 ripe plum tomatoes, chopped

1 large English cucumber, chopped

1 large red bell pepper, seeded
     and chopped

¼ small red onion, peeled and chopped

4 tablespoons chopped fresh cilantro

3 teaspoons fresh lemon juice

1 teaspoon minced garlic

Freshly ground black pepper, to taste

Hot pepper sauce

1 cup low-sodium prepared vegetable juice
     or fresh vegetable juice

1 ripe avocado, peeled and diced

1. In a food processor, combine all the ingredients except the juice and the avocado and process until well combined but still chunky.
2. Add the vegetable juice and pulse to combine to until the desired consistency is reached.
3. Store the soup in a sealed container in the refrigerator until you want to serve it.
4. Serve topped with chopped avocado.

Serves 4. Prep time 10 minutes. Cook time 30 minutes.

Calories **166** / Calories from fat **67** / Total fat **7.5g** / Saturated fat **1.0g** / Trans fat **0.0g** / Sodium **231mg** / Carbs **24.8g** / Sugars **13.7g** / Protein **5.0g**

Mango and Bean Salad

There is something decadent about ripe, luscious mango. Its texture is so silky and the flavor explodes in your mouth. Mango is high in fiber and vitamins A and C, and is also an excellent source of potassium and copper. This sunny fruit helps fight cancer, promotes great vision, and is excellent for the skin.

Shopping tip Prepared canned beans are usually a staple on clean eating diets because they are convenient, and there are many great organic sodium-free products available. You can certainly soak and cook your own, but the canned options will save time.

2 ripe mangoes, peeled, pitted, and diced

2 cups low-sodium black beans, rinsed well
   and drained

2 green onions, chopped finely

1 small red bell pepper, seeded and diced

1 large ripe tomato, seeded and diced

½ cup cooked barley

¼ cup chopped fresh cilantro

2 tablespoons fresh lime juice

Freshly ground black pepper, to taste

1. In a large bowl, combine all the ingredients.
2. Toss to mix and place in the refrigerator to chill for about 1 hour before serving.

Serves 6. Prep time 15 minutes.

Calories **239** / Calories from fat **49** / Total fat **5.4g** / Saturated fat **0.7g** / Trans fat **0.0g** / Sodium **207mg** / Carbs **38.0g** / Sugars **12.8g** / Protein **8.0g**

Low-sodium
Nightshade-free
Vegan
Vegetarian

SOUPS AND
SALADS

Moroccan Bulgur Salad

Texture and intense flavors are the hallmarks of this colorful, chunky main-dish salad that makes a filling, healthy lunch or snack. Bulgur is a wheat kernel that has been partially cooked and cracked. It is high in protein and fiber, low in sodium, and cholesterol-free.

Nutrition tip Bulgur is a fabulous substitute when you are tired of eating bowl after bowl of brown rice. It has twice the fiber and half the fat and calories of brown rice.

For the dressing:

3 tablespoons fresh lime juice

1 tablespoon olive oil

½ teaspoon ground cumin

¼ teaspoon ground coriander

¼ teaspoon ground cinnamon

Pinch of freshly ground black pepper

For the salad:

2 cups water

1½ cups uncooked bulgur, rinsed

2 cups canned low-sodium chickpeas, rinsed and drained

2 large carrots, peeled and shredded

½ cup dried cranberries

¼ cup slivered almonds

1 tablespoon chopped fresh mint

To make the dressing:

In a small bowl, whisk together all the dressing ingredients and set aside.

To make the salad:

1. In a medium saucepan over medium heat, combine the water and bulgur and bring to a boil.
2. Remove from the heat and cover the pot.
3. Let the bulgur sit for about 30 minutes until all the water is absorbed.
4. In a large bowl, combine the bulgur with the chickpeas, carrots, cranberries, almonds, and mint and toss.
5. Add the dressing and toss again until well mixed.
6. Cover the bowl and chill until you are ready to serve.

Serves 6. Prep time 15 minutes. Cook time 10 minutes.

Calories **239** / Calories from fat **49** / Total fat **5.4g** / Saturated fat **0.7g** / Trans fat **0.0g** / Sodium **40mg** / Carbs **56.3g** / Sugars **12.8g** / Protein **8.0g**

Shaved Asparagus Salad

There's a little extra prep here, but the effect is worth all the vegetable shaving involved in producing this salad. You want to try to get asparagus that is crisp and just thicker than a pencil. The thick asparagus might look easier to peel, but it can also be tough and bitter.

Cooking tip You can also grate your asparagus (on the coarsest grating surface) if you don't want to peel it. The salad will not have the same volume or elegant appearance as the shaved version, though.

3 bunches fresh asparagus,
   about 30 spears
1 tablespoon olive oil
1 small red onion, peeled and thinly sliced
2 tablespoons fresh orange juice

2 tablespoons fresh lemon juice
½ cup chopped pecans
½ cup shaved Parmesan cheese
2 tablespoons chopped fresh thyme
Freshly ground black pepper

1. Trim the woody ends off the asparagus.
2. Lay an asparagus stalk on a cutting board and shave off long ribbons with a vegetable peeler until the stalk is used up. Repeat with all the spears.
3. In a large bowl, toss the asparagus ribbons with the olive oil.
4. Add the onion, orange juice, and lemon juice and toss to combine.
5. Add the pecans, Parmesan cheese, and thyme.
6. Season with pepper.
7. Serve immediately or store the salad in an airtight container in the refrigerator for up to 6 hours.

Serves 6. Prep time 30 minutes.

Calories **145** / Calories from fat **98** / Total fat **10.9g** / Saturated fat **2.2g** / Trans fat **0.0g** / Sodium **117mg** / Carbs **7.7g** / Sugars **3.7g** / Protein **6.2g**

Cobb Salad

This main meal salad is high in protein but not too filling, so it is ideal before playing sports or engaging in an activity-packed afternoon. This recipe omits the bacon, cheese, and creamy dressing often found in the original Cobb salad, but none of the taste. Try different greens, such as spinach and peppery arugula, to create delicious variations.

Cooking tip You will find many uses for hardboiled eggs when eating clean. In the interest of saving time, boil a dozen at the beginning of the week and store them in the shells, in the egg carton, in your refrigerator until you need them.

For the dressing:
¼ cup balsamic vinegar
1 teaspoon honey
¼ cup olive oil
Freshly ground black pepper, to taste

For the salad:
6 cups chopped romaine hearts
2 large ripe tomatoes, chopped
2 large hardboiled eggs, peeled and sliced
One 6-ounce cooked boneless, skinless
    chicken breast, chopped
1 ripe avocado, peeled, pitted, and cut
    into ½ inch slices

To make the dressing:
In a small bowl, whisk together all the dressing ingredients and set aside.

To make the salad:
1. In a large bowl, combine all the salad ingredients and toss.
2. Arrange the salad on plates and drizzle with dressing.
3. Serve immediately.

Serves 6. Prep time 15 minutes.

Calories **243** / Calories from fat **163** / Total fat **18.1g** / Saturated fat **3.1g** / Trans fat **0.0g** / Sodium **72mg** / Carbs **8.3g** / Sugars **2.9g** / Protein **15.4g**

Asian Slaw

Gluten-free
Low-fat
Nightshade-free
Vegan
Vegetarian

SOUPS AND
SALADS

Jicama is an important ingredient in this salad because it has the most interesting crisp, juicy texture and a slightly sweet taste. It is a member of the potato family and can be eaten raw or cooked. Jicama is high in vitamin C, fiber, iron, potassium, and calcium, and extremely low in fat and sodium.

Shopping tip When purchasing jicama, look for medium-size vegetables, about three to four inches across, with no wet or soft spots. Never buy jicama that has been refrigerated or store them in the refrigerator, because temperatures lower than 50°F can reduce their shelf life.

1 small head red cabbage, shredded

2 medium carrots, peeled and shredded

1 jicama, peeled and shredded

2 apples, cored and diced

2 tablespoons fresh lemon juice

1 tablespoon sesame oil

1 tablespoon grated ginger

1 teaspoon minced garlic

½ cup toasted unsalted cashews

1. In a large bowl, combine the cabbage, carrots, jicama, and apples and toss until well mixed.
2. In a small bowl, whisk together the lemon juice, sesame oil, ginger, and garlic.
3. Add the dressing and cashews to the vegetables and toss again.
4. Put the slaw in the refrigerator for at least 1 hour before serving to let the flavors blend.

Serves 4. Prep time 20 minutes.

Calories **302** / Calories from fat **107** / Total fat **11.9g** / Saturated fat **2.2g** / Trans fat **0.0g** / Cholesterol **0mg** / Sodium **72mg** / Carbs **47.4g** / Sugars **20.4g** / Protein **6.3g**

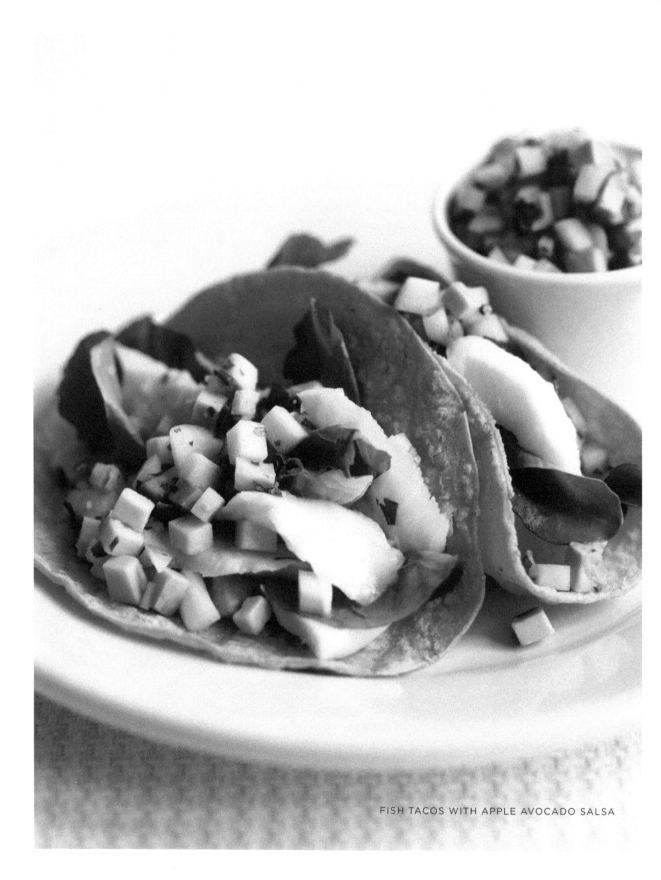

FISH TACOS WITH APPLE AVOCADO SALSA

CHAPTER EIGHT

Sandwiches and Wraps

Tabbouleh Pita

Tabbouleh is usually served as a salad, but it is a great sandwich stuffer. A main flavor component in this dish is parsley, and this herb also provides health benefits. Parsley is very high in vitamin K and flavonoids, especially luteolin, which helps fight free radicals in the body. This popular herb can help protect against heart disease, rheumatoid arthritis, and stroke.

Cooking tip Always chop parsley with a very sharp knife so you don't crush and bruise the tender leaves. Damaged parsley will smell like moldy grass in as little as a day, and will not taste nice, either.

4 whole-wheat pitas

1 cup uncooked bulgur, rinsed and drained

2 cups hot water

3 tablespoons olive oil

Juice of 1 lemon

1 teaspoon minced garlic

3 green onions, finely chopped

2 large tomatoes, diced

1 medium English cucumber, finely diced

1 large red bell pepper, seeded and diced

½ cup finely chopped fresh parsley

1. Cut the pitas in half and pry them open. Set aside.
2. Into a large bowl, add the bulgur first and then the hot water.
3. Soak for 15 minutes and then drain the remaining water out of the bowl.
4. Add the remaining ingredients to the bulgur and stir to thoroughly combine.
5. Divide the bulgur salad evenly among the pita halves and serve.

Serves 4. Prep time 15 minutes.

Calories **428** / Calories from fat **118** / Total fat **13.1g** / Saturated fat **1.9g** / Trans fat **0.0g** / Sodium **364mg** / Carbs **56.0g** / Sugars **5.1g** / Protein **12.7g**

Fish Tacos with Apple Avocado Salsa

Gluten-free
Low-fat
Low-sodium
Nightshade-free

SANDWICHES AND WRAPS

Traditional tacos are actually made with soft corn tortillas. If you prefer to buy hard taco shells, make sure you get ones that are low in sodium. Corn tortillas are high in fiber, phosphorus, copper, and manganese. They can also be a bit high in calories, and you won't want to use them for every sandwich and wrap.

Leftovers tip You will only be using half an avocado in this recipe, so it is important to preserve the other half for another recipe. Leave the skin on and the pit in the side of the fruit that you are storing. Place the avocado in an airtight container with a quarter of a peeled onion. The sulfur from the onion will keep the cut edges of the avocado from browning for up to three days in the fridge.

For the salsa:

1 small Macintosh apple, peeled, cored, and diced

½ avocado, peeled, pitted, and diced

¼ small sweet onion, diced

1 tablespoon chopped fresh cilantro

1 tablespoon freshly squeezed lime juice

Sea salt

Freshly ground black pepper

For the tacos:

2 tablespoons balsamic vinegar

2 tablespoons chopped fresh cilantro

Juice of ½ lime

1 teaspoon olive oil

1 teaspoon honey

6 ounces halibut fillets

Four 6-inch corn tortillas

¼ cup baby spinach

To make the salsa:

1. In a small bowl, stir together the apple, avocado, onion, cilantro, and lime juice.
2. Season with salt and pepper.
3. Set the salsa aside, covered in the fridge, until you need it.

continued ➤

To make the tacos:

1. In a small bowl, whisk together the balsamic vinegar, cilantro, lime juice, olive oil, and honey.
2. Add the fish to the balsamic mixture and marinate for 15 minutes.
3. In a small skillet over medium-high heat, cook the marinated fish (but not the extra marinade remaining in the bowl), turning once, until it flakes when cut with a fork, about 3 minutes per side.
4. Place the tortillas on a clean work surface and divide the salsa evenly between them.
5. Add the spinach to each tortilla.
6. Divide the fish evenly between the tortillas.
7. Fold the tortillas over the fish and serve warm.
8. Place the tortillas on a clean work surface and divide the slaw evenly between them. Divide the fish evenly between the tortillas.
9. Fold the tortillas over the fish and serve warm.

Serves 2. Prep time 15 minutes. Cook time 6 minutes.

Calories **409** / Calories from fat **144** / Total fat **16.0g** / Saturated fat **3.0g** / Trans fat **0.0g** / Sodium **206mg** / Carbs **41.9g** / Sugars **12.1g** / Protein **26.7g**

Baked Pita Pockets
with Tuna and Avocado

This is an extremely simple dish with few ingredients that can be thrown together in less than fifteen minutes. You don't have to bake this wrap if you are in a rush— simply stuff and run! Avocado provides a lovely creaminess to the tuna that is usually achieved in sandwiches with gobs of mayonnaise. You will love this healthier version of an old favorite.

Shopping tip Avocado is a fruit that does not ripen while on the tree. It ripens after it is picked, so you might buy an unripe one. When you get home, put it in a paper bag with an apple or a banana. These fruits naturally produce a fruit gas called ethylene, which will speed up the ripening process.

Four 6-inch whole-wheat pitas, halved and pried opened

1½ cups canned water-packed tuna, drained

1 large tomato, thinly sliced

½ avocado, peeled, pitted, and diced

4 ounces alfalfa sprouts

1. Preheat the oven to 350°F.
2. Place the pita bread on a clean work surface and spoon the tuna, divided evenly, into each of the halves.
3. Top each mound of tuna with a quarter of the tomato and avocado.
4. Place the pita halves on a baking sheet and bake about 5 minutes, or until lightly browned.
5. Add the sprouts and serve immediately.

Serves 4. Prep time 10 minutes. Cook time 5 minutes.

Calories **283** / Calories from fat **59** / Total fat **6.6g** / Saturated fat **1.1g** / Trans fat **0.0g** / Sodium **394mg** / Carbs **19.9g** / Sugars **2.4g** / Protein **30.3g**

Spinach and Bean Burrito Wraps

Beans and rice are a traditional food combination in many cultures around the world, because they are nutritious and relatively inexpensive. They are both high in iron and vitamin B, and when served together they create a complete protein with all nine essential amino acids. You can use other beans in this wrap, such as red beans and even lentils, if that is what is in your pantry.

Diet tip If you serve this wrap without the yogurt or substitute with an almond product, it can be a great vegan lunch or snack.

Four 8-inch whole-grain tortillas

4 cups shredded baby spinach

2 cups cooked black beans, rinsed
    and drained

1 cup cooked brown rice

½ cup chopped romaine lettuce

½ cup homemade salsa

¼ cup plain Greek yogurt

1. Preheat the oven to 250°F.
2. Place the tortillas in a stack and wrap them in in foil. Put them into the oven to warm.
3. In a large skillet over medium heat, heat the spinach and black beans, stirring, until the spinach and beans are warmed through, about 4 minutes.
4. Take the warm tortillas out of the oven and spread them out on a clean work space. Spoon the spinach mixture, divided evenly, in the center of each tortilla.
5. Spread the rice, lettuce, salsa, and yogurt, divided evenly, over the spinach mixture.
6. Roll up the wraps and serve warm.

Serves 4. Prep time 15 minutes. Cook time 5 minutes.

Calories **490** / Calories from fat **61** / Total fat **7.5g** / Saturated fat **2.1g** / Trans fat **0.0g** / Sodium **551mg** / Carbs **83.1g** / Sugars **4.0g** / Protein **25.2g**

Turkey and Sun-Dried Tomato Wraps

Turkey is sometimes passed over in favor of chicken because many people associate this bird with huge, gut-busting dinners and days spent in the gym to overcome overeating. Turkey breast is considerably lower in calories and fat than chicken breast and contains no saturated fat. The downside of turkey can be that it is also higher in sodium and lower in protein than chicken, but turkey is still a healthy clean eating option.

Cooking tip You can use up leftover turkey breast in this wrap after Thanksgiving and Christmas dinner.

1 large ripe tomato, chopped

1 cup fresh or frozen (and thawed) corn kernels

¼ cup chopped sun-dried tomatoes

Four 6-inch multigrain tortillas

Eight ¼-inch slices low-sodium deli turkey breast

2 cups shredded spinach

1. In a large bowl, stir together the tomato, corn, and sun-dried tomatoes until well mixed.
2. Place the tortillas on a clean work surface and top each one with two slices of turkey. Spoon the corn mixture, divided evenly, onto the turkey and top each tortilla with with ½ cup of spinach.
3. Roll up the wraps and serve.

Serves 4. Prep time 15 minutes.

Calories **203** / Calories from fat **30** / Total fat **3.4g** / Saturated fat **0.9g** / Trans fat **0.0g** / Sodium **543mg** / Carbs **36.2g** / Sugars **6.7g** / Protein **15.6g**

Chicken Caprese Wraps

Insalata Caprese is a simple salad of basil, fresh mozzarella cheese, and tomato served as an antipasto in Italy and other countries. This wrap takes those perfectly balanced components and adds chicken and a splash of balsamic vinegar to intensify the flavors. You can omit the chicken for a vegetarian meal and still have a filling and nutritious lunch.

Shopping tip Try fresh mozzarella cheese with this dish, if you can find a good source that uses whole milk. Keep in mind that fresh mozzarella should be eaten within a day of purchasing it because it is very perishable.

1 tablespoon balsamic vinegar

1 teaspoon minced garlic

Pinch of freshly ground black pepper

4 cups chopped romaine lettuce

2 cups cherry tomatoes, halved

Two 5-ounce cooked, skinless, boneless chicken breasts, shredded

2 tablespoons chopped or shredded fresh mozzarella cheese

½ cup chopped fresh basil

Four 6-inch gluten-free whole-wheat tortillas

1. In a large bowl, whisk together the balsamic vinegar, garlic, and pepper.
2. Add the lettuce, cherry tomatoes, chicken, cheese, and basil to the bowl and toss to combine.
3. Place the tortillas on a clean work space, and scoop about 1 cup of the chicken mixture onto each tortilla.
4. Roll up the tortillas and serve.

Serves 4. Prep time 15 minutes.

Calories **233** / Calories from fat **40** / Total fat **4.5g** / Saturated fat **1.4g** / Trans fat **0.0g** / Sodium **184mg** / Carbs **31.0g** / Sugars **3.1g** / Protein **22.1g**

Grilled Vegetable Buns

Low-fat
Low-sodium
Vegan
Vegetarian

SANDWICHES
AND WRAPS

This crusty, lightly toasted Italian bun is heaped with warm, slightly sweet grilled vegetables, along with ripe, juicy tomatoes and a splash of tart balsamic vinegar. The juices soak into the soft parts of the bread, and every bite is an explosion of flavor.

Cooking tip If you are in the mood for a salad instead of a sandwich, use this recipe for two portions and omit the bun. Or you can just use the bun to soak up all the juices on your plate.

1 small eggplant, cut into 8 slices about ¼-inch thick

2 red bell peppers, halved and seeded

1 small red onion, peeled and cut into ¼-inch-thick slices

1 green zucchini, cut lengthwise into 4 long pieces

Freshly ground black pepper, to taste

2 tablespoons olive oil, divided

2 tablespoons balsamic vinegar

4 ciabatta buns, split

2 ripe tomatoes, cut into 8 slices about ¼-inch thick

1. Preheat a barbecue grill to medium-high, or preheat the broiler.
2. In a large bowl, combine the eggplant, red pepper, red onion, zucchini, and black pepper with 1 tablespoon of the oil, and toss gently until well coated.
3. On the barbecue, grill the vegetables until tender and lightly charred on each side, about 6 minutes. Or in the oven, place the vegetables in a flat pan under the broiler, turning once, until tender and lightly charred, about 6 minutes.
4. In a large bowl, toss the grilled vegetables with the balsamic vinegar, and set aside.
5. Brush the bun halves with the remaining tablespoon of oil and place each half cut-side down on the grill, or cut-side up in the broiler.
6. Grill or broil for 1 minute and remove from the heat.
7. Top the bun bottoms with tomato slices and an assortment of the grilled vegetables, and top with the other half of the bun.
8. Serve warm.

Serves 4. Prep time 15 minutes. Cook time 7 minutes.

Calories **234** / Calories from fat **84** / Total fat **9.4g** / Saturated fat **1.0g** / Trans fat **0.0g** / Sodium **14mg** / Carbs **31.4g** / Sugars **9.3g** / Protein **7.4g**

FODMAP-free
Low-fat
Vegan
Vegetarian

SANDWICHES
AND WRAPS

Vegetarian Hummus Club Sandwiches

The club sandwich is more than one hundred years old and can be found in a dizzying range of dining establishments, from diners to four-star restaurants. There are many variations on the traditional chicken, bacon, tomato, and lettuce, including this tasty hummus club recipe. All real clubs have three pieces of bread stacked perfectly with other ingredient layers, all held together by toothpicks.

Shopping tip Look for reduced-calorie bread that is thinner and has air added during the production process, which produces slices that are about 50 calories each instead of 110 in standard bread slices.

Twelve 1-ounce slices whole-wheat or multigrain bread

1 cup homemade hummus

2 cups shredded Boston lettuce

2 large ripe tomatoes, sliced into 8 slices, about ¼-inch thick

1 small red onion, peeled and thinly sliced

1 large English cucumber, thinly sliced

1. Place 4 slices of bread on a clean work surface.
2. Spread 2 tablespoons of hummus evenly on each piece of bread.
3. Top the hummus with ¼ cup lettuce, 2 tomato slices, a couple of onion slices, and some sliced cucumber.
4. Place another piece of bread on top of the cucumber and spread 2 tablespoons of hummus on each piece of bread.
5. Top the second piece of bread with ¼ cup lettuce, 2 tomato slices, and a couple of onion and cucumber slices.
6. Top with the last pieces of bread and secure the sandwiches with toothpicks.
7. Cut each sandwich into four pieces diagonally, so that a toothpick is in each of the pieces, and serve.

Serves 4. Prep time 20 minutes.

Calories **262** / Calories from fat **35** / Total fat **3.9g** / Saturated fat **0.8g** / Trans fat **0.0g** / Sodium **361mg** / Carbs **58.0g** / Sugars **9.0g** / Protein **12.8g**

Tropical Chicken-Salad Wraps

The tart sweetness of the pineapple is lovely with chicken for a refreshing lunch or light dinner. Pineapple is not a single fruit but rather a bunch of small fruits around a core. You can see each fruit in the "eyes" that create the rough, scaly surface of the pineapple.

Cooking tip Make sure you squeeze out the pineapple very well or the wraps will be soggy. Reserve the pineapple juice for a smoothie, dressings, or marinades.

1 cup chopped, cooked chicken breast

½ cup crushed unsweetened canned pineapple, drained

3 tablespoons almond slivers

3 tablespoons Greek yogurt

1 tablespoon chopped green onion

Freshly ground black pepper

Two 8-inch whole-grain tortillas

½ cup shredded lettuce

1. In a medium bowl, mix the chicken, pineapple, almonds, yogurt, and green onion together.
2. Season the mixture with pepper.
3. Place the tortillas on a clean work surface and spoon the chicken filling into the center of each tortilla.
4. Top each tortilla with ¼ cup of shredded lettuce and roll the tortilla up.
5. Serve 1 tortilla per person.

Serves 2. Prep time 15 minutes.

Calories **320** / Calories from fat **87** / Total fat **9.7g** / Saturated fat **1.6g** / Trans fat **0.0g** / Sodium **275mg** / Carbs **26.1g** / Sugars **11.7g** / Protein **33.2g**

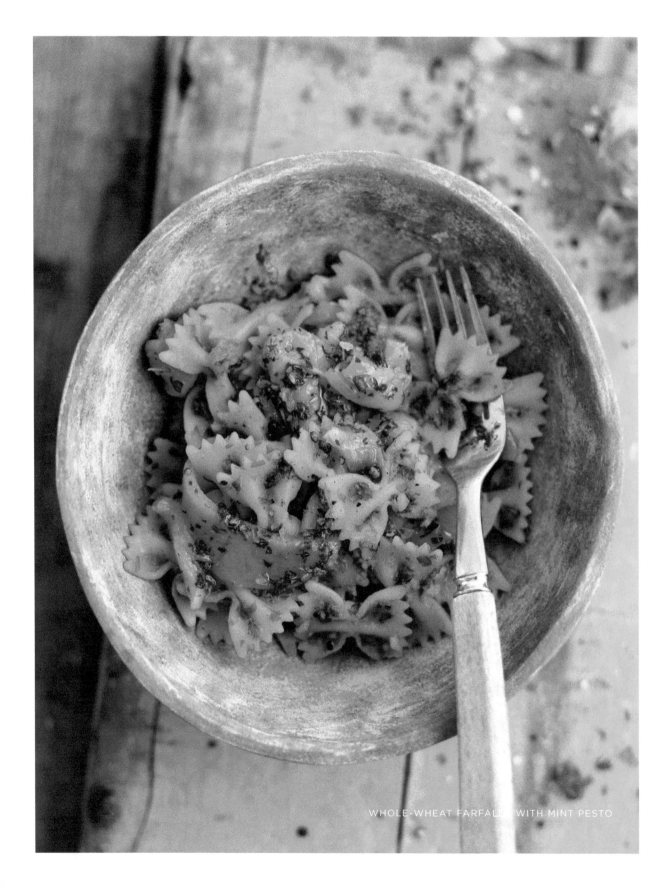

WHOLE-WHEAT FARFALLE WITH MINT PESTO

CHAPTER NINE

Side Dishes

Grilled Corn with Garlic

If you have never tried cooking corn on the barbeque, this recipe will be a revelation. Corn gets plump, juicy, and deliciously caramelized over open flames. If you don't have a grill, you can make corn in your broiler and it will still taste great. Corn has about 80 calories an ear, and is high in fiber and low in fat. Corn helps stabilize blood sugar, promotes healthy vision, and can help prevent heart disease.

Shopping tip If you shuck your corn before buying it in the supermarket, make sure you transfer it to a resealable plastic bag when you get home, to keep it fresh. You can keep corn in the refrigerator for up to five days if it is stored correctly.

4 teaspoons butter

2 teaspoons minced garlic

4 ears fresh corn on the cob, shucked

2 tablespoons grated Parmesan cheese

4 teaspoons chopped fresh parsley

Freshly ground black pepper

1. Preheat the barbecue to medium-high heat or preheat the broiler.
2. In a small saucepan over medium heat, melt the butter and sauté the garlic until soft, about 3 minutes.
3. Remove the pan from the heat and brush the garlic butter onto the corn.
4. On the barbecue, grill the corn, turning to grill all sides, until slightly charred and tender crisp, 10 to 20 minutes. Or in the oven, put the corn under the broiler for 15 to 20 minutes, turning about every 5 minutes.
5. Serve the corn topped with the cheese, parsley, and sprinkling of pepper.

Serves 4. Prep time 5 minutes. Cook time 15 minutes.

Calories **140** / Calories from fat **66** / Total fat **7.3g** / Saturated fat **4.5g** / Trans fat **0.0g** / Sodium **159mg** / Carbs **15.2g** / Sugars **2.3g** / Protein **6.6g**

Pico de Gallo Black Beans

This is a perfect side dish for a spicy grilled chicken or pork entrée. It can even be a main course if you are looking for a meat-free dish. The lovely citrusy and slightly nutty flavor of this dish comes from the cumin. Cumin is not just a fabulous seasoning; it is also a great source of iron, calcium, magnesium, and manganese. This means it can boost the immune system and promote healthy digestion.

Diet tip If you are following a vegan diet, leave out the feta cheese topping; this dish is already packed with protein.

1 cup dried black beans, rinsed and
    picked through

½ small sweet onion, finely chopped

1 teaspoon minced garlic

1 teaspoon ground cumin

1 teaspoon ground coriander

1 small ripe tomato, chopped

4 teaspoons finely chopped
    red bell pepper

4 teaspoons finely chopped red onion

¼ cup low-sodium feta cheese

1. In a medium bowl, cover the beans with water to about 1 inch above the level of the beans and soak in the refrigerator overnight. Drain the beans before using.
2. In a medium saucepan over medium-high heat, combine the beans with the onion, garlic, cumin, coriander, and 3 cups of water, and bring to a boil.
3. Reduce the heat to low and simmer until the beans are very tender, about 35 minutes.
4. While the beans are cooking, in a medium bowl make the pico de gallo by mixing together the tomato, red pepper, and red onion until well combined. Set aside.
5. Drain the beans and spoon them onto individual plates.
6. Serve topped with the pico de gallo and feta cheese.

Serves 4. Prep time 20 minutes, plus soaking time. Cook time 40 minutes.

Calories **186** / Calories from fat **17** / Total fat **1.9g** / Saturated fat **0.8g** / Trans fat **0.0g** / Sodium **110mg** / Carbs **33.1g** / Sugars **2.3g** / Protein **12.7g**

FODMAP-free
Gluten-free
Low-fat
Nightshade-free
Vegan
Vegetarian

SIDE DISHES

Roasted Vegetables with Thyme

The scent of gently caramelizing vegetables roasting in the oven will likely call your family to dinner long before you are ready to put it on the table. Try to cut the various root vegetables in similar sizes so they roast evenly, and make sure you toss them with the other ingredients thoroughly enough to coat every piece.

Shopping tip Don't be put off by the strange, dirty, bulbous appearance of the celery root (celeriac), because under the skin is a potato-like vegetable with a mild, pleasant celery taste. It is available year round, but is best in the late fall and winter months.

1 small butternut squash, peeled and cut into 1-inch cubes

2 carrots, peeled and cut into 1-inch chunks

3 parsnips, peeled and cut into 1-inch chunks

1 small celeriac root, peeled and cut into 1-inch chunks

1 large sweet potato, peeled and cut into 1-inch chunks

2 tablespoons olive oil

2 teaspoons chopped fresh thyme

Freshly ground black pepper, to taste

1. Preheat the oven to 400°F. Line a baking sheet with foil and set aside.
2. In a large bowl, toss together all the ingredients.
3. Transfer the vegetables to the prepared baking sheet and bake until they are tender and lightly browned, stirring occasionally, about 45 minutes.
4. Serve warm.

Serves 4. Prep time 10 minutes. Cook time 45 minutes.

Calories **231** / Calories from fat **68** / Total fat **7.5g** / Saturated fat **1.1g** / Trans fat **0.0g** / Sodium **75mg** / Carbs **42.3g** / Sugars **11.2g** / Protein **3.6g**

Spiced Squash Casserole

Gluten-free
Low-sodium
Nightshade-free
Vegetarian

SIDE DISHES

The prep is a bit more involved for this casserole than for many of the other recipes in this book—you double-process the squash—but the end result is smooth, luscious, and naturally sweet. Well worth the effort! Butternut squash is what's listed in the recipe, but any winter squash (except spaghetti) will do. Just make sure you have about eight cups of cubed squash.

Cooking tip Cutting winter squash in half can be a dangerous and difficult task, because it is so hard and the curved surface of the vegetable makes it likely to roll. Try placing the whole squash in the microwave about two minutes before cutting it, to make this process easier and safer.

Nonstick cooking spray

1 large butternut squash, cut in half
  and seeded

½ cup canned low-fat coconut milk

2 eggs

2 tablespoons pure maple syrup

4 teaspoons cornstarch

1 teaspoon ground cinnamon

¼ teaspoon ground nutmeg

¼ teaspoon ground cloves

1. Preheat the oven to 400°F. Line a baking sheet with foil and lightly coat the foil with cooking spray.
2. Place the squash cut-side down on the baking sheet and bake until the squash is tender and collapsed, about 30 minutes.
3. Remove the squash from the oven and let it cool for about 10 minutes.
4. Reduce the oven temperature to 350°F.
5. Scoop out the flesh of the squash with a spoon.
6. In a food processor, process the squash with the remaining ingredients until smooth, scraping down the sides of the bowl at least once.
7. Spoon the squash mixture into a casserole and bake until the mixture is set, about 35 minutes.
8. Serve warm.

Serves 8. Prep time 5 minutes. Cook time 1 hour and 10 minutes.

Calories **132** / Calories from fat **45** / Total fat **5.0g** / Saturated fat **3.6g** / Trans fat **0.0g** /
Sodium **25mg** / Carbs **22.2g** / Sugars **8.8g** / Protein **3.0g**

Gluten-free
Low-sodium
Nightshade-free
Vegan
Vegetarian

SIDE DISHES

Roasted Coconut Brussels Sprouts

Brussels sprouts are often overcooked in boiling water, which causes them to have a very unpleasant odor. Roasting them is a great way to make sure they are perfect. Brussels sprouts are low in fat and sodium, and are a rich source of fiber, which makes them a smart choice when eating clean. They also have a cancer-fighting chemical in them called sulforaphane, which can be destroyed by boiling but stays intact when these vegetables are roasted.

Shopping tip Make sure you get unsweetened shredded coconut rather than the sweetened product. Or better yet, shred your own coconut meat from a fresh coconut to ensure there's no added sugar.

2 pounds Brussels sprouts, trimmed and cut in half

2 teaspoons coconut oil, melted

¼ cup unsweetened toasted shredded coconut

1. Preheat the oven to 400°F. Line a baking sheet with foil and set aside.
2. In a large bowl, toss the Brussels sprouts with the melted coconut oil until the vegetables are well coated.
3. Spread the Brussels sprouts on the prepared baking sheet in one layer and roast until they are tender and browned, about 20 to 30 minutes.
4. Serve topped with toasted coconut.

Serves 4. Prep time 10 minutes. Cook time 30 minutes.

Calories **117** / Calories from fat **25** / Total fat **2.7g** / Saturated fat **2.0g** / Sodium **57mg** / Carbs **21.4g** / Sugars **5.1g** / Protein **7.8g**

Whole-Wheat Farfalle with Mint Pesto

You can put this lovely, simple side dish on the table in less than half an hour and enjoy the compliments. Try adding any vegetables, such as cherry tomatoes, asparagus, or tender green beans, if you have them on hand. You can also use whatever pasta is available, but these pretty bowties are quite festive and unusual.

Cooking tip You can make the mint pesto up to a week ahead of time. Store it in the refrigerator in an airtight container until you need it.

½ cup fresh mint leaves

½ cup fresh basil leaves

4 tablespoons pecans

2 tablespoons grated Parmesan cheese

1 tablespoon fresh lemon juice

1 tablespoon olive oil

Freshly ground black pepper, to taste

8 ounces dry whole-wheat farfalle

1 cup chopped artichoke hearts, cooked or canned

1 cup chopped roasted red peppers

1. Fill a large pot with water and bring to a boil over high heat.
2. Meanwhile, in a food processor, combine the mint, basil, pecans, Parmesan cheese, lemon juice, olive oil, and pepper and pulse until a chunky paste forms, about 2 minutes. Scoop the pesto into a bowl and set aside.
3. When the water is boiling, cook the pasta to al dente, according to the package directions.
4. Drain the pasta and return it to the pot. Add the pesto, artichoke hearts, and red peppers.
5. Stir to combine and heat through, about 5 minutes.
6. Serve immediately.

Serves 4. Prep time 10 minutes. Cook time 20 minutes.

Calories **333** / Calories from fat **115** / Total fat **12.7g** / Saturated fat **3.0g** / Trans fat **0.0g** / Sodium **174mg** / Carbs **49.9g** / Sugars **0.8g** / Protein **14.0g**

FODMAP-free
Gluten-free
Low-fat
Nightshade-free
Vegan
Vegetarian

SIDE DISHES

Grilled Carrots with Dill

Carrots seem like such a humble vegetable, but when you put them on the grill they get an exotic, slightly smoky taste that combines beautifully with fresh dill. Try not to cut your carrot sticks too small or thin, because you might lose them through the grill grates.

Shopping tip Although you can get dried dill year round, the best time to get fresh dill is in the early spring and summer.

1 pound carrots, washed and cut into batons about 3 inches long and ½ inch thick

1 teaspoon olive oil
1 tablespoon chopped fresh dill
1 tablespoon fresh lemon juice

1. Preheat the barbecue to medium-high heat or preheat the broiler.
2. On the barbecue, grill the carrots until softened and lightly charred, turning frequently, about 10 minutes. Or in the oven, broil the carrots, turning once, until tender, about 8 minutes.
3. In a large bowl, combine the carrots with the remaining ingredients and toss.
4. Serve warm.

Serves 4. Prep time 5 minutes. Cook time 10 minutes.

Calories **59** / Calories from fat **14** / Total fat **1.5g** / Trans fat **0.0g** / Sodium **80mg** / Carbs **11.4g** / Sugars **5.5g** / Protein **1.2g**

Rosemary Roasted Beets

The texture and color of the beets are ideal next to a lean, perfectly grilled steak or baked fish such as halibut. Rosemary also combines well with both red meat and fish, but you don't need very much to create a strong flavor. Rosemary is a good source of iron, calcium, and vitamins A, B_6, and C, which means it can help detoxify the liver, reduce the risk of cancer, and help provide some relief from arthritis-associated pain.

Diet tip If you want this dish to be low-sodium, simply omit the pinch of salt at the end and add a little freshly ground black pepper instead.

4 cups peeled and quartered beets

1 tablespoon olive oil

1 tablespoon chopped fresh rosemary

Pinch of sea salt

1. Preheat the oven to 400°F. Line a baking tray with foil and set aside.
2. In a large bowl, toss the beets with the oil until the beets are coated.
3. Spread the beets on the prepared baking sheet and roast in the oven until the vegetables are tender and lightly browned, about 25 to 35 minutes.
4. Remove the beets from the oven and sprinkle with the rosemary.
5. Season with salt and serve hot.

Serves 4. Prep time 10 minutes. Cook time 25 to 35 minutes.

Calories **91** / Calories from fat **35** / Total fat **3.9g** / Saturated fat **0.6g** / Sodium **165mg** / Carbs **14.6g** / Sugars **9.2g** / Protein **2.2g**

Gluten-free
Low-fat
Low-sodium
Vegetarian
Vegan

SIDE DISHES

Potato Fennel Bake

Fennel bulbs look a little like very fat celery bunches but taste like licorice. This flavor can be strong when the fennel is raw, but mellows when the vegetable is roasted, as in this dish. Fennel is rich in B vitamins, vitamin C, iron, potassium, and manganese. It can support healthy digestion and reduce the risk of heart disease and cancer.

Shopping tip The fennel fronds should never have any flowering buds, because that means it is past maturity and could be slightly bitter. Fennel is best in the winter and early spring.

2 large Yukon gold potatoes, skin on, washed and thinly sliced
1 tablespoon olive oil
Freshly ground black pepper
1 medium fennel bulb, trimmed and thinly sliced

2 teaspoons chopped fresh thyme
2 garlic cloves, thinly sliced
Zest and juice of 1 lemon
1 cup low-sodium, fat-free vegetable stock

1. Preheat the oven to 350°F.
2. In a medium bowl, toss the potatoes with the oil and season lightly with the pepper.
3. In a 9-by-11-inch baking dish, make an even layer of half the fennel slices.
4. Top the fennel with half the potatoes, half the thyme, and half the garlic.
5. Repeat the layering to use up all the fennel, potatoes, thyme, and garlic.
6. Sprinkle the casserole with lemon zest and juice.
7. Pour in the vegetable stock and cover the dish with foil.
8. Bake until the vegetables are very tender, about 45 minutes.
9. Remove the foil and bake for 5 more minutes to brown the potatoes.
10. Serve immediately.

Serves 4. Prep time 15 minutes. Cook time 50 minutes.

Calories **168** / Calories from fat **35** / Total fat **3.9g** / Saturated fat **0.6g** / Trans fat **0.0g** / Sodium **81mg** / Carbs **33.9g** / Sugars **1.8g** / Protein **4.2g**

Barley Kale Risotto

Risotto is usually prepared with a short- or medium-grain rice such as arborio, but it can also be prepared with most grains. Barley has a delightful chewy texture and nutty flavor, and it is an excellent source of fiber. Barley is also rich in manganese, selenium, copper, and vitamin B_1. It can help protect against heart disease, type 2 diabetes, and breast cancer.

Shopping tip You can usually find hulled barley in the bulk sections of major grocery stores. Make sure the containers of barley are tightly covered so there is no moisture, and that your grocery store has a rotation policy to ensure the freshness of the product.

1 medium butternut squash, peeled, seeded, and cut into ½ inch cubes

2 teaspoons olive oil, divided

Pinch of freshly ground black pepper

½ small sweet onion, peeled and finely chopped

1 teaspoon minced garlic

1 cup hulled barley, rinsed

4 cups chopped kale

2 tablespoons pine nuts

2 tablespoons chopped fresh thyme

1. Preheat the oven to 375°F. Line a baking sheet with foil.
2. Toss the squash with 1 teaspoon of the oil and the pepper.
3. Spread the squash on the prepared baking sheet and roast in the oven until the squash is tender and lightly browned, stirring several times, about 35 minutes.
4. While the squash is roasting, fill a medium saucepan with about 5 cups of water and bring to a boil.
5. Reduce the heat to keep the water warm but not simmering.
6. In a large saucepan over medium heat, add the remaining teaspoon of oil and sauté the onion and garlic in the oil until softened, about 3 minutes.
7. Add the barley and sauté, stirring, for about 2 minutes.
8. Add one cup of the hot water to the barley and stir until the water is absorbed.

continued ➤

Barley Kale Risotto *continued*

9. Repeat until you have added 3 cups of hot water to the barley.
10. Add the kale and stir until the kale is wilted and the water is absorbed.
11. Add more water, a small amount at a time, stirring often, until the barley is cooked through and tender.
12. Stir in the roasted squash and the pine nuts.
13. Serve the risotto topped with thyme.

Serves 4. Prep time 10 minutes. Cook time 1 hour.

Calories **323** / Calories from fat **75** / Total fat **8.3g** / Saturated fat **0.8g** / Trans fat **0.0g** / Sodium **37mg** / Carbs **58.5g** / Sugars **6.2g** / Protein **10.1g**

Tomato-Topped Spaghetti Squash

Gluten-free
Low-fat
Low-sodium
Nightshade-free
Vegetarian

SIDE DISHES

The pasta-like appearance of cooked spaghetti squash makes it popular for vegan, vegetarian, and gluten-free dishes. The texture is softer than pasta, so do not over-cook this vegetable if you want a firmer "noodle" for the side dish. You can also use a Clean Eating marinara sauce instead of fresh tomatoes to top the squash.

Shopping tip When picking your spaghetti squash, look for one with a firm dry stem because the stem can keep bacteria out of the inside of the squash.

1 spaghetti squash, cut in half lengthwise

1 tablespoon olive oil

Sea salt

Freshly ground black pepper

2 tomatoes, chopped

2 tablespoons chopped green onion

1 tablespoon chopped fresh basil or 3 teaspoons dried basil

3 tablespoons Parmesan cheese

1. Preheat oven to 350°F.
2. Line a baking tray with foil.
3. Scoop the seeds out of the squash and drizzle the cut sides with the olive oil.
4. Season the cut sides lightly with salt and pepper and lay the squash halves cut-side down on the baking sheet.
5. Bake the squash until it is tender, about 45 minutes. Let the squash cool on the tray for 10 minutes.
6. While the squash is baking, combine the tomatoes, green onion, and basil in a small bowl; set aside.
7. Use a fork to shred the squash strands into a medium bowl.
8. Top the shredded squash with the tomato mixture and Parmesan cheese and serve immediately.

Serves 2. Prep time 10 minutes. Cook time 45 minutes.

Calories **129** / Calories from fat **47** / Total fat **5.2g** / Saturated fat **1.6g** / Sodium **223mg** / Carbs **19.5g** / Sugars **3.3g** / Protein **4.8g**

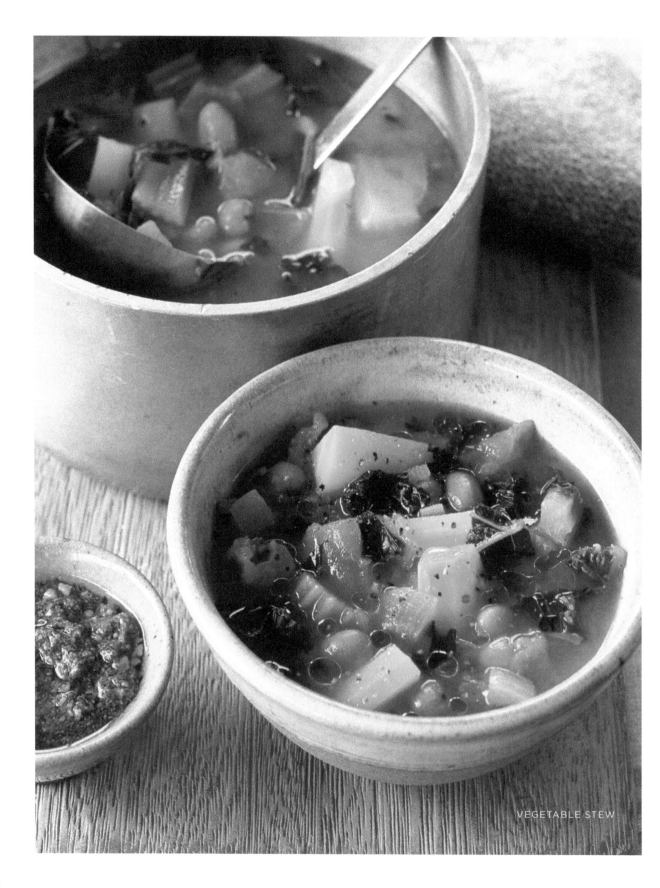

VEGETABLE STEW

CHAPTER TEN

Vegetarian Entrées

Bean Tostadas

Tostada is "toasted" in Spanish; this dish is a toasted tortilla topped with an array of delicious toppings. You can use any tortilla—corn, multigrain, or even gluten-free—for this dish. The jalapeño peppers in this recipe give a nice heat, which can be kicked up by using chipotle or even habañero peppers instead. Make sure you wash your hands thoroughly after handling the hot peppers, because the juices can severely irritate any mucus membranes they come in contact with.

Diet tip This recipe can easily be made gluten-free by using gluten-free tortillas instead of whole-wheat. Leave out the feta cheese and it's vegan.

Eight 6-inch whole-wheat tortillas
Nonstick cooking spray
3 cups canned sodium-free black beans, drained and rinsed
1 small sweet onion, peeled and coarsely chopped
1 red bell pepper, seeded and diced

2 jalapeño peppers, seeded and coarsely chopped
1 teaspoon ground cumin
4 tablespoons water
4 teaspoons chopped fresh cilantro
¼ cup crumbled low-sodium feta
1 large tomato, diced
1 cup shredded romaine lettuce

1. Preheat the oven to 400°F.
2. On two baking sheets, toast the tortillas in the oven until crisp, about 5 minutes.
3. Remove the tortillas from the baking sheets and set aside.
4. Lightly coat the baking sheets with cooking spray and spread the beans, onion, red pepper, and jalapeño peppers evenly on the sheets; roast the mixture in the oven for about 10 minutes.
5. In a food processor, combine the roasted beans and vegetables with the cumin and water and pulse until coarsely chopped.
6. On each tortilla, spread an equal amount of the bean mixture and sprinkle with the cilantro and feta.

7. Top each with the tomato and shredded lettuce.
8. Serve two tostadas per person.

Serves 4. Prep time 10 minutes. Cook time 15 minutes.

Calories **250** / Calories from fat **30** / Total fat **3.3g** / Saturated fat **0.7g** / Trans fat **0.0g** / Sodium **554mg** / Carbs **55.4g** / Sugars **2.4g** / Protein **10.6g**

Grilled Portobello Burgers with Goat Cheese

These large, meaty mushrooms are a favorite of many vegetarians. So why not use them as burger patties? Portobello mushrooms can be up to four inches in diameter, so they fit perfectly on most buns. They are a good source of fiber, protein, vitamin D, and potassium, and are low in calories and fat.

Cooking tip Make sure to brush your mushrooms evenly with oil, rather than tossing them, because these mushrooms can soak up the oil unevenly, creating dry sections when you grill them.

4 large Portobello mushroom caps, each
    about 4 inches in diameter

1 tablespoon olive oil

1 large red onion, cut into
    ¼-inch-thick slices

2 tablespoons balsamic vinegar

4 ciabatta buns, split

4 tablespoons crumbled goat cheese

1 large tomato, cut into ¼-inch-thick slices

1 cup shredded Boston lettuce

1. Preheat a barbecue to medium-high or preheat the broiler.
2. Brush the mushroom caps with the oil.
3. In a large bowl, combine the mushroom caps with the onion and toss with the balsamic vinegar.
4. On the barbecue, grill the mushroom caps and onion until they are tender, about 5 minutes per side. Or if using the oven, place the caps on a baking tray and broil until the mushrooms and onions are tender, about 5 minutes.
5. Remove from the heat and set aside on a plate.
6. Place the buns on the barbecue, cut-side down, and toast for about 1 minute. Or place them under the broiler, cut-side up, and broil for about 30 seconds.
7. Spread the goat cheese on the top bun halves.
8. Place a mushroom on each bun bottom and top with the onions.

9. Place a tomato slice on the onions and ¼ cup of the shredded lettuce for each bun.
10. Top with the top bun halves and serve.

Serves 4. Prep time 5 minutes. Cook time 15 minutes.

Calories **338** / Calories from fat **105** / Total fat **11.7g** / Saturated fat **5.0g** / Trans fat **0.0g** / Sodium **494mg** / Carbs **42.1g** / Sugars **5.9g** / Protein **14.8g**

Vegetable Stew

This recipe is only a guideline for the finished dish, because you can add any combination of vegetables and still have a delicious stew. The combination of vegetables in the ingredients provide an array of colors, textures, and tastes, giving you a complete culinary and nutrition experience in one bowl. Eating many different colors of produce means you are getting a full range of antioxidants and nutrients.

1 teaspoon olive oil

1 small sweet onion, peeled and chopped

1 teaspoon minced garlic

½ teaspoon ground cumin

½ teaspoon ground coriander

1 red bell pepper, seeded and chopped

2 large carrots, peeled and chopped

2 cups fat-free, low-sodium
    vegetable stock

2 large tomatoes, chopped

½ cup canned sodium-free white kidney
    beans, rinsed and drained

1 teaspoon fresh lemon juice

1 cup chopped kale

Pinch of crushed red pepper flakes

Freshly ground black pepper, to taste

1. In a large pot over medium heat, heat the oil and sauté the onion and garlic until softened, about 3 minutes.
2. Add the cumin, and coriander, and stir to coat, about 1 minute.
3. Add the red pepper and carrots and sauté for 5 minutes.
4. Stir in the vegetable stock, tomatoes, and kidney beans.
5. Bring the stew to a boil and then reduce the heat to low.
6. Simmer the stew until the vegetables are tender, stirring often, about 15 to 17 minutes.
7. Add the lemon juice and kale and heat until the kale is wilted, about 3 minutes.
8. Stir in the red pepper flakes and pepper.
9. Serve.

Serves 4. Prep time 15 minutes. Cook time 30 minutes.

Calories **101** / Calories from fat **16** / Total fat **1.8g** / Saturated fat **0.0g** / Trans fat **0.0g** / Sodium **63mg** / Carbs **17.7g** / Sugars **7.2g** / Protein **4.4g**

Simple Colcannon

Gluten-free
Low-fat
Vegan
Vegetarian

VEGETARIAN
ENTRÉES

Colcannon is a traditional Irish dish of cabbage and mashed potatoes with a history dating back hundreds of years. If you want to add a couple of cups of shredded green cabbage along with (or instead of) the kale, you will be in good culinary company, since that is the more traditional ingredient. Simply sauté the cabbage until it is tender, about ten minutes, before adding the kale.

Nutrition tip Let your chopped kale sit for about five minutes before cooking. This can increase the phytonutrient benefits because the "wounded" leaves produce anti-oxidants to repair the damage.

6 large russet potatoes, peeled and
    chopped into ½-inch chunks
1 teaspoon olive oil
1 small sweet onion, peeled and diced
3 teaspoons minced garlic

6 cups chopped kale
1 cup almond milk
Pinch of sea salt
Pinch of freshly ground black pepper

1. Bring a large pot of water to a boil over medium-high heat, and add the potatoes.
2. Boil until the potatoes are tender, about 15 minutes.
3. Drain and rinse the potatoes, and transfer them to a large bowl. Set aside.
4. In a large skillet over medium-high heat, heat the oil and sauté the onion and garlic until softened, about 3 minutes.
5. Add the kale and sauté until it is wilted, about 3 minutes.
6. Mash the potatoes with the almond milk, salt, and pepper until smooth.
7. Add the kale mixture to the mashed potatoes and stir until well combined.
8. Serve warm.

Serves 4. Prep time 15 minutes. Cook time 25 minutes.

Calories **370** / Calories from fat **22** / Total fat **2.4g** / Saturated fat **0.0g** / Trans fat **0.0g** / Sodium **189mg** / Carbs **77.4g** / Sugars **4.0g** / Protein **11.4g**

Baked Broccoli Rice Cakes

These are like golden savory muffins rather than cakes. Broccoli and cheese is a classic combination that works well with the rice in this dish. Broccoli is a vegetable you just can't eat often enough, because it is packed with nutrients and antioxidants. Broccoli can help boost the immune system and support healthy bones, as well.

Cooking tip Fresh broccoli can be stored in the refrigerator in a sealed plastic bag for as long as ten days if you leave it on the stalk and don't wash it until you're ready to cook it. If you cut it into florets before storing, the vitamin C content will start to diminish after a few days.

Nonstick cooking spray

2 cups chopped broccoli florets

2 cups cooked brown rice

¼ cup plain Greek yogurt

2 eggs, lightly beaten

½ cup grated sharp Cheddar cheese

¼ teaspoon ground nutmeg

Freshly ground black pepper

1. Preheat the oven to 350°F. Lightly coat 8 muffin cups with cooking spray and set aside.
2. Fill a medium saucepan with water and bring to a boil over medium-high heat.
3. Add the broccoli to the boiling water and blanch until it is tender-crisp, about 3 minutes. Drain the broccoli.
4. In a large bowl, combine the broccoli with the rice, yogurt, eggs, cheese, and nutmeg, and season with pepper to taste.
5. Portion the broccoli mixture evenly among the muffin cups and bake until golden, about 20 minutes.
6. Remove the cakes from the oven and let them stand for 5 minutes. Run a knife around the edges to loosen.
7. Serve two cakes per person with a green salad.

Serves 4. Prep time 10 minutes. Cook time 25 minutes.

Calories **461** / Calories from fat **93** / Total fat **10.3g** / Saturated fat **4.6g** / Trans fat **0.0g** / Sodium **142mg** / Carbs **76.3g** / Sugars **1.6g** / Protein **15.9g**

Market Quinoa Skillet

This packed skillet is a filling and satisfying choice on cold winter evenings when you crave comfort food. The quinoa provides bulk, along with many important nutrients, and is incredibly easy to prepare.

Diet tip Creating a vegan meal is as simple as leaving out the feta cheese or adding a favorite vegan cheese product in its place.

2 cups fat-free, low-sodium
   vegetable stock
1 cup uncooked quinoa, rinsed and drained
1 teaspoon olive oil
2 teaspoons minced garlic
2 cups fresh corn kernels
2 cups chopped green beans, cut into
   1-inch pieces
½ large zucchini, cut in half lengthwise and
   thinly sliced into half disks

1 red bell pepper, seeded and sliced
   into thin strips
2 green onions, thinly sliced
2 ripe tomatoes, chopped
½ cup crumbled low-sodium feta cheese
3 teaspoons chopped fresh basil
2 tablespoons fresh lemon juice
2 teaspoons lemon zest
Pinch of freshly ground black pepper

1. In a medium saucepan over medium heat, bring the vegetable stock to a boil and then add the quinoa.
2. Cover and reduce the heat to low.
3. Cook until the quinoa has absorbed all the stock, about 15 minutes.
4. Remove the quinoa from the heat and let it cool slightly.
5. In a large skillet over medium-high heat, heat the oil and sauté the garlic until softened, about 1 minute.
6. Add the corn, green beans, zucchini, red pepper, and green onions, and sauté until the vegetables are tender-crisp, about 5 minutes.
7. Add the quinoa and the remaining ingredients. Stir to combine.
8. Serve warm or cold.

Serves 4. Prep time 15 minutes. Cook time 30 minutes.

Calories **302** / Calories from fat **64** / Total fat **7.1g** / Saturated fat **2.1g** / Trans fat **0.0g** /
Sodium **606mg** / Carbs **51.9g** / Sugars **7.4g** / Protein **16.2g**

Broccolini Sauté

Broccolini looks like baby broccoli, but it is actually a hybrid of Chinese and regular broccoli, and tastes more like asparagus than broccoli. It has long, slender stalks and tight green buds that do not need much cooking time. Broccolini has all the health benefits of broccoli, as well, making this dish a wonderfully nutritious, light dinner for any vegetarian or vegan.

Nutrition tip This delicate vegetable is a naturally occurring hybrid rather than a genetically modified one.

3 teaspoons olive oil

4 cups chopped broccolini
(about 3 bunches)

3 green onions, chopped

4 roasted garlic cloves, sliced or
chopped (see page 190)

½ teaspoon freshly ground black pepper

¼ teaspoon crushed red pepper flakes

3 cups baby spinach

¼ cup chopped fresh parsley

Zest and juice of 1 lemon

1. In a large skillet over medium heat, heat the oil and sauté the broccolini, green onions, and roasted garlic until the broccolini is bright green but still crisp, about 5 minutes.
2. Add the black pepper and red pepper flakes and stir to combine.
3. Add the spinach, parsley, and lemon zest and sauté until the spinach is wilted, about 3 minutes.
4. Add the lemon juice to the skillet and stir.
5. Serve immediately.

Serves 4. Prep time 10 minutes. Cook time 10 minutes.

Calories **81** / Calories from fat **33** / Total fat **3.7g** / Saturated fat **0.5g** / Trans fat **0.0g** / Sodium **47mg** / Carbs **8.2g** / Sugars **2.5g** / Protein **4.2g**

Red Lentil Coconut Curry

Gluten-free
Low-sodium
Vegan
Vegetarian

VEGETARIAN
ENTRÉES

Curry is a staple dish in vegetarian cuisine because the grains and root vegetables in a typical curry really soak up the seasonings. Coconut is also a very popular addition in all forms, such as shredded meat, milk, and even coconut water as in this recipe. Coconut water is the liquid that is taken from young coconuts, and is not to be confused with coconut milk, which is made from squeezing the liquid out of the meat.

Nutrition tip Coconut water is fat free, cholesterol free, low fat, and low sodium. It also has four times the amount of potassium as bananas, so it's a great recovery drink after a workout. You can find this super drink in most health food stores or in the organic sections of major grocery stores.

1 tablespoon coconut oil

1 small sweet onion, peeled and diced

2 teaspoons minced garlic

2 medium carrots, peeled and diced

1 sweet potato, peeled and diced

2 teaspoons grated fresh ginger

1 tablespoon curry powder

3 large ripe tomatoes, diced

2 cups fat-free, low-sodium
    vegetable stock

1 cup coconut water

1 cup dried red lentils, rinsed and
    picked through

1 cup finely julienned spinach

1. In a large pot over medium heat, heat the coconut oil and sauté the onion and garlic until softened, about 3 minutes.
2. Add the carrots and sweet potato and sauté for 10 more minutes, stirring often.
3. Add the remaining ingredients except the spinach and stir to combine.
4. Bring the mixture to a boil and then reduce the heat to low.
5. Simmer the curry until most of the liquid is absorbed and the lentils and vegetables are tender, about 30 minutes.
6. Stir in the spinach and let the curry stand for about 10 minutes.
7. Serve plain or over rice.

Serves 6. Prep time 15 minutes. Cook time 45 minutes.

Calories **288** / Calories from fat **41** / Total fat **4.6g** / Saturated fat **3.1g** / Trans fat **0.0g** / Sodium **60mg** / Carbs **34.1g** / Sugars **8.7g** / Protein **16.2g**

Healthy Vegetable Chili

Making a spectacular chili is a mark of honor among many serious cooks, and there are serious competitions geared around this simple dish. This version is more than just a combination of beans, tomato, and spices; it is also packed with a nice assortment of healthy vegetables. If you want to substitute different vegetables, don't feel like you have to stick to the recipe. Chili is very accommodating of most ingredient choices.

Nutrition tip Chili powder is produced from dried chili peppers, and it can be mildly hot or it can sear your throat, depending on what chili pepper is used. Chili peppers contain a substance called capsaicin that creates this distinctive heat. It also can be an effective treatment for pain associated with osteoarthritis.

2 tablespoons olive oil

1 large sweet onion, peeled and
    finely chopped

3 teaspoons minced garlic

2 cups chopped button mushrooms

2 large carrots, peeled and diced

1 large red bell pepper, seeded and diced

1 large zucchini, diced

1 jalapeño pepper, seeded and chopped

¼ cup chili powder

1 tablespoon ground cumin

1 tablespoon dried oregano

1 teaspoon crushed red pepper flakes

4 large tomatoes, chopped

One 6-ounce can sodium-free
    tomato paste

1 cup fat-free, low-sodium
    vegetable stock

2 cups black beans, rinsed and drained

2 cups red kidney beans, rinsed
    and drained

2 cups navy beans, rinsed and drained

1. In a large pot over medium-high heat, heat the olive oil and sauté the onion, garlic, and mushrooms until softened, about 3 minutes.
2. Add the carrots, red bell pepper, and zucchini and sauté for an additional 8 minutes.
3. Add the remaining ingredients and stir to combine well.
4. Bring the chili to a boil and then reduce the heat to low.

5. Simmer the vegetables until they are fork tender and the flavors have mellowed, about 45 minutes.
6. Remove the chili from the heat and let it stand for about 10 minutes before serving.

Serves 12. Prep time 15 minutes. Cook time 1 hour.

Calories **408** / Calories from fat **51** / Total fat **5.7g** / Saturated fat **1.7g** / Trans fat **0.0g** / Sodium **54mg** / Carbs **69.1g** / Sugars **7.2g** / Protein **23.8g**

VEGETARIAN
ENTRÉES

Lentil Barley Burgers

The complexity of flavor found in these veggie burgers might surprise you if you are used to the bland, processed versions. Red lentils are the base for these burgers, but you can also use green, yellow, or brown lentils. The color will change and the flavor will also slightly change, because red lentils are the sweetest and nuttiest variety.

Shopping tip You can either cook your own lentils (they cook much faster than beans) or buy an organic, sodium-free cooked product to save time.

3 teaspoons olive oil, divided

½ small sweet onion, chopped

3 tablespoons grated carrot

1 teaspoon minced garlic

1 teaspoon ground cumin

1 teaspoon dried oregano

Pinch of chili powder

Pinch of salt

½ cup cooked lentils, rinsed and drained

½ cup cooked pearl barley

¼ cup panko breadcrumbs

3 tablespoons chopped fresh parsley

1 egg white

1 egg

1 large mango, peeled, pitted, and diced

1. In a medium skillet over medium heat, heat 1 teaspoon of the olive oil and sauté the onion, carrot, and garlic until the vegetables are softened.
2. Add the cumin, oregano, chili powder, and salt and stir to combine. Remove from the heat.
3. In a large mixing bowl, combine the onion mixture with the remaining ingredients, except for the mango.
4. Stir until the mixture holds together well, adding more panko if the mixture is too wet.
5. Cover the burger mixture and refrigerate until firm, about 1 hour.
6. Divide the burger mixture into four portions, and press them into four ½-inch-thick patties.

7. In a large skillet over medium-high heat, heat the remaining 2 teaspoons of olive oil and cook the patties until both sides are golden brown, about 3 minutes per side.

8. Serve topped with mango.

Serves 4. Prep time 15 minutes. Cook time 11 minutes.

Calories **355** / Calories from fat **89** / Total fat **9.9g** / Saturated fat **2.3g** / Trans fat **0.0g** / Sodium **147mg** / Carbs **49.9g** / Sugars **10.0g** / Protein **17.6g**

Mushroom Cashew Rice

The cashews in this hearty rice dish provide an interesting crunch and richness that is very pleasing to the palate. Cashews are heart-healthy, can help reduce the risk of cancer, and promote bone health. Despite the bad reputation nuts usually have because of their fat content, cashews actually support weight loss as well. They contain healthy fats and are an energy-dense choice for dieters.

Shopping tip When buying cashews, especially in bulk, it is important to smell them to make sure they aren't rancid. Cashews can be stored in the refrigerator in a sealed container for up to six months.

1 tablespoon olive oil

3 celery stalks, chopped

½ small sweet onion, peeled and chopped

2 teaspoons minced garlic

1 cup sliced button mushrooms

2 cups uncooked brown basmati rice

3½ cups fat-free, low-sodium
    vegetable stock

Freshly ground black pepper

½ cup chopped cashews

1. In a large saucepan over medium-high heat, heat the oil and sauté the celery, onion, garlic, and mushrooms until they are softened.
2. Add the rice and sauté for an additional minute.
3. Add the stock and bring to a boil, then reduce the heat to low and cover the pot.
4. Simmer the rice until the liquid is absorbed and the rice is tender, about 35 to 40 minutes.
5. Season with pepper to taste.
6. Top with cashews and serve.

Serves 6. Prep time 10 minutes. Cook time 15 minutes.

Calories **341** / Calories from fat **80** / Total fat **8.9g** / Saturated fat **1.7g** / Trans fat **0.0g** / Sodium **458mg** / Carbs **51.1g** / Sugars **1.7g** / Protein **9.5g**

Lemon Artichoke Pesto with Zucchini Noodles

Gluten-free
Low-sodium
Vegan
Vegetarian

VEGETARIAN
ENTRÉES

This is a truly gorgeous example of everything that is wonderful about vegetarian cuisine. It is colorful, fresh, and packed with flavor. The artichokes add a richness and bulk to the pesto and finished dish, as well as some important health benefits. Artichokes are extremely high in antioxidants, which means they are super disease fighters. Artichokes can cut your risk of cancer, reduce cholesterol, and support effective liver function.

Leftovers tip You might not use up all the pesto in this recipe. Spoon the extra into ice cube trays, cover the whole tray in plastic wrap, and freeze it for up to six months.

1 cup chopped artichoke hearts

½ cup packed fresh basil leaves

½ cup chopped pecan halves

2 teaspoons minced garlic

Zest and juice of 1 lemon

Pinch of freshly ground black pepper

¼ cup olive oil

2 large zucchini, julienned

2 cups cherry tomatoes, halved

Pinch of crushed red pepper flakes

1. In a food processor, combine half the artichoke hearts with the basil, pecans, garlic, lemon zest, lemon juice, and black pepper; pulse until very finely chopped.
2. Add the olive oil and pulse until blended.
3. In a large bowl, toss the zucchini "noodles" with the remaining artichoke hearts, cherry tomatoes, and red pepper flakes until well mixed.
4. Add the pesto by tablespoons until you have the desired flavor and texture.
5. Store any leftover pesto in a sealed container in the refrigerator for up to 2 weeks.
6. Serve immediately.

Serves 4. Prep time 30 minutes.

Calories **259** / Calories from fat **203** / Total fat **22.6g** / Saturated fat **2.7g** / Trans Fat **0.0g** / Sodium **106mg** / Carbs **14.1g** / Sugars **5.4g** / Protein **5.4g**

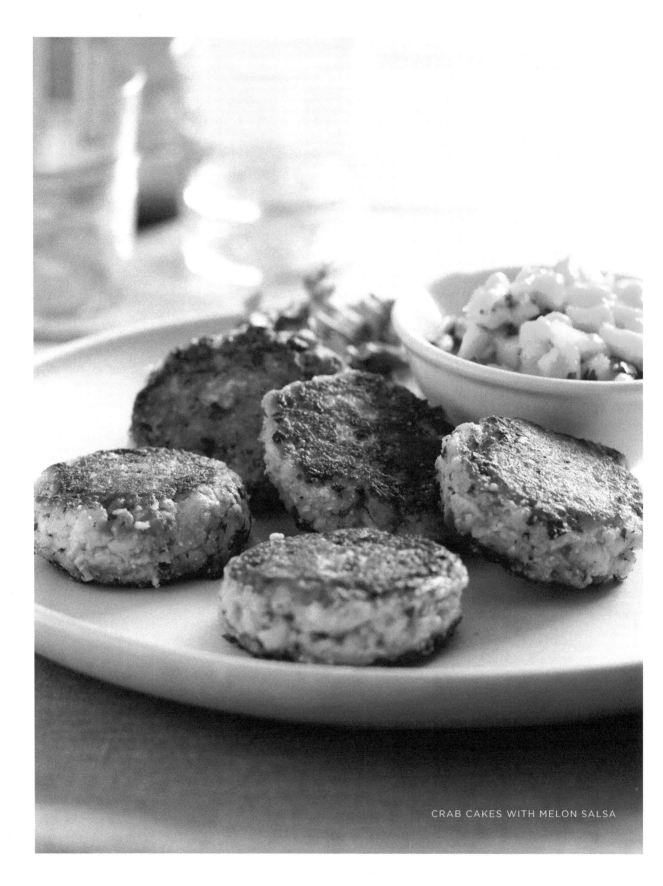

CRAB CAKES WITH MELON SALSA

CHAPTER ELEVEN

Seafood

Cod with Cucumber Mint Sauce

This dish is spring on a plate—snowy, tender fish topped with delicate pastel green cucumber and cool mint. It is a delight to the taste and light on the stomach. Mint is high in vitamins A and C, and is also a good source of copper, calcium, potassium, and magnesium. It can stimulate digestion, boost the immune system, and cleanse the blood.

Shopping tip Whenever possible, buy Pacific cod because the Atlantic cod population is diminishing. This white fish should be firm and slightly springy to the touch with a very mild fish scent.

Nonstick cooking spray

Four 5-ounce cod fillets

Sea salt

Freshly ground black pepper

4 tablespoons fat-free plain Greek yogurt

¼ English cucumber, grated, liquid squeezed out

2 teaspoons chopped fresh mint

2 tablespoons chopped green onion

1. In a large skillet over medium-high heat, add a light coat of cooking spray.
2. Season the fish with salt and pepper to taste and pan fry the fish in the skillet, turning once, until it is just cooked through, about 4 minutes per side. Remove the fish from the heat and transfer the fillets to individual plates.
3. In a small bowl, stir together the yogurt, cucumber, mint, and green onion until well mixed.
4. Serve the fish topped with the yogurt sauce.

Serves 4. Prep time 10 minutes. Cook time 8 minutes.

Calories **127** / Calories from fat **12** / Total fat **1.3g** / Saturated fat **0.0g** / Trans fat **0.0g** / Sodium **96mg** / Carbs **1.0g** / Sugar **0.0g** / Protein **27.0g**

Kale Quinoa Topped with Halibut

Gluten-free
Low-fat
Low-sodium
Nightshade-free

SEAFOOD

This recipe produces a side dish and main course in one. Kale is one of those super greens that are now available in most grocery stores and markets. It is rich in calcium, beta-carotene, chlorophyll, and vitamins A, C, and K. Kale can support a healthy digestive system, improve eyesight, and reduce the risk of heart disease, cancer, and type 2 diabetes.

Shopping tip Fresh halibut is usually best between March and November. If you buy frozen halibut, it takes about one-third less cooking time than fresh. Cook the fish after it has thawed.

1 cup uncooked quinoa, rinsed

2 cups water

Nonstick cooking spray

½ small sweet onion, peeled and chopped

1 cup diced cooked sweet potato

2 cups chopped kale

Four 4-ounce halibut fillets

Sea salt

Freshly ground black pepper

1. In a medium saucepan, combine the quinoa and water.
2. Bring the quinoa to a boil over medium-high heat and then reduce the heat to low so the liquid simmers.
3. Cover and cook the quinoa until all the liquid is absorbed, about 15 minutes.
4. Transfer the quinoa to a large bowl and set aside.
5. In a large nonstick skillet, add a light coat of cooking spray and heat over medium-high heat.
6. Add the onion and sauté until it is softened, about 3 minutes.
7. Stir in the cooked sweet potato and sauté until heated through, about 5 minutes.
8. Add the kale and stir until it is wilted, about 3 minutes.
9. Add the quinoa mixture to the kale and stir to mix well.

continued ➤

10. Preheat the oven to broil.
11. Place the halibut on a small baking sheet and season with salt and pepper to taste.
12. Broil the fish, turning once, until the fish flakes when pressed with a fork, about 4 minutes per side.
13. Serve the fish over the quinoa.

Serves 4. Prep time 10 minutes. Cook time 35 minutes.

Calories **401** / Calories from fat **87** / Total fat **9.6g** / Saturated fat **1.3g** / Trans fat **0.0g** / Sodium **111mg** / Carbs **39.8g** / Sugars **4.4g** / Protein **38.4g**

Ginger Salmon in
Foil Packets

Gluten-free
Low-sodium

SEAFOOD

This is similar to cooking fish "en papillote" (in parchment), so go ahead and create parchment-paper packets if you are familiar with that culinary technique. This dish has some definite Asian flavors, using cut vegetables, sesame, and ginger.

Nutrition tip Bean sprouts are crunchy and sweet, but they are also very heart-friendly due to their high potassium and vitamin K content. Bean sprouts are also a good source of fiber, which can help lower cholesterol levels.

4 cups bean sprouts

1 large red bell pepper, seeded and thinly sliced into strips

1 cup snow peas, stringed and halved

Four 4-ounce salmon fillets, skin removed

¼ cup fat-free, low-sodium vegetable stock

2 teaspoons grated fresh ginger

1 green onion, chopped finely

½ teaspoon minced garlic

1 teaspoon sesame oil

2 tablespoons sesame seeds

1. Preheat the oven to 400°F. Cut four pieces of foil, each about 12 inches square.
2. Evenly divide the bean sprouts, red pepper, and snow peas into quarters and place onto the middle of each piece of foil.
3. Place a salmon fillet on top of each pile of vegetables.
4. In a small bowl, stir together the vegetable stock, ginger, green onion, garlic, and oil until well mixed.
5. Drizzle the sauce evenly over the salmon.
6. Fold the foil up into sealed packets and place them on a baking sheet.
7. Bake until the fish flakes when pressed with a fork, about 20 minutes.
8. Remove the salmon and vegetables from the foil and top each serving with sesame seeds.

Serves 4. Prep time 10 minutes. Cook time 20 minutes.

Calories **276** / Calories from fat **104** / Total fat **11.6g** / Saturated fat **1.6g** / Trans fat **0.0g** / Sodium **91mg** / Carbs **14.9g** / Sugars **3.8g** / Protein **32.6g**

Crab Cakes with Melon Salsa

This salsa elevates what is a very nice dish to something truly special. Crab and fruit are a naturally good combination, especially with the addition of a little acid such as lemon juice. Cantaloupe and watermelon are very well known for their health benefits, but the often underused honeydew is also a nutritional prize. It is high in fiber, potassium, and vitamins B_6 and C.

Shopping tip When picking honeydew, sniff the melon to make sure it is ripe. You will be able to smell the flesh right through the pale, creamy skin if it is ready to eat.

For the salsa:
1 cup finely diced honeydew
½ cup finely diced watermelon
½ cup finely diced cantaloupe
1 green onion, finely chopped
2 tablespoons fresh lemon juice
Pinch of sea salt

For the crab cakes:
1 pound cooked lump crabmeat, drained and picked over
¼ cup whole-wheat panko breadcrumbs
2 teaspoons Dijon mustard
2 green onions, finely chopped
1 tablespoon chopped fresh parsley
1 teaspoon freshly grated lemon zest
1 teaspoon smoked paprika
2 egg whites
4 tablespoons whole-wheat flour
Nonstick cooking spray

To make the salsa:
1. In a medium bowl, combine all the salsa ingredients and mix well.
2. Store the salsa in a sealed container in the refrigerator until serving the crab cakes.

To make the crab cakes:

1. In a large bowl, combine the crabmeat, panko, mustard, green onions, parsley, lemon zest, paprika, and egg whites and mix very well.
2. Divide the crab mixture into 8 equal portions and form each portion into a patty about 1 inch thick.
3. Transfer the crab cakes to a plate, cover, and chill them in the refrigerator for at least an hour or overnight to firm up.
4. Put the flour on a plate and dredge the chilled crab cakes in the flour until they are lightly coated.
5. In a large skillet over medium heat, add a light coat of cooking spray and cook the crab cakes until they are golden brown, turning once, about 5 minutes per side.
6. Serve the crab cakes with the salsa.

Serves 4. Prep time 30 minutes. Cook time 10 minutes.

Calories **216** / Calories from fat **26** / Total fat **2.9g** / Trans fat **0.0g** / Sodium **554mg** / Carbs **36.4g** / Sugars **7.2g** / Protein **27.4g**

Spicy Lime Tilapia

Tilapia is a very popular fish because it is inexpensive and has a pleasant, mild taste that combines well with many other ingredients. Tilapia is rich in protein and omega-3 fatty acids, which are considered to be very heart-friendly. Because most tilapia is farmed, try to limit your consumption to one meal a week even though the fish is classified as a low-mercury fish. Farmed fish can sometimes have a high concentration of antibiotics, pesticides, and other contaminants such as PCBs. Fish is still considered to be a clean eating choice, but wild caught is preferred.

Leftovers tip This spicy fish is fabulous cold and tucked into a pita, or wrapped in a tortilla the next day with a little shredded spinach.

Four 6-ounce tilapia fillets

1 teaspoon chili powder

1 teaspoon garlic powder

½ teaspoon freshly ground black pepper

¼ teaspoon cayenne pepper

Nonstick olive oil cooking spray

Juice of 1 lime

1. Preheat the oven to 450°F. Line a baking sheet with foil and set aside. Pat the fish fillets dry with paper towels and place them on the prepared baking sheet. Set aside.
2. In a small bowl, stir together the chili and garlic powders, pepper, and cayenne until well mixed.
3. Sprinkle half of the spice mixture evenly over the fish and use your fingertips to lightly rub it in.
4. Spray a little olive oil over the fish and then sprinkle half of the lime juice over the fillets.
5. Flip the fish fillets over and repeat steps 3 and 4 on the other sides.
6. Bake in the oven until the fish flakes, about 8 minutes.

Serves 4. Prep time 15 minutes. Cook time 8 minutes.

Calories **145** / Calories from fat **15** / Total fat **1.7g** / Saturated fat **0.7g** / Trans fat **0.0g** / Sodium **67mg** / Carbs **1.1g** / Sugar **0.0g** / Protein **31.9g**

Salmon with Herbed Yogurt Sauce

Salmon is often found in clean eating plans because it is rich in omega-3 fatty acids, calcium, selenium, and vitamins A, B, and D. Salmon is very heart-smart, helps prevent Alzheimer's disease, and can boost your metabolism. Salmon can also support healthy hair, glowing skin, and clear eyes.

Nutrition tip Greek yogurt is packed with gut-friendly probiotics, which are beneficial bacteria. Probiotics help support a healthy immune system and stabilize the balance of flora in your digestive tract.

½ cup plain Greek yogurt

2 tablespoons fresh lime juice

1 tablespoon chopped fresh cilantro

1 teaspoon chopped fresh dill

1 teaspoon chopped fresh thyme

Freshly ground black pepper

Nonstick olive oil cooking spray

Four 6-ounce salmon fillets, skinned

1. In a small bowl, stir together the yogurt, lime juice, cilantro, dill, and thyme and then season with pepper to taste.
2. Store the sauce in a sealed container in the refrigerator until you are ready to serve the salmon; the sauce will keep for up to 2 days.
3. In a large skillet over medium-high heat, add a light coat of olive oil spray.
4. Season the salmon with pepper to taste and cook in the preheated skillet, turning once, until the fish flakes when pressed, about 4 minutes per side.
5. Serve with the herbed yogurt sauce.

Serves 4. Prep time 5 minutes. Cook time 8 minutes.

Calories **256** / Calories from fat **105** / Total fat **11.7g** / Saturated fat **2.3g** / Trans fat **0.0g** / Sodium **86mg** / Carbs **3.3g** / Sugars **1.5g** / Protein **35.7g**

Lemon Tuna Patties

Canned tuna becomes a sophisticated, citrusy patty in this dish that also has a generous herb flavoring. Lemon is very high in limonene and vitamin C, and is a good source of citric acid, calcium, vitamin A, and potassium. It is a great detoxifier and can help reduce the risk of cancer.

Leftovers tip Try these tuna patties on a nice crusty bun for lunch or freeze them in resealable plastic bags for a later meal.

Three 5-ounce cans tuna packed
    in water, drained
1 green onion, finely chopped
½ teaspoon minced garlic
3 eggs, beaten

Juice of ½ large lemon
1 tablespoon chopped fresh parsley
1 teaspoon chopped fresh dill
Nonstick cooking spray

1. In a large bowl, combine all the ingredients except the cooking spray.
2. Form the mixture into 12 equal patties, each about 2 inches in diameter.
3. Place the patties on a plate, cover, and chill in the refrigerator until firm, about 1 hour.
4. In a large skillet over medium-high heat, add a light coat of cooking spray and cook the tuna patties, turning once, until lightly browned, about 4 minutes per side.
5. Serve 3 tuna cakes per portion.

Serves 4. Prep time 15 minutes. Cook time 8 minutes.

Calories **200** / Calories from fat **43** / Total fat **4.8g** / Saturated fat **1.4g** / Trans fat **0.0g** / Sodium **116mg** / Carbs **1.0g** / Sugars **0.0g** / Protein **36.5g**

Shrimp with Roasted Tomatoes and Feta Cheese

Shrimp is a low-fat and low-calorie seafood. It is very high in selenium, vitamin B_{12}, protein, and phosphorus, as well as antioxidants that are usually associated with produce. This popular crustacean can cut the risk of cancer, heart disease, and type 2 diabetes. Try to buy wild-caught shrimp to avoid issues sometimes found in farmed shrimp, such as parasites and virus contamination.

Nutrition tip If you are on a low-cholesterol diet, shrimp may not be the best choice for you. A four-ounce portion of shrimp contains 220 milligrams of cholesterol.

6 large tomatoes, cut into eighths

3 teaspoons olive oil

3 teaspoons minced garlic

Freshly ground black pepper

42 medium shrimp, peeled and deveined

½ cup chopped fresh parsley

4 teaspoons lemon juice

½ cup crumbled low-sodium feta cheese

1. Preheat the oven to 450°F.
2. In a large bowl, toss the tomatoes with the oil and garlic until well coated.
3. Transfer the tomatoes to a 9-by-13-inch glass baking dish and season with pepper to taste.
4. Bake the tomatoes in the oven for 20 minutes.
5. Add the shrimp, parsley, and lemon juice to the tomatoes and stir to combine, then sprinkle the feta over the top.
6. Return the dish to the oven and bake until the shrimp are cooked through, about 15 minutes. Serve hot.

Serves 6. Prep time 15 minutes. Cook time 35 minutes.

Calories **374** / Calories from fat **91** / Total fat **10.1g** / Saturated fat **3.1g** / Trans fat **0.0g** / Sodium **793mg** / Carbs **11.3g** / Sugars **7.3g** / Protein **58.9g**

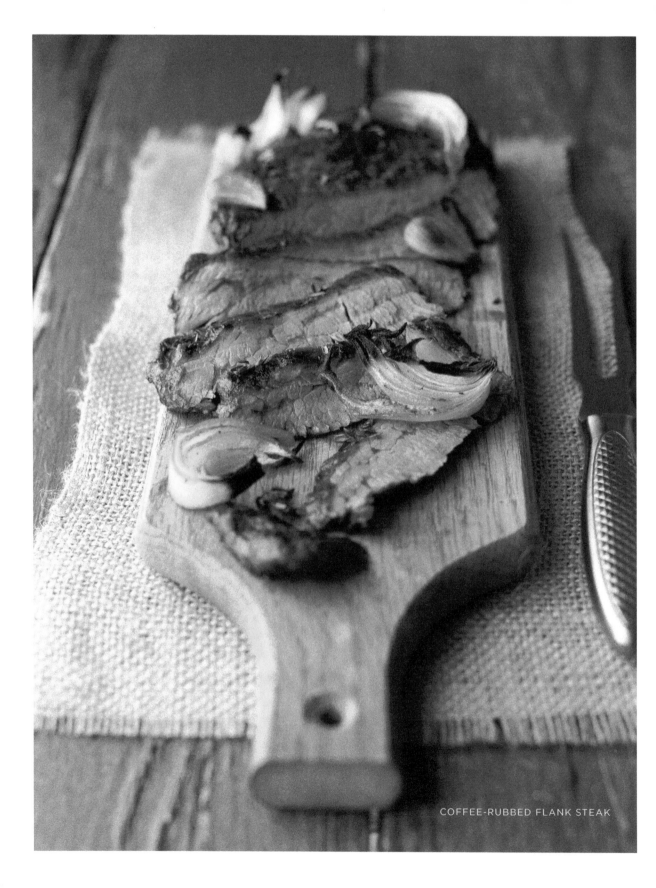

COFFEE-RUBBED FLANK STEAK

CHAPTER TWELVE

Meat and Poultry

Chicken Ratatouille

Zucchini is a vegetable that people either love or hate. It is often the texture that gets the thumbs down, because it can be unpleasantly soft and spongy if the vegetable is too ripe. Although winter squashes seem starchier than summer squashes, both get about 85 percent of their calories from carbohydrates. Summer squash (zucchini and yellow summer squash) is an excellent source of manganese, copper, magnesium, and vitamins A and C, as well as fiber.

Shopping tip When choosing your zucchini, look for vegetables that seem heavy for their size and have an unmarked, shiny skin. Do not purchase larger zucchini thinking you will need less of them, because the big ones are usually fibrous and have tough seeds.

1 teaspoon olive oil

Two 6-ounce boneless, skinless chicken breasts, diced

1 small sweet onion, peeled and sliced

2 teaspoons minced garlic

2 zucchini, unpeeled, sliced lengthwise, then cut into half moons

1 small eggplant, diced

2 red bell peppers, seeded and diced

4 large tomatoes, chopped

2 tablespoons chopped fresh basil

1 tablespoon chopped fresh thyme

Pinch of crushed red pepper flakes

1. In a large skillet over medium heat, heat the oil and sauté the chicken breast pieces until browned and cooked through, about 5 minutes.
2. Add the onion and garlic and sauté until softened, about 3 minutes.
3. Stir in the zucchini, eggplant, and bell peppers, and cook for 15 minutes, stirring occasionally.
4. Stir in the tomatoes, basil, thyme, and red pepper flakes, combining well, and cook for 5 more minutes.
5. Serve the ratatouille plain or over rice.

Serves 6. Prep time 15 minutes. Cook time 30 minutes.

Calories **285** / Calories from fat **75** / Total fat **8.4g** / Saturated fat **2.0g** / Sodium **93mg** / Carbs **13.2g** / Sugars **13.2g** / Protein **30.3g**

Jerk Chicken

This style of seasoning is Jamaican and was developed to preserve meat with spices, salt, and peppers. This recipe does not use as much salt as some, but the flavoring is pungent. Chilies and allspice are traditional ingredients in jerk marinades. Be careful, because habañeros are very hot. You can adjust the heat by using milder or hotter chilies depending on your preference.

Shopping tip Turbinado is a less processed variety of cane sugar. It is brown and comes in large crystals—the color comes from its molasses content. It's turning up in more and more supermarkets, sometimes packaged as "sugar in the raw."

Four 5-ounce boneless, skinless
   chicken breasts

1 small sweet onion, peeled and cut
   into chunks

3 habañero peppers, halved lengthwise
   and seeded

3 teaspoons minced garlic

3 tablespoons fresh lime juice

1 tablespoon olive oil, plus more to
   oil the grill

1 tablespoon turbinado sugar

1 tablespoon chopped fresh thyme

1 tablespoon ground allspice

1 teaspoon freshly ground black pepper

½ teaspoon ground nutmeg

½ teaspoon ground cinnamon

1. Put two chicken breasts each in two large, zipper-top plastic bags and set them aside.
2. In a food processor, combine all the remaining ingredients and pulse until the marinade is very well blended, about 1 minute.
3. Divide the jerk marinade evenly between the two bags of chicken, squeeze as much air as possible out of the bags, and seal them. Squeeze and shake the bags to distribute the marinade evenly on the surface of the chicken breasts.
4. Put the bags in the refrigerator for at least 4 hours or overnight.
5. Preheat a barbecue to medium-high heat and brush the grill lightly with olive oil. Or preheat your oven to 400°F and grease a heavy, ovenproof skillet with olive oil.

continued ➤

Jerk Chicken *continued*

6. Take the chicken out of the refrigerator about 15 minutes before cooking and then remove the chicken from the bags.

7. On the barbecue, grill the chicken, turning at least once, until cooked through, about 6 minutes per side. Or on the stovetop, heat the greased ovenproof skillet over medium-high heat and brown the chicken in the skillet, turning once, about 4 minutes per side. Then put the skillet in the oven and roast until the chicken is cooked though, about 10 minutes. Let the chicken rest for about 5 minutes before serving.

Serves 4. Prep time 30 minutes, plus marinating time. Cook time 20 minutes.

Calories **374** / Calories from fat **160** / Total fat **17.8g** / Saturated fat **4.0g** / Trans fat **0.0g** / Sodium **132mg** / Carbs **9.0g** / Sugars **1.4g** / Protein **41.6g**

Greek Chicken Breasts

Stuffed chicken breasts look like they are incredibly hard to make, but this simple recipe takes only about 15 minutes to put together. The Kalamata olives give this dish a nice briny flavor, and they are also a good source of fiber, iron, and vitamin E. Olives are heart-friendly, promote good digestion, and boost the immune system.

Shopping tip When selecting olives, make sure they are firm with no softness or mushiness. Olives purchased in jars can be kept in the refrigerator for several months, but those bought from open olive bars in the supermarket will only keep for about two weeks. Make sure there is enough brine or liquid in your storage container to cover the olives.

1 large red bell pepper

1 teaspoon olive oil, plus more for the grill

4 tablespoons crumbled low-sodium
    feta cheese

3 Kalamata olives, pitted and finely chopped

2 tablespoons chopped fresh basil

Pinch of freshly ground black pepper

Four 5-ounce skinless, boneless
    chicken breasts

1. Preheat the oven to 400°F. Lightly coat the red pepper in 1 teaspoon of olive oil.
2. In a small baking dish, roast the red pepper in the oven until tender, about 30 minutes.
3. Remove the pepper from the oven and transfer it to a small bowl. Cover the bowl tightly with plastic wrap and set aside for about 10 minutes to loosen the pepper's skin.
4. Peel and seed the pepper using your fingers, then dice it.
5. In a small bowl, combine the roasted pepper, feta, olives, basil, and pepper until well mixed.
6. Chill the filling in the refrigerator for about 10 minutes.
7. Preheat a barbecue to medium-high heat and brush the grill rack with olive oil. Or place a large, heavy skillet over medium-high heat on the stove and lightly oil the skillet with olive oil.

continued ➤

Greek Chicken Breasts *continued*

8. Cut a slit horizontally in each chicken breast, creating a pocket in the middle.
9. Spoon about 2 tablespoons of the filling into each breast pocket and secure the opening with a wooden toothpick.
10. On the barbecue, grill the chicken until completely cooked through, about 10 minutes per side. Or on the stovetop, place the chicken breasts in the skillet and pan fry the breasts until cooked through, turning once, about 10 minutes per side.
11. Remove the chicken from the heat and let stand for 10 minutes.
12. Remove the toothpicks and serve.

Serves 4. Prep time 15 minutes. Cook time 50 minutes.

Calories **188** / Calories from fat **58** / Total fat **6.4g** / Saturated fat **2.6g** / Trans fat **0.0g** / Sodium **184mg** / Carbs **2.7g** / Sugar **0.0g** / Protein **33.5g**

Chicken Florentine

When you see the word "Florentine" in a recipe, it usually means that spinach is a key ingredient. Spinach is a super food, meaning it is packed with healthy nutrients and antioxidants. Spinach is rich in beta-carotene, protein, lutein, calcium, folic acid, potassium, iron, and vitamins A, C, and E.

Nutrition tip Spinach can promote overall healing as well as specifically reduce the pain associated with arthritis and the risk of high blood pressure and cancer. Spinach is also an efficient liver cleanser.

1 teaspoon olive oil

Four 4-ounce boneless, skinless
   chicken breasts

3 large tomatoes, finely chopped

1 tablespoon chopped fresh basil

1 tablespoon chopped fresh oregano

1 teaspoon minced garlic

2 cups packed baby spinach

4 teaspoons grated Parmesan cheese

1. In a large skillet over medium-high heat, heat the olive oil and brown the chicken breasts in the skillet, about 6 minutes per side. Add the tomatoes, basil, oregano, and garlic, and reduce the heat to medium.
2. Cover the skillet and cook the chicken for about 15 minutes.
3. Add the spinach and cover the skillet again. Cook for 5 more minutes or until the spinach is wilted.
4. Top with Parmesan cheese and serve.

Serves 4. Prep time 10 minutes. Cook time 30 minutes.

Calories **336** / Calories from fat **142** / Total fat **15.8g** / Saturated fat **5.5g** / Trans fat **0.0g** / Sodium **415mg** / Carbs **4.0g** / Sugars **1.6g** / Protein **43.2g**

Turkey with Apricot Chutney

The easiest description of chutney is that it is a spicy cooked salsa that can be savory, but is usually more on the sweet side. Apricots are a great ingredient for a chutney because they have a firm texture that does not break down completely, and a hint of natural acid to cut the sweetness. Apricots are a lovely rosy gold color, which means they are high in antioxidants—the deeper the color, the greater the concentration of antioxidants. Apricots have powerful cancer-fighting properties due to their high lycopene content.

Leftovers tip If you have chutney left over after your meal, try it as a spread on sandwiches, a dipping sauce, or as a glaze on roasted pork or chicken. Store the chutney in the refrigerator in a sealed container for up to a week.

6 ripe apricots, pitted and diced
¼ cup unsweetened apple juice
¼ small sweet onion, finely chopped
2 tablespoons honey
1 tablespoon grated fresh ginger
1 tablespoon chopped fresh thyme
1 tablespoon balsamic vinegar

1 teaspoon freshly grated lemon zest
Juice of 1 lime
1 pound whole boneless turkey breast, skin removed, trimmed of visible fat
1 teaspoon smoked paprika
½ teaspoon ground cumin
1 teaspoon olive oil

1. In a small saucepan, combine the apricots, apple juice, onion, honey, ginger, thyme, vinegar, lemon zest, and lime juice.
2. Cook over medium heat, stirring constantly until the apricots become soft and mushy, about 10 minutes.
3. Remove the chutney from the heat and set aside.
4. Preheat the oven to 375°F.
5. Season the turkey breast with the paprika and cumin.
6. In a large ovenproof skillet over medium-high heat, heat the oil and pan sear the turkey on all sides, about 5 minutes per side.

7. Put the skillet in the oven and roast the turkey until the breast is cooked through and the internal temperature reaches 165°F, about 45 minutes.
8. Let the turkey breast rest for about 10 minutes before carving it into slices.
9. Serve with the chutney.

Serves 4. Prep time 15 minutes. Cook time 1 hour and 5 minutes.

Calories **204** / Calories from fat **32** / Total fat **3.5g** / Saturated fat **0.6g** / Trans fat **0.0g** / Sodium **1154mg** / Carbs **24.2g** / Sugars **19.5g** / Protein **20.5g**

Pork Tenderloin with Squash Salsa

Pork is a very healthy clean eating choice, but is often forgotten in favor of chicken and fish. Pork is a red meat, but it does not have the same nutritional profile as beef. Pork tenderloin is actually as lean as a skinless chicken breast and has fewer calories. Lean cuts of pork, such as chops and tenderloins, also have less total fat and calories than lean beef.

Cooking tip The days of cooking pork until it was dry and an unappetizing gray are gone, because trichinosis is no longer a risk. Pork can actually be served with a hint of pink in the middle, especially if the cut is thick, such as a pork tenderloin.

½ small butternut squash, peeled and diced into ¼-inch cubes

2 tablespoons olive oil, divided

1 apple, peeled, cored, and diced

1 small red bell pepper, seeded and finely chopped

1 green onion, finely chopped

1 tablespoon fresh lime juice

1 teaspoon chopped fresh thyme

1 teaspoon honey

½ teaspoon nutmeg

Freshly ground black pepper

Two 10-ounce pork tenderloins, trimmed of fat

1. Preheat the oven to 400°F. Line a baking sheet with foil and set it aside.
2. In a small bowl, toss the squash with 1 tablespoon of the olive oil.
3. Transfer the squash to the prepared baking sheet and bake until cooked but not mushy, about 20 minutes.
4. Transfer the squash to a large bowl and let it cool for about 15 minutes.
5. Add the apple, bell pepper, onion, lime juice, thyme, honey, and nutmeg to the squash and stir to combine well. Season the salsa with black pepper to taste.
6. Store the salsa in the refrigerator until you are ready to serve the pork.
7. In a large skillet over medium-high heat, heat the remaining tablespoon of oil.

8. Season the pork lightly with pepper and pan fry the meat, turning to brown each side, until it is cooked through and the internal temperature is 160°F, about 20 minutes total.
9. Let the pork rest for about 10 minutes before cutting each one in half.
10. Transfer each half to an individual plate and top with salsa. Serve immediately.

Serves 4. Prep time 15 minutes. Cook time 40 minutes.

Calories **417** / Calories from fat **169** / Total fat **18.8g** / Saturated fat **5.2g** / Trans fat **0.0g** / Sodium **96mg** / Carbs **17.6g** / Sugars **8.9g** / Protein **43.4g**

Marinated Pork Chops with Grilled Peaches

The marinade for these thick chops is the perfect blend of sweetness and acid. Many marinades use acids to break the protein bonds in the meat, creating a tender finished product. You have to be careful not to marinate meats such as chicken and pork in an acidic marinade for too long, because time can cause the bonds to tighten up again and your meat will be dry and tough.

Cooking tip Reserve about 3 tablespoons of the marinade before adding the pork chops to the bag, and brush the extra marinade on the peaches before grilling them.

¼ cup balsamic vinegar

¼ cup olive oil, plus more for the grill

2 tablespoons honey

1 tablespoon chopped fresh
   thyme, divided

½ teaspoon chopped fresh
   rosemary, divided

Four 5-ounce boneless pork chops,
   trimmed of visible fat

2 ripe peaches, halved and pitted

Freshly ground black pepper

1. In a large zipper-top plastic bag, combine the vinegar, olive oil, honey, half of the thyme, and half of the rosemary, and shake to blend.
2. Add the pork chops to the vinegar mixture and squeeze the bag to coat all the sides of the meat with marinade.
3. Squeeze as much air out of the bag as possible, seal it, and place the bag in the refrigerator to marinate for at least 1 hour and no more than 4 hours.
4. Preheat a barbecue to medium-high heat and brush the grill lightly with olive oil. Or preheat the broiler and lightly oil a broiler pan.
5. On the barbecue, grill the peaches cut-side down until very tender. Or in the oven, broil them for 2 minutes per side.
6. Remove the peaches from the heat to a medium bowl and set aside to cool for 5 minutes.

7. Chop the peaches and add the remaining thyme and rosemary. Season with pepper to taste and set aside. Take the pork chops out of the bag and shake off any excess marinade.

8. On the barbecue, grill the pork until cooked through but still juicy (160°F on a meat thermometer), about 5 minutes per side. Or in the oven, broil the pork until it is cooked through, about 6 minutes per side.

9. Remove the chops from the heat and let them sit for 5 minutes.

10. Serve topped with the grilled peaches.

Serves 4. Prep time 10 minutes, plus marinating time. Cook time 15 minutes.

Calories **367** / Calories from fat **160** / Total fat **17.8g** / Saturated fat **3.5g** / Trans fat **0.1g** / Sodium **82mg** / Carbs **14.0g** / Sugars **12.8g** / Protein **37.7g**

Sweet Pepper Sauté with Sirloin

Sweet bell peppers are the supporting ingredient of the lean sirloin, but they more than hold their own with respect to nutrition. This recipe features every color of pepper except green, and each color has different phytonutrients. All the sweet bell peppers are high in potassium, zinc, calcium, magnesium, and vitamins A, B, C, and E. They can help boost the immune system, prevent cataracts, and reduce the risk of heart disease, blood clots, and cancer.

Leftovers tip The pepper sauté makes a delicious, healthy pasta sauce, especially if you add a bit of blue cheese to the finished dish.

1 pound boneless top sirloin steak, about 1 inch thick, trimmed of visible fat

1 tablespoon olive oil, plus more for brushing the steak

Salt and freshly ground black pepper

1 small red onion, peeled and thinly sliced

2 teaspoons minced garlic

2 yellow bell peppers, seeded and thinly sliced

2 red bell peppers, seeded and thinly sliced

1 orange bell pepper, seeded and thinly sliced

1 cup baby spinach

1 cup halved cherry tomatoes

½ cup crumbled blue cheese

1. Preheat a barbecue to medium-high heat or preheat the broiler.
2. Lightly brush the steak on both sides with the olive oil and season with salt and pepper to taste.
3. On the barbecue, grill the steak, turning once, until it reaches the desired doneness, about 5 minutes per side for medium (160°F). Or in the oven, broil the steak, turning once, until it reaches the desired doneness. For medium, broil the meat 6 minutes per side or until a meat thermometer reads 160°F.
4. Transfer the steak to a cutting board and let it rest for at least 10 minutes before slicing it against the grain into 16 slices.

5. In a large skillet on the stove over medium heat, heat the remaining tablespoon of oil and sauté the onion and garlic until softened, 3 minutes.
6. Add the peppers and sauté until they are tender but still crisp, about 5 minutes.
7. Add the spinach and cherry tomatoes and stir until the spinach is wilted, about 2 minutes.
8. Season the mixture with pepper to taste.
9. Divide the sautéed peppers among 4 plates and top with about 4 steak pieces each and a sprinkle of blue cheese.

Serves 4. Prep time 15 minutes. Cook time 20 minutes.

Calories **364** / Calories from fat **144** / Total fat **16.0g** / Saturated fat **6.4g** / Sodium **324mg** / Carbs **13.2g** / Sugars **8.1g** / Protein **40.2g**

Coffee-Rubbed Flank Steak

If you are a meat-eater, you might be surprised to discover that coffee is a great marinade for steaks. It imparts a lovely smoky taste to the meat without any chemicals or preservatives. This recipe uses ground coffee beans as a base; if you like the taste of the coffee-accented meat, you could also try soaking your beef in brewed coffee. Make sure you don't use hot coffee for your marinade or you will cook the meat.

Shopping tip Flank steak is an ideal, inexpensive grilling choice if you are marinating your meat. Keep in mind that the tougher cuts of meat, like flank steak, are also more flavorful than the tender cuts, like tenderloin.

3 teaspoons minced garlic

¼ cup whole espresso coffee beans

2 tablespoons chopped fresh parsley

2 tablespoons chopped fresh rosemary

2 teaspoons freshly ground black pepper

3 tablespoons balsamic vinegar

2 tablespoons turbinado sugar

1 tablespoon olive oil, plus more
    for the grill

1 pound flank steak, trimmed of visible fat

1. In a food processor, combine the garlic, espresso beans, parsley, and rosemary and pulse until the beans are coarsely ground.
2. Add the pepper, vinegar, sugar, and olive oil and pulse until the marinade is well blended.
3. Pour the coffee marinade into a large zipper-top plastic bag, add the flank steak, and squeeze the excess air out of the bag and seal it.
4. Marinate the steak in the refrigerator for at least 4 hours or overnight, turning the bag occasionally.
5. Preheat a barbecue to medium-high heat and brush the grill with olive oil. Or preheat the broiler and brush a broiler pan with olive oil.
6. Remove the steak from the bag and shake off the excess marinade.
7. On the barbecue, grill the steak, turning once, until it reaches the desired doneness, about 5 minutes per side for medium (160°F). Or in the oven, broil the steak, turning once, until it is the desired doneness, about 6 minutes per side.

8. Transfer the steak to a cutting board and let the meat rest for at least 10 minutes before slicing it against the grain.
9. Serve the steak with a mixed green salad or your favorite side dish.

Serves 4. Prep time 20 minutes, plus marinating time. Cook time 10 minutes.

Calories **312** / Calories from fat **151** / Total fat **16.7g** / Saturated fat **5.0g** / Trans fat **0.0g** / Sodium **68mg** / Carbs **7.1g** / Sugars **4.5g** / Protein **31.9g**

Beef Tenderloin with Onion Marmalade

This marmalade is outrageously flavorful, and it has a surprisingly sweet taste that pairs well with the tenderloin. The trick to a perfectly balanced and delicious onion marmalade is slow cooking the onions until all the natural sugars are released, so don't rush the process. You can use any onion in this recipe rather than the red ones—such as the fancy Vidalia or the plain yellow ones—but the color will be lighter.

Cooking tip You can leave out the honey entirely if your marmalade is already sweet and rich after caramelizing.

1 teaspoon olive oil, plus more for the grill

2 large red onions, peeled and diced

2 tablespoons unsweetened apple juice

3 teaspoons red wine vinegar

2 tablespoons honey

1 tablespoon chopped fresh thyme

Pinch of salt

Pinch of freshly ground black pepper

Four 4-ounce beef tenderloin steaks, each about 1 inch thick and trimmed of fat

1. In a large saucepan over medium-low heat, heat the oil and sauté the red onion until it is very soft and lightly caramelized, about 1 hour, stirring frequently.
2. Add the juice, vinegar, honey, thyme, salt, and pepper.
3. Reduce the heat to low and continue to cook, stirring frequently, until most of the liquid evaporates and the marmalade is sticky and thick, about 10 minutes. Remove the pan from the heat and set it aside.
4. Preheat a barbecue to medium-high heat and brush the grill with olive oil. Or preheat the broiler and lightly oil a broiling pan.
5. On the barbecue, grill the tenderloin, turning once, until it is the desired doneness, about 5 minutes per side for medium (160°F). Or in the oven, broil the tenderloin until is it the desired doneness, turning once, about 6 minutes per side.

6. Transfer the tenderloin to a cutting board and let it rest for at least 10 minutes.
7. Serve topped with the onion marmalade.

Serves 4. Prep time 30 minutes. Cook time 1 hour and 20 minutes.

Calories **291** / Calories from fat **75** / Total fat **8.3g** / Saturated fat **2.9g** / Trans fat **0.0g** / Sodium **223mg** / Carbs **17.1g** / Sugars **12.7g** / Protein **35.0g**

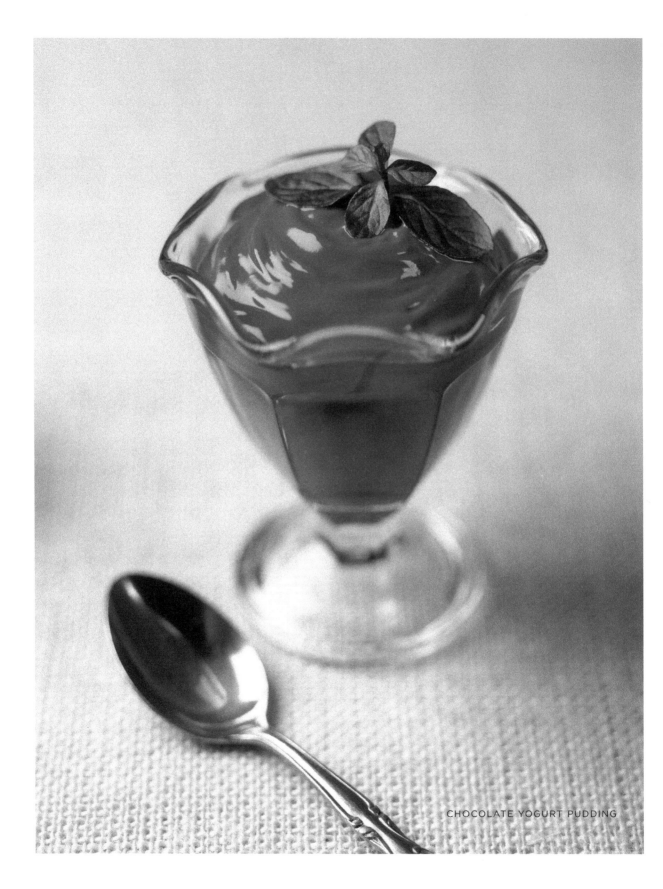

CHOCOLATE YOGURT PUDDING

CHAPTER THIRTEEN

Desserts

Citrus Coconut Mousse

This dessert is like an infusion of the tropics, with lemon, orange, and coconut. Coconut is a high-calorie and high-fat addition to the recipe, but it is also packed with fiber and contains no trans fats. Shredded coconut can help improve digestion, and it is a delicious energy booster.

Diet tip This dish is not appropriate for a vegetarian or vegan diet because it contains gelatin, which is an animal-based product. But there are vegan gelling agents: agar-agar and carrageen are both derived from seaweed. Many kosher gelatins use these products, and are vegan.

3 teaspoons fresh lemon juice

1 teaspoon fresh orange juice

1 teaspoon unflavored gelatin

1 cup unsweetened almond milk

3 tablespoons turbinado sugar

½ teaspoon pure vanilla extract

3 pasteurized egg whites

1 small mango, peeled, pitted, and diced

¼ cup unsweetened shredded coconut

1. In a small bowl, mix the lemon and orange juices and then sprinkle the gelatin over them. Let the mixture stand for 5 minutes.
2. In a small saucepan over medium heat, heat the almond milk.
3. When the milk starts to bubble around the sides of the pan, add the sugar and vanilla extract and stir until the sugar is completely dissolved.
4. Remove the mixture from the heat and whisk in the gelatin mixture.
5. Transfer the almond milk mixture to a large bowl and chill in the refrigerator for about 15 minutes.
6. In a medium bowl, beat the egg whites with an electric beater or whisk until soft peaks form.
7. Remove the almond milk mixture from the refrigerator and fold in the beaten egg whites in three increments, keeping as much volume as possible.

8. Divide the mousse among four serving dishes and place them in the refrigerator to set for at least 2 hours or overnight.
9. Serve with the mango and coconut.

Serves 4. Prep time 30 minutes, plus setting time. Cook time 10 minutes.

Calories **100** / Calories from fat **17** / Total fat **1.9g** / Saturated fat **1.5g** / Sodium **49mg** / Carbs **14.8g** / Sugars **15.1g** / Protein **4.7g**

Chocolate Yogurt Pudding

This decadent pudding tastes a little like a rich chocolate cheesecake and is much simpler to make. Be sure to use dark chocolate, at least 70 percent cocoa, for this dessert because it is very healthy in small amounts. Dark chocolate is much lower in fat and sugar than milk chocolate, and may lower cholesterol levels, reduce the risk of heart disease, and prevent cognitive decline. Serve this pudding topped with antioxidant-rich berries for a super healthy dessert.

Shopping tip Choose the highest quality chocolate possible for this dessert because the taste and texture will be superior. If you can find it, try single-plantation chocolate because the taste of chocolate can be affected by where the beans come from, similar to wine and grapes.

2 cups vanilla Greek yogurt

4 ounces dark chocolate,
    coarsely chopped

½ teaspoon pure vanilla extract

1. Line a medium fine-mesh sieve with cheesecloth.
2. Place the sieve over a bowl and spoon the yogurt into the cheesecloth.
3. Put the bowl and sieve in the refrigerator for about 1 hour to drain.
4. Transfer the drained yogurt to a medium bowl and whisk the yogurt for about 30 seconds.
5. Let the yogurt sit on the counter for about 15 minutes to come to room temperature.
6. Place the chocolate in a small heatproof bowl and melt it in the microwave or over a pan of simmering water.
7. Whisk the melted chocolate and vanilla into the yogurt until very well blended.
8. Spoon the chocolate pudding into 4 serving bowls, cover them, and put them in the refrigerator until you are ready to serve them. They will keep overnight.

Serves 4. Prep time 15 minutes. Cook time 5 minutes.

Calories **271** / Calories from fat **94** / Total fat **11.4g** / Saturated fat **7.1g** / Trans fat **0.0g** / Sodium **73mg** / Carbs **33.5g** / Sugars **30.7g** / Protein **11.2g**

Simple Banana Strawberry Ice Cream

Gluten-free
Low-fat
Low-sodium
Nightshade-free
Vegan
Vegetarian

DESSERTS

You do not need an ice cream maker to create this creamy cold dessert—just a blender. Bananas are a very good source of potassium, fiber, manganese, and vitamins B_6 and C. They also contain tryptophan, which can improve your mood. Bananas help improve digestion and protect against cardiovascular disease, type 2 diabetes, and cancer.

Cooking tip For best results, take the frozen bananas out of the freezer and let them sit at room temperature for about 30 minutes, until they are soft enough to blend into a creamy dessert.

2 frozen bananas, peeled before freezing
½ cup frozen strawberries, cut in half
    before freezing

1 teaspoon pure vanilla extract

1. In a food processor, combine the bananas and strawberries and pulse until smooth and creamy, about 2 minutes.
2. Add the vanilla and pulse until well combined.
3. Serve immediately or store the ice cream in the freezer in a sealed container for up to 1 week.

Serves 4. Prep time 15 minutes.

Calories **62** / Calories from fat **2** / Total fat **0.2g** / Trans fat **0.0g** / Sodium **1mg** / Carbs **15.3g** / Sugars **8.5g** / Protein **0.7g**

Strawberry Crisp

Strawberries are very high in ellagic acid, vitamin C, beta-carotene, iron, folic acid, and potassium. They can boost the immune system, help stabilize blood sugar, and cut the risk of heart disease, cognitive decline, and some types of cancer. They are truly a nutritional powerhouse.

Shopping tip Strawberries have a very short shelf life and can start losing vitamin C after sitting in your refrigerator for two days. Try to find local organic berries in the early summer for the best taste and quality.

Nonstick cooking spray

½ cup rolled oats

¼ cup unsweetened shredded coconut

¼ cup finely chopped raw pecans

¼ cup turbinado sugar, divided

¼ teaspoon ground cinnamon

¼ teaspoon ground nutmeg

2 tablespoons pure maple syrup

1 tablespoon coconut oil, melted

4 cups sliced strawberries

1 tablespoon fresh lemon juice

1 tablespoon arrowroot powder

1. Preheat the oven to 350°F. Lightly coat a 9-by-13-inch glass baking dish with cooking spray and set aside.
2. In a medium bowl, mix together the oats, coconut, pecans, half of the turbinado sugar, cinnamon, and nutmeg until well mixed.
3. Stir in the maple syrup and coconut oil and toss together until the mixture resembles coarse crumbs.
4. In a large bowl, toss together the strawberries, lemon juice, remaining sugar, and arrowroot until well mixed.
5. Spoon the strawberry mixture into the baking dish and top evenly with the oat mixture.
6. Bake for 15 minutes.
7. Serve warm.

Serves 6. Prep time 20 minutes. Cook time 15 minutes.

Calories **274** / Calories from fat **126** / Total fat **14.0g** / Saturated fat **7.6g** / Trans fat **0.0g** / Sodium **6mg** / Carbs **24.5g** / Sugars **14.0g** / Protein **3.6g**

Pumpkin Pie Mousse

Pumpkin and warm spices are a traditional combination found in pies, cakes, and breads. This mousse is a little like pumpkin pie without the crust, and is a great deal healthier. Pumpkin is often thought of as a vegetable, but it is actually a fruit. Pumpkin is a wonderful source of beta-carotene, vitamins B, C, D, and E, and iron, potassium, and copper. It can cut the risk of developing quite a few diseases, including strokes, kidney stones, cancer, heart disease, and insomnia.

Cooking tip Silken tofu is a fabulous, fat-free way to create creamy, thick desserts that have the lightness associated with whipped cream and beaten egg whites.

One 15-ounce can plain pumpkin purée
One 10½-ounce package silken tofu,
    well drained
⅓ cup pure maple syrup
1 teaspoon ground cinnamon

¼ teaspoon ground nutmeg
¼ teaspoon ground ginger
Pinch of ground cloves
¼ cup plain Greek yogurt

1. In a food processor, combine the pumpkin and tofu and pulse until smooth, about 30 seconds.
2. Add the remaining ingredients except the yogurt and pulse until very smooth, about 30 seconds.
3. Put the mousse in the refrigerator in a sealed container for at least 4 hours.
4. Drain any liquid from the top of the mousse and spoon the mousse into serving dishes.
5. Top with a little Greek yogurt and serve.

Serves 5. Prep time 10 minutes, plus setting time.

Calories **97** / Calories from fat **11** / Total fat **2.1g** / Saturated fat **0.7g** / Trans fat **0.0g** / Sodium **10mg** / Carbs **24.8g** / Sugars **16.5g** / Protein **4.7g**

Pecan Fruit Salad

What is a perfect clean eating dessert? Fruit salad, of course! Fresh, delicious fruit is a sweet end to a meal, and this version adds a tiny surprise crunch of spicy caramelized nuts to enhance the flavor and texture. You can use any fruit for this dish, depending on your own personal preference, but try to get a nice assortment of colors for visual impact.

Leftovers tip Store any remaining fruit salad in the refrigerator in a sealed container. It will make for a great breakfast the next morning and an energy-packed start to the day.

1 cup halved strawberries

1 kiwi, peeled and sliced

1 peach, pitted and diced

1 cup raspberries

1 mango, peeled, pitted, and diced

1 teaspoon honey

¼ teaspoon cayenne pepper

¼ cup chopped pecans

1. Preheat the oven to broil.
2. In a large bowl, toss the strawberries, kiwi, peach, raspberries, and mango together, and set aside.
3. In a small bowl, stir together the honey and cayenne pepper.
4. Add the pecans to the honey mixture and stir to coat.
5. On a small baking sheet, spread the nuts and broil until they are toasted and lightly caramelized, about 1 minute.
6. Stir the toasted nuts into the fruit salad and serve.

Serves 4. Prep time 15 minutes. Cook time 1 minute.

Calories **137** / Calories from fat **49** / Total fat **5.5g** / Saturated fat **0.0g** / Trans fats **0.0g** / Sodium **2mg** / Carbs **22.8g** / Sugars **16.4g** / Protein **1.9g**

Oatmeal Maple Cookies

Desserts don't have to be fancy or elaborate to be successful. Sometimes a simple, rich cookie served with an herbal tea is the best end to a good meal. These cookies will remind you of your grandmother's recipe because they have a melt-in-your-mouth texture and a hint of maple sweetness. If you are watching your fat consumption, you can omit the coconut oil in the ingredients and double the applesauce, but this will change the texture a little.

Diet tip If you want a gluten-free cookie, substitute almond flour for the whole-wheat flour, and make sure your oats are gluten-free as well.

3 cups rolled oats

1½ cups whole-wheat flour

1 teaspoon ground cinnamon

½ teaspoon baking soda

Pinch of sea salt

½ cup pure maple syrup

½ cup unsweetened applesauce

¼ cup coconut oil

1 teaspoon pure vanilla extract

1 large banana, mashed

1. Preheat the oven to 375°F. Line a baking sheet with foil or parchment paper and set it aside.
2. In a large bowl, stir together the oats, flour, cinnamon, baking soda, and salt.
3. In a medium bowl, stir together the remaining ingredients until there are no banana lumps.
4. Add the wet ingredients to the dry ingredients and stir to combine well.
5. Drop the batter by tablespoons onto the baking sheet, about 12 per batch.
6. Bake the cookies until golden brown, about 10 minutes.
7. Repeat with the remaining batter.
8. Store the cookies in a sealed container for up to 1 week.

Makes 24 cookies. Prep time 10 minutes. Cook time 20 minutes.

Calories **112** / Calories from fat **27** / Total fat **3.1g** / Saturated fat **2.1g** / Trans fat **0.0g** / Sodium **41mg** / Carbs **19.3g** / Sugars **5.2g** / Protein **2.2g**

Low-fat
Low-sodium
Nightshade-free
Vegan
Vegetarian

DESSERTS

Rhubarb Apple Brown Betty

Rhubarb looks a little like reddish green celery, but it is cooked more like a fruit in pies, stews, and cakes. Rhubarb can be incredibly tart. This recipe mellows the flavor with the addition of sweet apple and apple juice. If you want the fruit layer of this crisp to be less tart, add a couple tablespoons of maple syrup to the stewed mixture. Rhubarb is very low in calories and is a great source of lutein, calcium, and vitamin K.

Shopping tip Buy your rhubarb from late spring to late summer and always remove the leaves because they contain oxalic acid, which can be toxic.

For the filling:
4 cups diced rhubarb
2 large apples, peeled, cored, and diced
½ cup unsweetened apple juice
1 teaspoon ground cinnamon
½ teaspoon ground nutmeg
1 tablespoon cornstarch

For the topping:
¾ cup rolled oats
¼ cup chopped pecans
½ cup uncooked quinoa, rinsed
4 dates, chopped

To make the filling:

1. In a large saucepan over medium heat, combine all the filling ingredients and bring to a boil.
2. Reduce the heat to low and simmer the mixture, stirring frequently, for about 1 hour, until the filling is thick and stewed.

To make the brown betty:

1. While the rhubarb filling is stewing, in a food processor combine all the topping ingredients and pulse until it resembles coarse crumbs. Set aside.
2. Preheat the oven to 350°F.
3. When the filling is cooked, pour it into a 9-by-13-inch glass baking dish and sprinkle the topping over the filling.
4. Bake the brown betty until golden and bubbly, about 20 minutes.
5. Remove the dessert from the oven, and let it cool on a wire rack for about 30 minutes, and serve warm or cool.
6. Store any leftovers in a sealed container in the refrigerator for up to 5 days.

Serves 6. Prep time 15 minutes. Cook time 1 hour and 20 minutes.

Calories **207** / Calories from fat **45** / Total fat **5.0g** / Saturated fat **0.6g** / Trans fat **0.0g** / Sodium **6mg** / Carbs **24.1g** / Sugars **14.7g** / Protein **4.5g**

Simple Chocolate Fudge

This is an incredibly rich, creamy fudge that can be stored in the refrigerator for up to three weeks—but will probably not make it past the first week because it is addictive. The sweetness in this recipe comes from dates, so if you want to adjust the level of sweetness add or subtract the number of dates. Dates help prevent and relieve digestion problems such as constipation, and can help prevent anemia and osteoporosis.

Cooking tip This fudge can also be stored in the freezer for up to 2 months, so make a double batch. Let your fudge sit at room temperature out of the freezer for about 10 minutes to soften up before eating it.

½ cup coconut oil

¾ cup unsweetened cocoa powder

1 large ripe banana

8 dates, chopped

1 teaspoon pure vanilla extract

1. Line a 9-by-13-inch baking dish with parchment paper and set it aside.
2. In a large saucepan over medium heat, melt the coconut oil.
3. Remove the oil from the heat and stir in the cocoa powder until there are no lumps.
4. In a food processor, combine the banana, dates, and vanilla and pulse until they form a smooth paste.
5. Add the cocoa mixture to the processor and pulse until smooth and blended, scraping down the sides at least once.
6. Spoon the fudge mixture into the baking dish, cover the dish with plastic wrap, and refrigerate until the fudge is firm, about 3 hours.
7. Cut the fudge into pieces and store it in a sealed container in the refrigerator for up to 3 weeks.

Makes 24. Prep time 10 minutes. Cook time 1 minute, plus setting time.

Calories **58** / Calories from fat **44** / Total fat **4.9g** / Saturated fat **4.1g** / Trans fats **0.0g** / Sodium **1mg** / Carbs **4.9g** / Sugars **2.5g** / Protein **0.6g**

Lime Pots de Crème

This is a smooth, tart treat that can be topped with fresh berries to create a gorgeous dessert for family or guests. Buttermilk might sound heavy, but it has no butter in it. It is actually the liquid that remains after the fat is taken out of the milk to make butter. That means buttermilk has less fat than regular milk, and it's good for you because it is also a great source of calcium, phosphorus, potassium, and vitamin B_{12}.

Leftovers tip Try a tablespoon or two of buttermilk on baked potatoes (unless you are on a nightshade-free diet) to get a rich sour cream taste without all the added fat and calories.

1 cup skim milk

1 teaspoon pure vanilla extract

1 tablespoon unflavored gelatin

1 cup Greek yogurt

1 cup low-fat buttermilk

½ cup honey

Zest and juice of 1 lime

1. In a medium saucepan over medium-high heat combine the milk and vanilla.
2. Let the milk warm for about 1 minute and whisk in the gelatin.
3. Remove the milk mixture from the heat when it starts to bubble around the edges of the pan, after about 5 minutes.
4. Remove the pan from the heat and set it aside to cool for about 15 minutes.
5. In a large bowl, whisk together the remaining ingredients until very well blended.
6. Whisk the slightly cooled milk mixture into the lime mixture.
7. Spoon the mixture into four 6-ounce ramekins, cover them with plastic wrap, and put them in the refrigerator to set completely, for at least 4 hours or overnight.
8. Serve chilled.

Serves 4. Prep time 10 minutes. Cook time 7 minutes, plus setting time.

Calories **222** / Calories from fat **14** / Total fat **1.5g** / Saturated fat **1.1g** / Trans fat **0.0g** / Sodium **118mg** / Carbs **43.0g** / Sugars **42.9g** / Protein **10.7g**

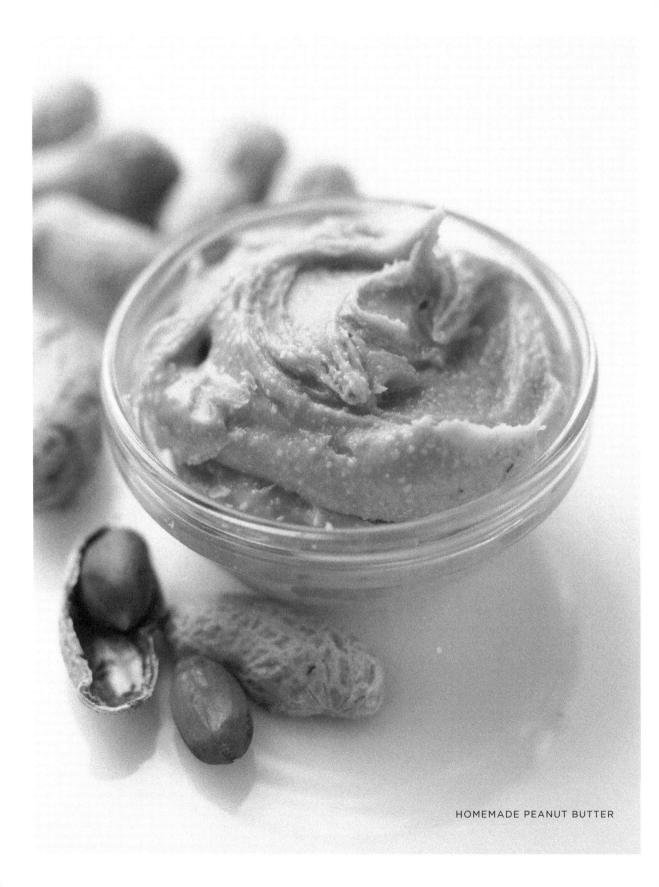

HOMEMADE PEANUT BUTTER

Kitchen Basics

Blueberry Chia Jam

This is not really a jam, but since you can spread it on toast and use it as a dessert topping, calling it jam does not seem like much of a culinary stretch. Blueberries are a wonderful choice for this spread, but any berry would be nice. Blueberries are very high in phytonutrients, folic acid, calcium, iron, potassium, and vitamins B_1, B_3, B_6, and C. This jam is the perfect way to start the day off with a nutritional jump.

Diet tip If your blueberries are sweet enough naturally, you can omit the maple syrup and create a lovely FODMAP-appropriate jam.

4 cups fresh blueberries

½ cup chia seeds

¼ cup pure maple syrup

1. In a food processor, combine all the ingredients and process until well blended.
2. Transfer the mixture to a medium bowl and put in the refrigerator until thickened, about 4 hours.
3. Store the jam in a sealed container in the refrigerator for up to 1 week.

Makes 16 servings. Prep time 5 minutes.

Calories **48** / Calories from fat **13** / Total fat **1.4g** / Saturated fat **0.0g** / Trans fat **0.0g** / Sodium **1mg** / Carbs **10.1g** / Sugars **6.5g** / Protein **1.0g**

Homemade Peanut Butter

Peanut butter has long been on the list for healthy eaters and people who work out or play sports, because of its high protein content. Unfortunately, processed peanut butters also contain a fair bit of sugar, salt, and preservatives. Natural peanut butter does not have to be anything other than roasted peanuts. Making it yourself will take a fair bit of time, so be patient and you will enjoy a wonderful, creamy, flavor-packed, healthy spread.

Diet tip Peanuts are certainly not a low-fat food, but the fat found in peanuts is monounsaturated fat and oleic acid, which are the same healthy fats found in olive oil.

2 cups roasted unsalted peanuts

1. In a food processor, pulse the peanuts for about 30 seconds.
2. Continue to process the peanuts in 1-minute intervals with a couple of seconds rest in between each minute to let the oils come out of the peanuts.
3. Continue to process until the peanut butter is creamy and smooth, about 20 minutes.
4. Store the peanut butter in a sealed container in the refrigerator for up to 2 weeks.

Makes 32 tablespoons. Prep time 20 minutes.

Calories **52** / Calories from fat **41** / Total fat **4.5g** / Saturated fat **0.6g** / Trans fat **0.0g** / Sodium **2mg** / Carbs **1.5g** / Sugars **0.0g** / Protein **2.4g**

Roasted Garlic

Roasted garlic is a superb addition to many clean eating recipes, as well as mashed up with potatoes or root vegetables. It has a mild, rich, almost nutty flavor. This recipe lightly blanches the garlic in milk before roasting it, to remove any bitterness that might be present. This step can be skipped with no ill effects and then the roasted garlic will be vegan.

Cooking tip You can roast the garlic in the bulb by slicing off the top to expose a little of the cloves and drizzling the whole clove with a little olive oil. Roast in the oven until the cloves are softened and then squeeze the garlic out of the papery bulb.

2 cups peeled garlic cloves

½ cup milk

1 tablespoon olive oil

1. Preheat the oven to 350°F.
2. In a small ovenproof skillet on medium-high heat, combine the garlic cloves and milk and bring to a boil.
3. Reduce the heat to low and simmer the garlic and milk for about 5 minutes, stirring occasionally.
4. Drain the milk from the skillet and stir in the olive oil.
5. Cover the skillet with foil, transfer it to the oven, and roast the garlic until it is very tender and golden, about 20 minutes.
6. Store the roasted garlic in a sealed container in the refrigerator for up to 1 week.

Serves 8. Prep time 5 minutes. Cook time 30 minutes.

Calories **25** / Calories from fat **19** / Total fat **2.1g** / Saturated fat **0.0g** / Trans fat **0.0g** / Sodium **25mg** / Carbs **1.0g** / Sugars **0.7g** / Protein **0.5g**

Spicy Lime Cilantro Dressing

Cilantro has a bright, fresh taste, and combines nicely with lime and jalapeño pepper to create a distinctive Southwestern dressing. This herb is a staple of both Latino and Asian cuisine. Cilantro is also high in many vitamins and minerals, including iron, calcium, and vitamins A, B_6, C, and K. Cilantro is used to detox the body of heavy metals, as well as to stabilize blood sugar.

Cooking tip This dressing would make a delicious marinade for fish, but remember that fish should not be marinated longer than an hour or the flesh can become tough.

¼ cup chopped fresh cilantro

2 garlic cloves

½ jalapeño pepper

¼ cup fresh lime juice

¼ cup water

Pinch of sea salt

Pinch of freshly ground black pepper

Pinch of cayenne pepper

½ cup olive oil

1. In a blender, combine all the ingredients except the oil and blend until very smooth and well combined.
2. Add the olive oil in a thin stream, and continue to blend until the dressing emulsifies.
3. Store the dressing in a sealed container in the refrigerator for up to 2 weeks.

Serves 12. Prep time 10 minutes.

Calories **73** / Calories from fat **73** / Total fat **8.4g** / Saturated fat **1.2g** / Trans fat **0.0g** / Sodium **20mg** / Carbs **0.2g** / Sugar **0.0g** / Protein **0.1g**

Yogurt Cheese

This versatile cheese should be at the top of the list of your clean eating staples. It ends up the consistency of cream cheese, and you can use it as a base for many other recipes. Add a vast assortment of other ingredients to the yogurt cheese to vary the flavor, including herbs, fruit, and chocolate.

Nutrition tip Yogurt is an excellent source of magnesium, calcium, potassium, and vitamins B_2 and B_{12}. It can help reduce the risk of high blood pressure, promote a healthy digestive system, and make you feel full.

8 cups Greek yogurt   Pinch of salt

1. Place a fine mesh sieve over a large bowl.
2. Line the sieve with 4 layers of damp cheesecloth and pour the yogurt into the sieve.
3. Cover the sieve with plastic wrap and allow the yogurt to drain overnight in the refrigerator.
4. Remove the soft cheese from the cheesecloth and store it in the refrigerator in a sealed container for up to 1 week.

Serves 8. Prep time 5 minutes, plus draining time.

Calories **169** / Calories from fat **41** / Total fat **4.5g** / Saturated fat **3.4g** / Trans fat **0.0g** / Sodium **93mg** / Carbs **9.0g** / Sugars **9.0g** / Protein **22.5g**

Cilantro Herb Salsa

Gluten-free
Low-fat
Low-sodium
Vegan
Vegetarian

KITCHEN
BASICS

Salsa is one of the most versatile staples in clean eating because you can use it for any type of meal, from breakfast to lunch wraps, and with any meat for an entrée. This is a standard mild tomato salsa with a healthy amount of pungent cilantro for flavoring. Tomatoes are available year round in most grocery stores. Try to get organic on-the-vine tomatoes for better taste and superior quality.

Cooking tip If you want a salsa that can keep for longer, try seeding your tomatoes before chopping them and reserve the scooped-out pulp for soups, sauces, and stews.

6 medium tomatoes, chopped

2 tablespoons minced garlic

1 small red onion, peeled and chopped

1 red bell pepper, seeded and
  finely chopped

1 small jalapeño pepper, finely chopped

½ cup chopped fresh cilantro

1. In a large bowl, mix all the ingredients together.
2. Store the salsa in a sealed container in the refrigerator for up to 3 days.

Serves 4. Prep time 10 minutes.

Calories **57** / Calories from fat **5** / Total fat **0.5g** / Saturated fat **0.0g** / Trans fat **0.0g** / Sodium **12mg** / Carbs **12.1g** / Sugars **7.0g** / Protein **2.4g**

Gluten-free
Low-sodium
Nightshade-free
Vegetarian

KITCHEN
BASICS

Lemon Garlic Vinaigrette

This vinaigrette might become your new favorite for any salad, and even an interesting dressing for a pasta dish. It has the smallest touch of honey to balance the tartness of the lemon. Honey has been a valuable culinary and medicinal ingredient for several thousand years, and continues to be used today for its warm sweetness and health benefits. It was even thought to help people live longer—and maybe it can!

Shopping tip The flavor of the honey will depend on what flowers the bees collect nectar from to make it. Try the different types to see what flavor appeals to your palate.

2 teaspoons minced garlic

¼ cup fresh lemon juice

2 tablespoons red wine vinegar

1 tablespoon chopped fresh oregano

½ teaspoon honey

Pinch of freshly ground black pepper

½ cup olive oil

1. In a small bowl, whisk together all the ingredients except the oil until well blended.
2. Whisk in the olive oil until the dressing emulsifies.
3. Store the vinaigrette in a sealed container in the refrigerator for up to 1 week.

Makes 12 tablespoons. Prep time 5 minutes.

Calories **60** / Calories from fat **57** / Total fat **6.3g** / Saturated fat **0.9g** / Trans fat **0.0g** / Sodium **16mg** / Carbs **0.7g** / Sugars **0.6g** / Protein **0.1g**

Ranch Dressing

Gluten-free
Nightshade-free
Vegetarian

KITCHEN
BASICS

You can use this dressing for salads and as a tasty dip for cut vegetables. The chives in this recipe add a slightly peppery taste to the dressing. Chives are one of the easiest herbs to grow and are perennials, so they continue to grow year round with a nice healthy root system. Try keeping a big pot on a sunny counter and simply snip off what you need for your recipes with a sharp pair of scissors.

Cooking tip If you want a less dense dressing, add some more buttermilk or thin it out with a touch of water.

⅔ cup low-fat buttermilk

⅓ cup plain Greek yogurt

2 tablespoons minced sweet onion

1 tablespoon chopped fresh parsley

1 tablespoon chopped fresh chives

1 teaspoon chopped fresh dill

Pinch of freshly ground black pepper

1. In a medium bowl, stir together all the ingredients until well blended.
2. Store the dressing in a sealed container in the refrigerator for up to 1 week.

Makes 16 tablespoons. Prep time 5 minutes.

Calories **8** / Calories from fat **1** / Total fat **0.1g** / Saturated fat **0.0g** / Trans fat **0.0g** / Sodium **15mg** / Carbs **0.9g** / Sugars **0.9g** / Protein **0.7g**

Tomato Pesto Vinaigrette

This is a basic vinaigrette that is perfect for everyday use on any salad. The best pesto to use in the recipe is a nice homemade one, so you know exactly what ingredients are in it. Use your own pesto recipes, or try Sun-Dried Tomato Pesto in this chapter. Use a dairy-free pesto and the vinaigrette works for vegan diets.

Cooking tip This vinaigrette is also delicious with balsamic vinegar instead of apple cider vinegar, just note that the finished product will be darker in color.

12 sun-dried tomatoes

3 tablespoons fresh lemon juice

1 tablespoon basil pesto

1 tablespoon apple cider vinegar

2 teaspoons minced garlic

Pinch of freshly ground black pepper

½ cup olive oil

1. In a blender, combine all the ingredients except the olive oil and blend into a smooth paste.
2. Add the olive oil in a thin stream while the blender is running.
3. Store the dressing in a sealed container in the refrigerator for up to 1 week.

Makes 12 tablespoons. Prep time 5 minutes.

_____

Calories **40** / Calories from fat **38** / Total fat **4.2g** / Saturated fat **0.6g** / Trans fat **0.0g** / Sodium **21mg** / Carbs **1.4g** / Sugar **0.0g** / Protein **0.2g**

Sun-Dried Tomato Pesto

Gluten-free
Vegetarian

KITCHEN
BASICS

Pesto is one of the best ways to get an intense flavor into a dish without too much added fat, salt, or calories. This sun-dried tomato variation uses pecans instead of the traditional pine nuts, for a unique taste. Pecans are extremely high in antioxidants, protein, and fiber.

Leftovers tip Basil is a very delicate herb with high water content. It needs to be frozen instead of dried if you have extra. Simply put whole stems of basil in the freezer for several hours until completely frozen and then transfer them to a sealed container. Do not pack them in, because basil bruises easily.

1 cup packed fresh basil leaves

2 tablespoons chopped sun-dried tomatoes

2 tablespoons pecans

2 tablespoons grated Parmesan cheese

1 teaspoon minced garlic

Pinch of freshly ground black pepper

2 tablespoons olive oil

1. In a food processor, combine all the ingredients except the olive oil and pulse until they are well combined and form a thick paste, scraping down the sides of the bowl at least once with a spatula.
2. Add the olive oil and pulse until the oil is incorporated.
3. Store the pesto in a sealed container in the refrigerator for up to 1 week.

Makes 16 tablespoons. Prep time 10 minutes.

Calories **34** / Calories from fat **28** / Total fat **3.1g** / Saturated fat **0.8g** / Trans fat **0.0g** / Sodium **41mg** / Carbs **0.6g** / Sugar **0.0g** / Protein **1.3g**

Gluten-free
Low-fat
Low-sodium
Vegan
Vegetarian

KITCHEN
BASICS

Simple Marinara Sauce

Basil and oregano are traditional herbs in Italian cuisine, and they impart a pleasant sweetness that is mirrored in the ripe tomatoes. Basil is a great choice for this sauce; the herb has antibacterial properties.

Cooking tip Marinara sauce freezes beautifully, so whip up a double batch and store it in resealable zipper-top bags or sealed containers for up to a year in the freezer.

½ small sweet onion, peeled and chopped

1 tablespoon minced garlic

1 teaspoon olive oil

6 large tomatoes, coarsely chopped

½ cup water

1 small bay leaf

3 tablespoons chopped fresh basil

1 tablespoon chopped fresh oregano

Pinch of freshly ground black pepper

1. In a large saucepan over medium heat, sauté the onion and garlic in the oil until softened and lightly browned, about 10 minutes.
2. Add the tomatoes, water, and bay leaf and bring the mixture to a gentle boil.
3. Reduce the heat to low and simmer, covered, for about 15 minutes.
4. Remove the pan from the heat and take out the bay leaf.
5. Stir in the basil, oregano, and pepper.
6. Serve immediately or chill and store the sauce in the refrigerator in a sealed container for up to 1 week.

Serves 4. Prep time 5 minutes. Cook time 25 minutes.

Calories **70** / Calories from fat **17** / Total fat **1.9g** / Saturated fat **0.0g** / Trans fat **0.0g** / Sodium **14mg** / Carbs **13.0g** / Sugars **7.6g** / Protein **2.8g**

Tzatziki Sauce

Gluten-free
Low-fat
Nightshade-free
Vegetarian

If you have ever tried gyros or souvlaki, you've tasted this tangy, rich sauce. It's a great complement to both meats and vegetables. The garlic, a common ingredient in almost every cuisine in the world, adds a wonderful pungent flavor. To get the freshest garlic, try to buy bulbs that feel heavy, because this means they are not old and dried out.

Cooking tip Sometimes it is impossible to get the scent of garlic off your hands after you mince it. Try rubbing something stainless steel over your hands, like a spoon or the side of a bowl, to remove the smell. Or simply run your hands along your stainless steel sink.

2 cups plain Greek yogurt

1 large English cucumber, grated, with all the liquid squeezed out

3 tablespoons chopped fresh dill

1 teaspoon minced garlic

Pinch of sea salt

1. In a medium bowl, stir together all the ingredients until they are well blended.
2. Store the sauce in a sealed container in the refrigerator for up to 4 days.

Makes 32 tablespoons. Prep time 5 minutes.

Calories **14** / Calories from fat **5** / Total fat **0.6g** / Saturated fat **0.0g** / Trans fat **0.0g** / Sodium **13mg** / Carbs **1.1g** / Sugar **0.6g** / Protein **1.4g**

FODMAP-free
Gluten-free
Nightshade-free
Vegetarian

KITCHEN
BASICS

Clean Eating Mayonnaise

This is not a truly healthy recipe, but it is much better than processed mayonnaise, which has additives and preservatives. Eating clean is all about food choices that are not processed, and this tangy dressing fits those guidelines. Eat this spread and dressing sparingly with sandwiches or wraps, and use it as a base for your favorite dips as a rare treat.

Shopping tip While traditional mayonnaise is made with raw egg yolks, that's not really a safe option due to the risk of salmonella infection. Eggs can be pasteurized in the shell or sold in cartons of liquid pasteurized egg. Pasteurization involves nothing but heat, so it does not alter the egg's nutrition.

2 yolks from pasteurized eggs or ⅓ cup
   pasteurized liquid eggs
2 teaspoons white wine vinegar
2 teaspoons Dijon mustard

½ teaspoon sea salt
¼ teaspoon freshly ground black pepper
1 cup olive oil

1. In a blender, combine the eggs, vinegar, mustard, salt, and pepper until well mixed.
2. Run the blender on low speed and slowly add approximately one-third of the oil in a thin stream, until the mixture is creamy.
3. Add the remaining oil in a thin stream until it is completely incorporated and the mayonnaise is thick.
4. Transfer the mayonnaise to a sealed container and store it in the refrigerator for up to 2 weeks.

Makes 32 teaspoons. Prep time 5 minutes.

Calories **58** / Calories from fat **58** / Total fat **6.6g** / Saturated fat **1.0g** / Trans fat **0.0g** / Sodium **35mg** / Carbs **0.1g** / Sugar **0.0g** / Protein **0.2g**

Cinnamon Applesauce

Gluten-free
Low-fat
Low-sodium
Nightshade-free
Vegan
Vegetarian

KITCHEN
BASICS

Most of the applesauce found on grocery store shelves doesn't really taste like apples and has an incredible array of added ingredients. Since making your own is so simple, there is no need to ever use store-bought again for your breakfast, snacks, desserts, and baked goods. Make a big batch, because this applesauce keeps well in the freezer.

Cooking tip If you have a slow cooker, one of the best ways to cook applesauce is to place all your ingredients into the slow cooker, and cook them on low until you have the desired texture.

6 apples, peeled, cored, and chopped into
    ½-inch chunks
½ cup water

1 teaspoon fresh lemon juice
1 teaspoon ground cinnamon

1. In a medium saucepan over medium-high heat, combine the apples, water, and lemon juice and bring to a boil.
2. Reduce the heat to low and simmer until the apples are tender, about 15 minutes.
3. Remove the mixture from the heat and either mash the apples with a potato masher or use an immersion blender to purée, depending on how chunky you want the finished product.
4. Stir in the cinnamon and serve either warm or cold.
5. Store the applesauce in the refrigerator in a sealed container for up to 1 week.

Serves 4. Prep time 5 minutes. Cook time 15 minutes.

Calories **144** / Calories from fat **0** / Total fat **0.0g** / Saturated fat **0.0g** / Trans fat **0.0g** / Sodium **4mg** / Carbs **32.8g** / Sugars **28.4g** / Protein **0.0g**

Appendix

Grab 'n Go: Thirty-Five Clean Eating Snack Ideas

1. Nuts, dried fruit, seeds, and trail mix
2. Fresh fruit (plain, or with Greek yogurt)
3. Fresh vegetables
4. Hardboiled eggs
5. Greek yogurt with granola or nuts
6. Smoothies
7. Frozen grapes
8. Homemade unsweetened applesauce
9. Apple slices with natural nut butters
10. Air-popped popcorn
11. Edamame
12. Celery sticks topped with natural peanut butter and raisins
13. Homemade fruit popsicles
14. Medjool dates
15. Dried fruit or vegetable chips
16. Mixed green salad
17. Steel-cut oatmeal with a little homemade applesauce
18. Homemade baked sweet potato fries
19. Homemade protein bar

20. Baked pita bread with honey and dried fruit

21. Rye melba toast with low-fat cream cheese and dried cranberries

22. One ounce of great quality dark chocolate

23. Half a whole-wheat English muffin with nut butter

24. Wraps stuffed with leftovers

25. Apples with cheese

26. Whole-wheat pretzels

27. Homemade fruit leathers

28. 100 percent shredded wheat with low-fat almond milk

29. Homemade clean eating cookies or muffins

30. One can of water-packed tuna with a drizzle of homemade dressing

31. Half an avocado with homemade salsa

32. Chickpeas, either plain or roasted

33. Wraps and pitas stuffed with lean meats, veggies, and beans

34. Homemade beef jerky

35. Olives and low-sodium pickles

The Dirty Dozen Plus

As you probably already know, not all produce is created equal, but some fruits and vegetables are cleaner than others. The dirty dozen are fruits and vegetables the Environmental Working Group (EWG) has identified as being the most contaminated. To steer clear of hazardous pesticides, choose organic when buying the produce on this list. Visit the Environmental Working Group's website at www.ewg.org for updates to this list.

- Apples
- Celery
- Cherry tomatoes
- Cucumbers
- Grapes
- Hot peppers

- Kale/collard greens
- Nectarines (imported)
- Peaches
- Potatoes

- Snap peas (imported)
- Spinach
- Sweet bell peppers
- Strawberries

The Clean Fifteen

The clean fifteen are nonorganic fruits and vegetables the EWG has identified as having the least amount of contamination. If you're watching your food budget, the clean fifteen are the best produce to buy nonorganic. Visit the Environmental Working Group's website at www.ewg.org for updates to this list.

- Asparagus
- Avocados
- Cabbage
- Cantaloupe
- Eggplant
- Grapefruit
- Kiwis
- Mangoes

- Mushrooms
- Onions
- Papayas
- Pineapple
- Sweet corn
- Sweet peas (frozen)
- Sweet potatoes

Glossary

amino acids there are twenty amino acids, which are the building blocks of protein. The body uses the protein from food by breaking it down into amino acids.

antioxidants the vitamins, minerals, and phytonutrients that protect your body from free radicals and are crucial for good health.

artificial sweeteners laboratory-created sweeteners created to replace sugar. These are not on the clean eating plan.

blood glucose or blood sugar the glucose (sugar) level in the blood.

calories a unit of energy. With respect to food, calories are the amount of energy in the food; the higher the number, the more energy the food contains.

carbohydrates organic compounds comprised of sugars, starches, and cellulose. The body breaks down carbohydrates into blood sugar, which is used as energy. Carbohydrates can be simple or complex. Simple carbohydrates are not recommended on a clean eating diet because they are broken down very quickly, creating spikes in blood sugar. Complex carbohydrates include many of the foods found in the clean eating diet, such as vegetables, fruit, whole grains, and legumes. These healthy carbs break down more slowly, for more stable blood sugar.

chia seeds nutritious seeds with the highest level of omega-3 fatty acids found in a plant source. They are a member of the mint family, and are often used in sauces or puddings because they can soak up about nine times their volume in liquid.

coconut oil an oil that comes from coconut milk. It is high in saturated fat but also has many health benefits, so it is part of the clean eating plan. Coconut oil supports a healthy digestive system, boosts immunity, and helps lower cholesterol.

complete proteins proteins that contain all nine essential amino acids. Essential amino acids cannot be produced in the body so they need to come from foods such as dairy, meats, poultry, and seafood.

diet the food you eat—although the word is often applied to weight loss or health oriented eating plans.

essential amino acids the nine amino acids that the body cannot produce in the quantities required, or at all.

essential fatty acids the most well-known essential fatty acids are omega-3s and omega-6s. These fats are not produced in the body and need to be taken from food, because they are crucial for proper physical functioning.

fiber the indigestible component in plants that sweeps through the body like a broom. It is crucial for a healthy, efficient digestive system. A diet high in fiber can help prevent some types of cancer, diabetes, heart disease, and other health problems.

flavonoids natural pigments found in plants that function as antioxidants to help protect human cells from damage.

flaxseed the seeds of the flax plant; they are a great plant source of omega-3 fatty acids, and are very high in fiber and other nutrients.

free radicals oxygen or nitrogen molecules that are missing electrons, so they try to take electrons from the cells in the body, causing damage. Unchecked, free radicals can damage cells in all kinds of ways.

gluten a cereal grain protein that can cause health problems in people with gluten sensitivity.

glycemic index a measure of how fast a food causes the blood sugar to rise after consuming it.

grass-fed meat the recommended meat on the clean eating plan because it is not factory-farmed and comes from pasture-raised animals that are allowed to graze.

insulin the hormone that moves glucose from the blood into the cells.

lactose a sugar in milk that can be an allergen for many people.

macronutrients main groups of nutrients that your body uses for essential tasks; they include protein, carbohydrates, and fat.

omega-3 fatty acid a family of three fats (ALA, EPA, and DHA) that are not produced in the body but are essential for health because omega-3s help with almost every type of cell activity.

omega-6 fatty acid unsaturated fatty acids that aren't made by the body but are crucial for good health.

phytonutrients beneficial compounds found only in plants and may help prevent disease and keep your body functioning smoothly.

prebiotics indigestible carbohydrates that serve as food for probiotics.

probiotics the bacteria that live in your digestive system that help digestion and aid in eliminating bad bacteria from the body.

processed foods products treated with additives, chemicals, and preservatives; these foods are not recommended when eating clean.

protein essential nutrient made from amino acids that is used for many body functions, and maintaining and building cells.

References

Collins, Sonya. "The Truth About Belly Fat." WebMD. Accessed March 9, 2014. http://www.webmd.com/diet/features/the-truth-about-belly-fat.

dLife. "12 Best Fiber Foods." Accessed March 9, 2014. http://www.dlife.com/dlife_media /diabetes_slideshows/12-best-fiber-foods?index=9.

Environmental Working Group. "EWG's 2013 Shopper's Guide to Pesticides in Produce." Accessed March 9, 2014. http://www.ewg.org/foodnews/summary.php.

Environmental Working Group. "PCBs in Farmed Salmon." Accessed March 9, 2014. http://www.ewg.org/reports/farmedpcbs.

Goto, K., et al. "Effects of resistance exercise on lipolysis during subsequent submaximal exercise." *Medicine & Science in Sports & Exercise.* February 2007; 39(2): 308–15.

Harvard School of Public Health. "Fiber: Start Roughing It!" The Nutrition Source. Accessed March 9, 2014. http://www.hsph.harvard.edu/nutritionsource/what-should-you-eat /fiber-full-story/.

Hensrud, Donald, MD. "Sleep and Weight Gain: What's the Connection?" Mayo Clinic. Accessed March 9, 2014. http://www.mayoclinic.com/health/sleep-and-weight-gain /AN02178/.

Hyman, Mark, MD. *The Blood Sugar Solution.* New York: Little, Brown and Company, 2012.

Jacob, Agalee. "Damaging Effects of Too Much Sugar in the Diet." SF Gate, Healthy Eating. Accessed March 9, 2014. http://healthyeating.sfgate.com/damaging-effects-much-sugar -diet-1508.html.

Mayo Clinic Staff. "Exercise: 7 benefits of regular physical activity." Accessed March 9, 2014. http://www.mayoclinic.com/health/exercise/HQ01676.

Mckee, G. *Guide to Food Additives.* Chicago: The Learning Seed, 2008.

MediResource Canada. "High Cholesterol." Accessed March 9, 2014. http://bodyandhealth
.canada.com/channel_condition_info_details.asp?disease_id=148&channel_id
=41&relation_id=10852.

National Cancer Institute. "Cruciferous Vegetables and Cancer Prevention." Accessed March
9, 2014. http://www.cancer.gov/cancertopics/factsheet/diet/cruciferous-vegetables.

Natural Resources Defense Council. "Consumer Guide to Mercury in Fish." Accessed March
9, 2014. http://www.nrdc.org/health/effects/mercury/guide.asp.

Reno, Tosca. *The Eat-Clean Diet: Fast Fat-Loss That Lasts Forever!* Mississauga, Ontario:
Robert Kennedy Publishing, 2007.

Teicholz, Nina. "What If Bad Fat Is Actually Good for You?" *Men's Health.* October 10, 2007.
Accessed March 9, 2014. http://www.menshealth.com/health/saturated-fat?fullpage=true.

Tomiyama, Janet A., et al. "Low Calorie Dieting Increases Cortisol," *Psychosomatic Medicine.*
May 2010; 72(4): 357–364.

Venuto, Tom. *The Body Fat Solution.* New York: Avery, 2009.

WebMD. "Portion Control and Weight Loss." Accessed March 9, 2014. http://www.webmd.com
/diet/control-portion-size.

Wedro, Benjamin, MD. "High Cholesterol." eMedicine Health. Accessed March 9, 2014.
http://www.emedicinehealth.com/high_cholesterol/article_em.htm.

Women Fitness. "Ugly Truths About White Flour." Accessed March 9, 2014.
http://www.womenfitness.net/ugly_truths.htm.

Worden, Jeni, GP. "Carbohydrates." NetDoctor. Accessed March 9, 2014. http://www.netdoctor
.co.uk/focus/nutrition/facts/lifestylemanagement/carbohydrates.htm.

Recipe Index

Subject Index

CPSIA information can be obtained
at www.ICGtesting.com
Printed in the USA
LVHW071307231222
735850LV00016B/231

Step 3: Create an outline

When designing a website, content is king – not only in terms of providing visitors with quality material and media but also in driving the structure of the site – see Figure 1-1. Content influences all aspects of the design, including its appearance, structure and navigation.

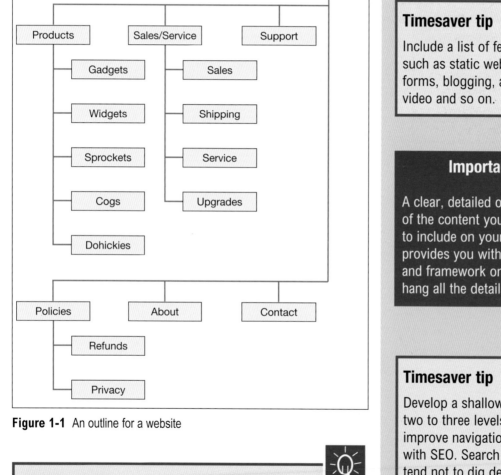

Figure 1-1 An outline for a website

Jargon buster

SEO (search engine optimisation): Techniques designed to attract search engines and enable them to properly index a site's content and assign the site the highest possible search engine ranking.

Timesaver tip

Include a list of features, such as static web pages, forms, blogging, audio, video and so on.

Important

A clear, detailed outline of the content you plan to include on your site provides you with a vision and framework on which to hang all the details.

Timesaver tip

Develop a shallow outline, two to three levels deep, to improve navigation and help with SEO. Search engines tend not to dig deeper than a few levels.

Understanding the web design process (cont.)

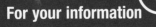

Step 4: Establish the layout (wireframing)

Creating wireframes or line drawings of pages free of content, colours and fonts allows you to establish a layout for your pages without the distraction of text, graphics and other objects.

With wireframes, you determine how much screen space the heading consumes, where your navigation bar or menu bar will appear (usually at the top or on the left), the size of the footer, the number of columns to be used on each page and so on. Figure 1-2 gives an example.

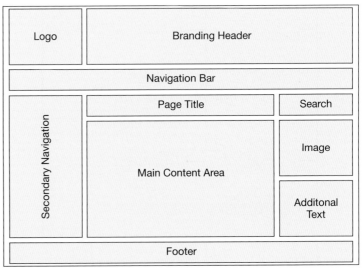

Figure 1-2 Using wireframes to define a layout

See also

For more about wireframing, see Chapter 4, 'Designing your website structure'.

Step 5: Design the appearance

Using your wireframes as a guide, you are ready to begin the serious business of actually designing the site – placing the header, navigation bar or menu bar, establishing the content areas, choosing colours and fonts, and so on – see Figure 1-3.

At this stage, professional designers often rely on high-end graphics programs, such as CorelDRAW, to establish the overall look and feel of the pages.

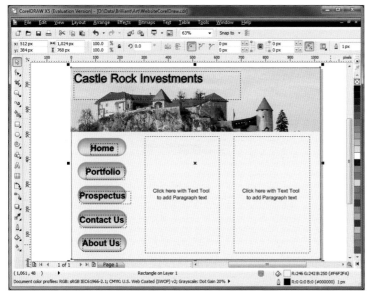

Figure 1-3 Designing a website

See also

For more about designing the site's appearance, see Chapter 5, 'Adding colour', Chapter 6, 'Designing the text elements', Chapter 7, 'Accenting your website with graphics' and Chapter 8, 'Putting your design in motion'.

Did you know?

Some professionals and do-it-yourselfers may rely on predesigned templates or may begin with a template and then customise it.

For your information

You may already have a web design program on your computer and not even know it. Some desktop publishing programs, including Microsoft Publisher, feature templates to help you get started with designing your own custom site.

Understanding the web design process (cont.)

Jargon buster

Content management system (CMS): A tool for facilitating the collaborative development and maintenance of a website.

WYSIWYG (What You See Is What You Get): A technology that displays pages on your screen as they will appear upon publication, either on paper or when viewed in a web browser.

Step 6: Create web pages

When you have the design in place, you can begin creating the individual pages, which will ultimately comprise your site, as in Figure 1-4. This is the stage at which you dig into your web toolbox and pull out your web page authoring tools.

Professional designers often rely on high-end programs, such as Dreamweaver, which is like a desktop publishing program for the web. You create your pages using a WYSIWYG interface, and the program handles all the complex HTML and CSS tagging behind the scenes.

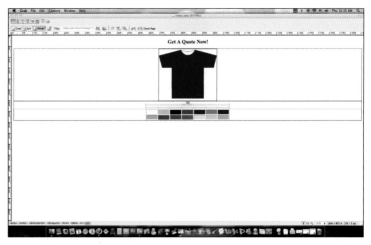

Figure 1-4 Professional web design application

Jargon buster

HTML (HyperText Markup Language): A system of codes used to format web pages.

CSS (Cascading style sheets): A web page formatting system that helps keep content and formatting separate, so designs can change the appearance of an element throughout the site simply by editing the site's style sheet.

Step 7: Test your site

Prior to unveiling your website to the public, you should always test it thoroughly. Read through all the text for misspellings, typos or grammatical errors; check the appearance of every page from top to bottom; click all the links and buttons to determine whether they do what they are supposed to do; and so on. Then, when you've all finished that, check your website on other platforms (Windows, Mac OS and Linux) and in other web browsers (such as Internet Explorer, Mozilla Firefox and Google Chrome).

Step 8: Launch your site

If you created the website on your computer, launching it consists of uploading the pages and any other essential files to the server on which your website will reside. However, with modern custom management systems, you may actually create the website online, in which case uploading the files is unnecessary. Another part of your launch may consist of promoting the website, so people will know it is ready for visitors and know where to find it.

Understanding the web design process (cont.)

1

!

Important

Beware. Your website may appear and function perfectly on your computer in the web browser you normally use, but look and operate terribly on someone else's computer or in a different web browser.

!

Important

Website development culminates in the launch, but that does not mean your job is done. You must continuously monitor your site to ensure it is accomplishing its goals, keep the site content fresh and update it occasionally to keep pace with current technology. The web is constantly evolving and so should your website.

See also

For more about testing your site, refer to Chapter 11, 'Designing for different platforms, browsers and screen resolutions'

Exploring the fundamentals of good web design

▶

Jargon buster

Front end: The website visitors see, as opposed to the back end that works behind the scenes to control the site's appearance and functionality.

You can find plenty of poorly designed web pages and blogs on the internet and most of these poor designs can be attributed to the fact that the creators chose not to adhere to the fundamentals of good web design. They broke the rules either out of ignorance or in a vain attempt to be creative. We are not censoring creativity, but you can be creative within certain parameters. Know the rules – and then break them only when you have a very good reason to do so.

In the following sections, we introduce you to the fundamentals of good web design for both the front and back end and explain the reasoning behind each guideline.

Front end

On the front end, the focus is on the user. Your goal is to meet or exceed your audience's expectations in terms of content while making that content as attractive and easily accessible as possible. An attractive design with few distractions and intuitive navigation is far more important than packing the site with dazzling graphics and a rainbow of colours.

Keep it simple

Simplicity is key in keeping visitors focused, as Figure 1-5 illustrates. An overabundance of colours, fonts, graphics, buttons, animations and other elements distracts and confuses visitors. If you are not quite sure whether a particular item is necessary, omit it.

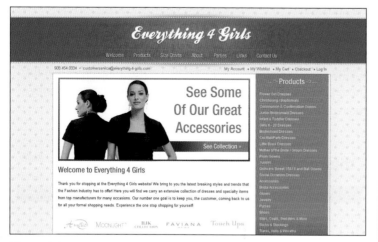

Figure 1-5 A simple design keeps visitors focused

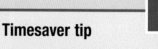

Timesaver tip

When in doubt, leave it out. An overly cluttered design tends to overwhelm and confuse visitors.

Exploring the fundamentals of good web design (cont.)

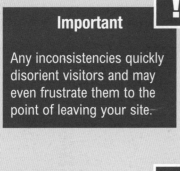
Strive towards unity

Unity holds a page together. All elements on the page contribute to its overall appearance and effect. In the same way, all pages on a site contribute to making the site as usable as possible. Without unity, a site becomes a loose collection of independent elements, which dilutes its impact.

Be consistent

A consistent design reduces the learning curve for your visitors. Soon after reaching a site, most visitors quickly orient themselves to the navigation system. They develop a feel for the layout and the navigation system, so they can efficiently move around the site, as in Figure 1-6.

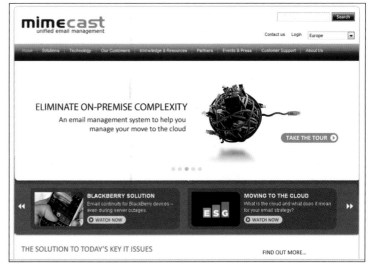

Figure 1-6 Consistency helps visitors navigate the site

Maintain balance

A balanced design such as that in Figure 1-7 makes visitors feel more comfortable by giving equal weight to both sides of the page. You can establish balance through various designs, including symmetrical, asymmetrical and intentionally off-balance or discordant designs.

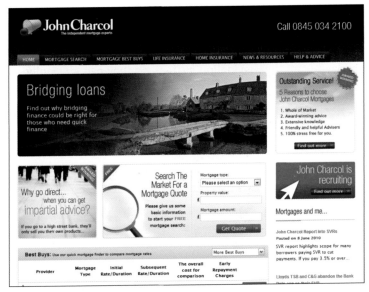

Figure 1-7 A balanced design appeals to visitors

Important

One of the biggest challenges is to maintain the balance as the user scrolls down the page, bringing different elements into view. Make sure each page is balanced from top to bottom.

Exploring the fundamentals of good web design (cont.)

1 Add a consistent menu bar.

2 Chunk information.

Timesaver tip

Having a few key redundant links at the very bottom of the page, in the footer, is acceptable and often warranted, because it allows visitors quick access to important information without having to scroll back up to the top.

Make navigation intuitive

Visitors should not have to think twice about where to go to find something, especially what you really want them to find. A navigation or menu bar near the top of every page or running along the left side is essential. Avoid redundancy: having a menu bar at the top with the same options in a navigation bar on the left can cause confusion. See Figure 1-8 for an example.

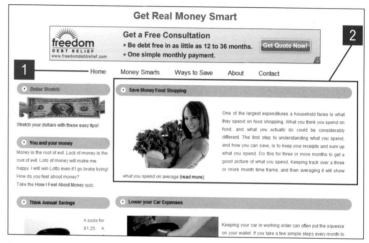

Figure 1-8 Make navigation intuitive

Position key information above the fold

The concept of a fold harks back to the days of newspapers (remember those?) where the important headlines and information of the day were printed to attract readers' attention. For web pages, 'above the fold' references content that appears on the screen when a visitor first accesses a page. The fold in this case is the bottom of the browser window, as in the lower section of Figure 1-9.

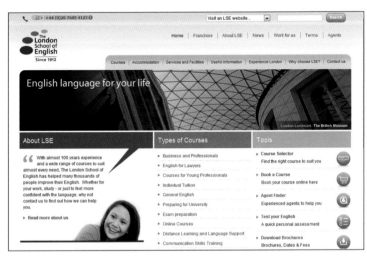

Figure 1-9 Important content should be 'above the fold'

Provide relevant and compelling content

Content is not exactly part of the site's design, but it is one of the main reasons people visit a site and keep coming back. In your zest to create an attractive, usable site, do not overlook the fact that people do not visit your site to be dazzled by the design. They come and come back for the content the site offers.

Timesaver tip

By positioning key information above the fold, you instantly provide visitors with what they are looking for; they do not have to scroll down to view it.

Important

Keep in mind that the purpose of the front-end design is to facilitate the delivery of content to visitors. Whatever hinders access to what a visitor is looking for functions as a barrier. Barriers can range from a background that makes the text difficult to read, to a poorly placed link, to a popup window that pesters the visitor into buying something. Remove all the barriers and your design should be right on target.

Back end

Behind every website or blog is a back end that visitors never see. It functions as the puppet master responsible for all of the site's functionality and features. The back end does not need to look pretty, but it must function correctly and efficiently.

Cross-platform friendly

The site must look good and function properly whether it is accessed from a Windows PC or a Mac, or using Internet Explorer, Mozilla Firefox, or other popular web browsers. Figure 1-10 shows the same site opened in different browsers.

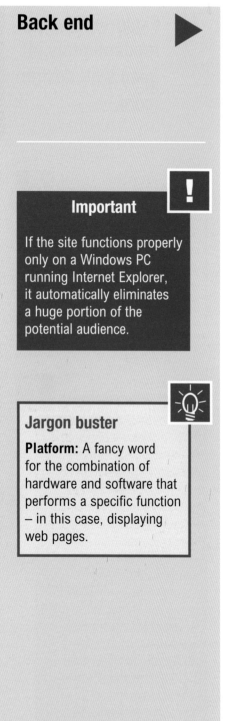

Important !

If the site functions properly only on a Windows PC running Internet Explorer, it automatically eliminates a huge portion of the potential audience.

Jargon buster

Platform: A fancy word for the combination of hardware and software that performs a specific function – in this case, displaying web pages.

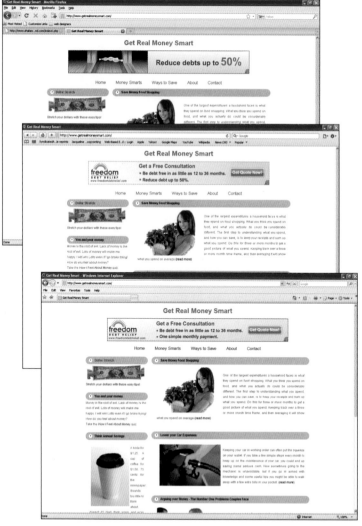

Figure 1-10 A site needs to be attractive and function properly in all web browsers

SEO optimised

Unless people already know where to find a particular site, most visitors will discover it through a search engine. Search engine optimisation makes a site a bigger target for search engines, including Google, Yahoo! and Bing.

To optimise a site, you typically use a combination of descriptive, relevant text on pages throughout your site along with meta tags and a linking strategy – internal and external links that establish the site's relevance as it relates to a particular topic. See Figure 1-11.

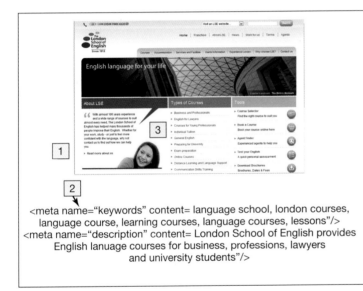

```
<meta name="keywords" content= language school, london courses,
language course, learning courses, language courses, lessons"/>
<meta name="description" content= London School of English provides
English lanuage courses for business, professions, lawyers
and university students"/>
```

Figure 1-11 Use meta tags to optimise a site

1 Add descriptive, relevant text.

2 Insert meta tags to describe contents to search engines.

3 Create internal links.

4 Establish external links from relevant websites.

Jargon buster

Meta tags: Codes that enable web developers to insert descriptive text about a site and about pages that can help search engines properly index content on the site. This descriptive text does not appear when the page is opened in a web browser.

Back end (cont.)

Performance enhanced

The web is an on-demand medium, meaning data is served when a visitor requests it. Because of this, web users typically expect to receive what they request instantly. Sites must not only look pretty, they must also perform to web users' expectations, which can be fairly high.

Easy to maintain

Content management systems have made websites incredibly easy to maintain. After logging on to the site, you can quickly add or delete pages, edit text, apply formatting, insert pictures or video, and perform other site-maintenance tasks simply by typing text and clicking buttons, as shown in Figure 1-12.

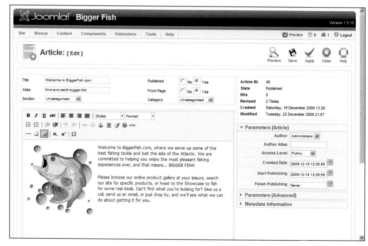

Figure 1-12 Content management systems make it easy to maintain a site

E-commerce-enabled (if applicable)

If a site's purpose is to allow customers to order products or services online, the site must be e-commerce-enabled to allow customers to enter order and payment information. In addition, any e-commerce features must be easy to access and use. As a general rule, accessing an order form, such as the one in Figure 1-13, should never require more than two clicks.

Address Details		
First Name:	Sally	*
Last Name:	Rogers	*
Street Address:	192 Gray's Inn Road	*
Address Line 2:		
Town/City:	London	*
County:		
Post/Zip Code:	WC1X 8AA	*
Country:	United Kingdom	*
Additional Contact Details		
Telephone:		
Login Details		
Email Address:	srogers@sample.co.uk	*
Password:	●●●●●●●●●●●●●●●●	* (at least 5 characters)
Confirm Password:	●●●●●●●●●●●●●●●●	*
Newsletter and Email Details		
☐ Subscribe to Our Newsletter.		
	SUBMIT	

Figure 1-13 An online order form on an e-commerce site

Secure

No website or blog is completely secure, but the site should be reasonably secure, particularly if it enables users to submit sensitive information, such as their address, phone number or credit card number. Sites must also have some built-in protection to keep hacker vandals at bay.

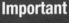

Jargon buster

E-commerce: Short for electronic commerce, various technologies and techniques that enable people to buy and sell goods and services on the internet.

Important !

If a hacker can log into a site, he can delete files, post unacceptable content and even redirect forms to send any data users enter to himself.

Timesaver tip

Although users may never step behind the curtain to see the back end, never lose sight of its importance. The back end plays a key role in how easy it is for visitors to find your site, navigate it and feel that any information they enter is secure. In addition, building CMS into a site can save hundreds of hours later in reconfiguring the site and refreshing its contents.

Exploring common web page building blocks

1 Container
2 Header
3 Navigation bar

Jargon buster

Container: The outer boundaries of each page within which everything else appears.

Header: Graphic, text or a combination of the two at the top of the page, typically including a logo for businesses and organisations.

Navigation bar or menu: The narrow band, typically above, below or inside the header or along the left margin, that contains links that visitors click to move around the site.

Up to this point, we have been looking at the big picture – the process and principles of brilliant web design. However, web design also applies on a smaller scale to individual web pages. By understanding the components of a web page, you can grasp the overall structure of a page and begin to envision page layouts. Just about every web page you encounter comprises six components or building blocks (shown in Figures 1-14 and 1-15).

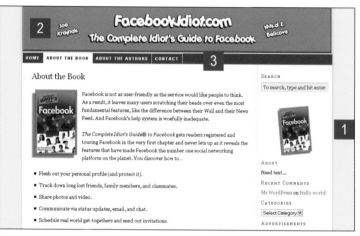
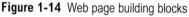

Figure 1-14 Web page building blocks

Timesaver tip

Regardless of where the navigation bar appears, ideally all navigation buttons or links should appear above the fold, so visitors do not have to scroll down to bring them into view.

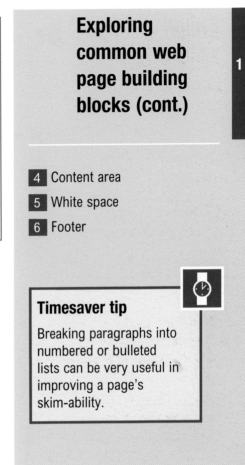

The following building blocks appear in the figure:

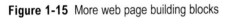
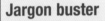

Figure 1-15 illustrates:

```
■ Share photos and video.
■ Communicate via status updates, email, and chat.
■ Schedule real world get-togethers and send out invitations.       4
■ Share common interests in groups.
■ Play games.
■ Buy and sell stuff in the Facebook Marketplace.

You also learn how tap the power of Facebook for more than simply personal use – such as
personal branding; marketing a business, product, service, or non profit; or promoting a worthy
cause.

Where to buy...

Amazon                                                              5

Borders

 Share / Save

                      Copyright © 2009-Present by Joe Kraynak, Mikal E. Belicove, and Marie Butler-Knight
              6       Designed with the Thesis WordPress Theme from DIYthemes.
                      Hosted by Bluehost.
```

Figure 1-15 More web page building blocks

4 Content area
5 White space
6 Footer

Jargon buster

Content area: The body of each web page, where text, graphics, video clips, animations and other content appear. This is typically the largest area of each page.

White space: Appears throughout the page to give everything else on the page some breathing room and facilitate a visitor's ability to skim the page for information.

Footer: Text that appears at the bottom of every page.

Timesaver tip

Breaking paragraphs into numbered or bulleted lists can be very useful in improving a page's skim-ability.

Exploring website types

▶

Surf the web and you're likely to find all sorts of sites – personal, corporate, static, dynamic, sites designed to share content including photos or video, e-commerce sites for selling goods and services, blogs designed to share information and insights and build community, and more.

While all sites are unique, grouping them into categories can help you identify certain types and choose the right type for the purpose you have in mind.

Standard CSS/HTML websites

Standard websites use a combination of CSS and HTML to format all the text and graphics that comprise the site. You can build a standard website by typing your text and any formatting tags into your documents in any text editor or by using an HTML/CSS editor, which functions as a desktop publishing program for the web. You format the document as you would in a word-processing program and the editor inserts the formatting tags behind the scenes. Standard CSS/HTML sites tend to be static – more like pages in a book than anything else.

Flash sites

Flash sites such as the one shown in Figure 1-16 are more dynamic, featuring video and animation. They also tend to take more time to load and are not very search engine friendly. Flash sites are used primarily to razzle and dazzle visitors, making them the website of choice for movies and various types of interactive entertainment, including games.

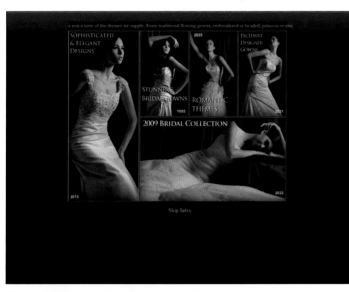

Figure 1-16 Flash sites razzle and dazzle

Jargon buster

Flash: A multimedia development platform for creating rich, interactive, animated web pages and web-based content. Flash is commonly used to add animation, interactivity and advertisements to websites.

Exploring website types (cont.)

Blogs

Blogs are sites that enable individuals, organisations, businesses and others to quickly and easily post content to the web on a regular basis and allow visitors to comment.

Posts are typically displayed in reverse chronological order – most recent first. Because content is posted regularly, blogs tend to be search engine friendly and are most effective in building community around a topic, cause or product that's likely to generate plenty of questions and opinions. See Joe's blog in Figure 1-17.

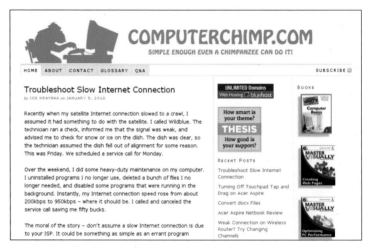

Figure 1-17 Blogs are a popular way to post fresh content to a site regularly

CMS-based

Sites built with a content management system in place, such as Joomla! or Drupal, are a sort of cross between blogs and standard CSS/HTML websites. They look and function like a website, but they are easier to customise, edit and update like a blog.

Many website designers use blog platforms, including WordPress, as their primary CMS for building websites, regardless of whether the site includes a blog component. See Figure 1-18.

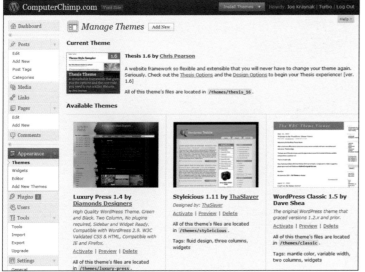

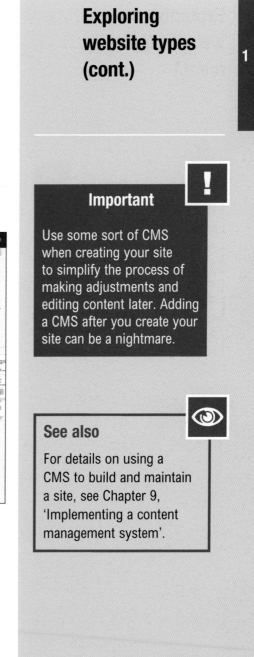

Figure 1-18 Using a CMS makes it easier to manage a site

Important

Use some sort of CMS when creating your site to simplify the process of making adjustments and editing content later. Adding a CMS after you create your site can be a nightmare.

See also

For details on using a CMS to build and maintain a site, see Chapter 9, 'Implementing a content management system'.

Exploring website types (cont.)

Another, perhaps more practical, way to categorise sites is by examining the purpose of the site – whether it is to communicate with friends and family, establish a corporate presence on the internet, showcase a product, build a community or sell products or services.

Personal

A personal website or blog is best for individuals who want to establish a home on the web and perhaps share their knowledge, experiences, insights and interests with others, such as the one shown in Figure 1-19.

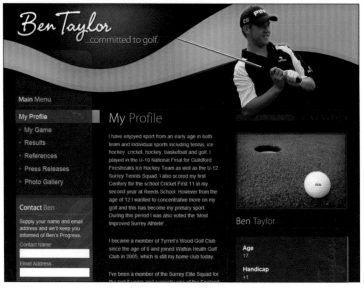

Figure 1-19 Blogs can convey all sorts of personal information

Photo sharing

Photo sharing sites are just what their name implies – the site is essentially a photo album or several albums designed to share digital photos with others on the web, such as the one shown in Figure 1-20.

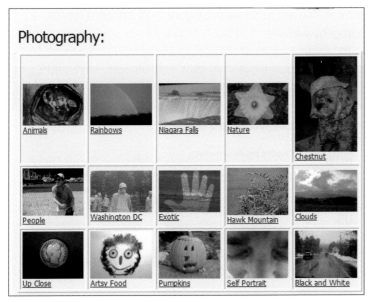

Figure 1-20 Sites can be designed specifically for sharing photos

Exploring website types (cont.)

Company

Like companies themselves, websites can range from large corporate sites to small business sites that provide information about the company, its management and employees, the products and services it offers, and any news that's applicable to the company or its industry. Most company websites also provide contact information. Figure 1-21 shows a typical company website.

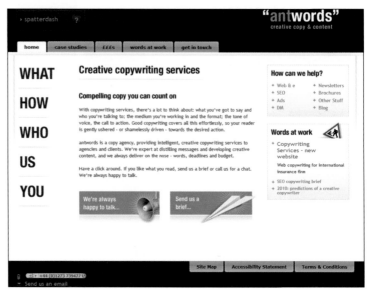

Figure 1-21 A typical company website

E-commerce

E-commerce sites enable people to do business online, including shopping for and buying goods and services, and managing accounts. These sites require a higher level of security. Many are simply online catalogues (see Figure 1-22) that include secure forms for placing orders.

Some common uses for e-commerce sites include:

- order products online
- pay for products online
- transfer funds electronically
- process business-to-business transactions
- buy and sell services online, such as freelance editing, writing or marketing.

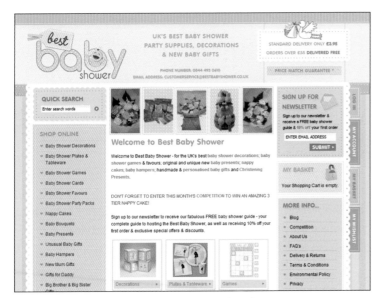

Figure 1-22 E-commerce sites let you shop from home

Exploring website types (cont.)

1

See also

To learn how to integrate an e-commerce component into a website, see Chapter 15, 'Developing an e-commerce site'.

Exploring website types (cont.)

Community

Community sites (commonly referred to as social networking sites) are primarily designed to facilitate communication among members of a community who share a common interest or goal. Community sites such as Facebook and MySpace (for personal use) and LinkedIn (for professional use) are examples of large sites that can host thousands of communities. Other community sites can be rather small and even exclusive – members-only clubs.

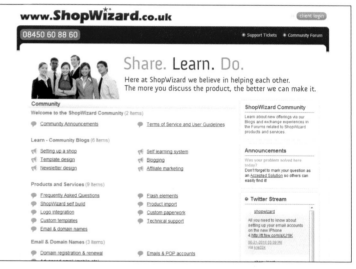

Figure 1-23 The ShopWizard site provides information and resources to the ShopWizard community

The ShopWizard site shown in Figure 1-23 provides ShopWizard customers with access to valuable information, services and discussion forums where they can exchange information.

Some common uses for community sites include:

■ facilitate communication among a group of people with shared interests or goals

■ social media marketing for enlisting community members to become brand evangelists

- market research – monitoring what customers say about a company and its brands, products and services

- professional or social networking to meet new people and establish connections.

Intranet

Intranets look and function like the internet but are internal – for company use only – see Figure 1-24. Intranets are commonly set up to function as business networks to facilitate communication, and file and resource sharing among employees of a company or members of an organisation. They aim to do the following:

- facilitate communication among employees via email and other technologies

- improve and simplify data sharing and distribution

- enable the sharing of expensive resources, including computer equipment and storage

- encourage professional or social networking to meet new people and establish connections.

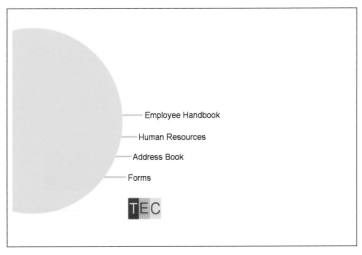

Figure 1-24 A company intranet facilitates communication

Understanding visual web design principles

When people land on any website, they need to know where to look for the most important information. We know, for example, that when visitors access a website, their eyes tend to look first at the upper left quadrant of the page before drifting to the middle and then skimming down the page. Because of this, placing the most important content on the right would be a mistake.

One way to simplify navigation for visitors is to follow web design principles that apply to the overall layout and appearance of the site.

See in thirds

You can usually tell when the objects in a painting, drawing or other graphic design are properly proportioned and positioned just by looking at it.

Many people simply chalk this up to artistic talent, but mathematics plays a role in graphic design just as it does in music. The miracle of music is the octave – the interval between one musical pitch and another of half or double its frequency. The miracle of graphic design is the golden ratio – roughly 1.62.

Divide a line in two, with one segment equal to the length of the line divided by 1.62, and the result is two line segments with one two-thirds as long as the other, as demonstrated in Figure 1-25.

$$1000 \text{ pixels} \div 1.62 = 617 \text{ pixels}$$

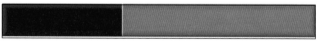

Figure 1-25 The golden ratio is the key to great website design

Explore the design grid

Ultimately, you may not want your web design to look boxy, but using a grid to guide the overall layout helps your design remain true to the golden ratio.

Form a grid with three equally spaced columns and three equally spaced rows, so you have something that looks like a tic-tac-toe grid, as in Figure 1-26.

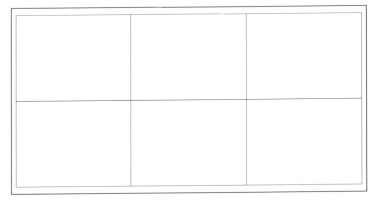

Figure 1-26 A design grid

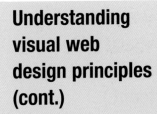

Understanding visual web design principles (cont.)

1

For your information

While the lines may make this grid approach seem too rigid, you still have a great deal of flexibility in where you position various elements.

Timesaver tip

You can further divide each row and column to create smaller divisions, if necessary for your design, while retaining the overall design grid that meets the rule of thirds guideline.

Understanding visual web design principles (cont.)

Balance your design

In addition to being visually pleasing, a balanced design facilitates skimming by distributing content somewhat evenly on the page. You can achieve balance in a variety of ways.

Horizontal symmetry

The content is either centred on the page or evenly distributed among the columns, as in Figure 1-27.

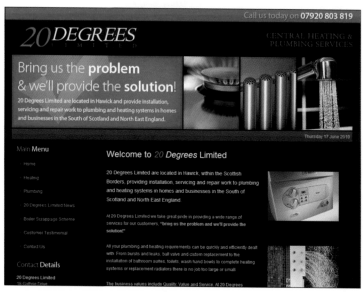

Figure 1-27 An example of horizontal symmetry

Bilateral symmetry

The content is distributed evenly across two axes, which rarely comes into play when designing a web page but may play a role when designing certain elements, such as a graphic header or a logo. You may need to balance the left and right sides of the image, as in Figure 1-28, and the bottom and top.

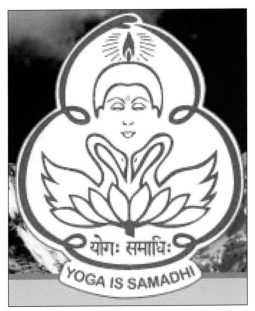

Figure 1-28 An example of bilateral symmetry

Understanding visual web design principles (cont.)

Radial symmetry

With radial symmetry, objects on a page are spaced equally around a centre point. A sunflower or a daisy provides a clear example of radial symmetry, as does Figure 1-29.

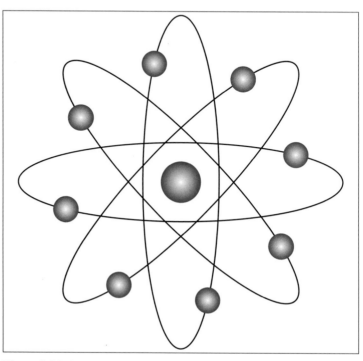

Figure 1-29 An example of radial symmetry

Asymmetry

An asymmetrical design may space objects unevenly on a page but still attain a sense of balance through the various weights of different objects. For example, three small objects on the left of the page may be counterbalanced by one large object on the right.

The design shown in Figure 1-30 is slightly asymetrical, with a larger image on the left than on the right, but the three images across the bottom help hold the design together.

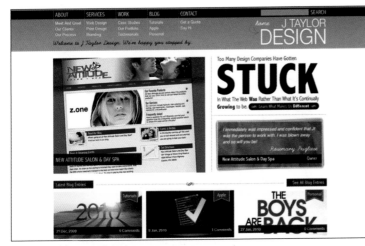

Figure 1-30 An example of asymmetry

Understanding visual web design principles (cont.)

Establish visual unity

Unity holds a page or a website together and makes the site appear and function as a unit rather than as a loose collection of mismatched pieces. You can achieve a sense of unity through the various components of your web design.

Header

Having the same header on every page is a very basic and effective way to establish unity throughout your site.

Fonts

Sticking with a single font family and merely adjusting the type size for headers and body text is the easiest way to establish unity through fonts.

Colours

Use a colour scheme consistently throughout your site.

See Figure 1-31 for an example of all these elements.

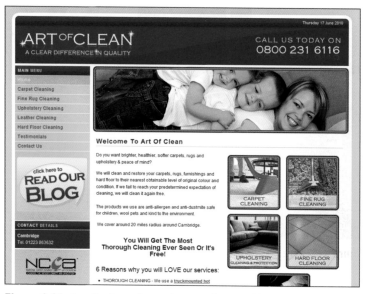

Figure 1-31 An effective colour scheme pulls everything together and sets the right tone

Structure

A consistent structure among pages leaves visitors with a sense that all the pages belong together, while providing a more intuitive interface for navigating the site.

Proximity

Keeping elements close enough so they appear together is key to establishing a unified design. This is particularly true in making sure that headlines are visually connected to the text that follows them.

Repetition

Repeating an object on a page or throughout a site establishes a sense of unity, just as consistency of colours, fonts and structure serves to pull everything together.

Figure 1-32 is a good example of visual unity.

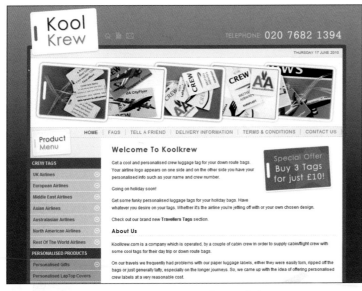

Figure 1-32 Visual unity is very important for a website

Keying in on your audience ▶

Both beauty and usability are in the eye of the beholder. Just because you think your site is well designed with intuitive navigation does not mean it actually achieves those goals. You need to key in on your audience and focus the design on meeting their needs and fulfilling their expectations.

- Remain aware of why visitors are coming to your site and what they expect to find when they arrive.

- Keep in mind that visitors click and skim, and rarely read.

- Realise that visitors have little patience. They are on your site to find something specific, so help them find it as quickly as possible.

- Test your site with real people. If possible, test it while watching the person so that you can observe their behaviour for yourself. Sometimes what people report does not reflect their actual experience.

Important !

Unity is important not only in pulling everything together and providing visitors with a consistent interface to navigate, but also in establishing a baseline from which you can emphasise certain objects. If everything is razzle-dazzle brilliant, visitors will not know where to look first. By setting the stage with consistent elements, you can use emphasis to make certain objects really pop out on a page.

Defining your goal and vision

2

Introduction

The web offers no one-size-fits-all design to serve every site's needs, so the first step in web design is to define the site's purpose and goal. The purpose and goal influence everything else, including the type of site (for example, static website or blog), the type of content (text, photos, video, animation) and the site's features (for example, whether the site requires forms, a discussion forum, live chat or other components).

In this chapter, we show you how to develop a clear purpose for a website, gather existing assets that can help focus the site's content, set measurable goals to define success and choose the right site type to achieve those goals. By the end of this chapter, you should have a clear vision for the site and what you want it to achieve.

What you'll do

Conduct a client survey

Gather existing assets

Set measurable goals

Choose the right site type

Conducting a client survey

▶

1 Business name.

2 Business type.

3 Contact name and title.

4 Contact email address.

5 Contact phone number.

Whether you are designing a site for yourself or a client, start with a client survey, like the one in Figures 2-1-2-4.

Brilliant Web Design

Client Survey

Business name: _____

Business type: _____

Mailing address: _____

Contact name: _____ Title: _____

Contact email address: _____

Contact phone number: _____

Contact name: _____ Title: _____

Contact email address: _____

Contact phone number: _____

Contact name: _____ Title: _____

Contact email address: _____

Contact phone number: _____

Figure 2-1 Client survey: name and contact details

For your information

When choosing a contact, ask for the person who will make the final decision about the site design and contents. Otherwise, you are likely to face an entire new round of changes just when you begin to think the site is complete.

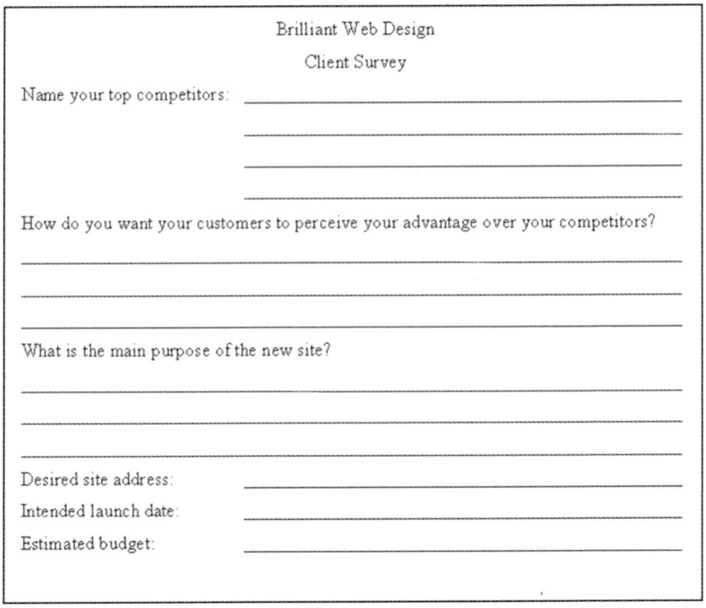

Figure 2-2 Client survey: competitors and purpose

6 Top competitors.

7 Difference from competitors.

8 Site's purpose.

9 Current or desired site address.

10 Intended launch date.

11 Estimated budget.

2

For your information

By recognising the top competitors in a field, you can begin to determine how you want to differentiate yourself from the pack.

Conducting a client survey (cont.)

---

12 Targeted audience demographic.

13 Call to action.

14 Desired tone or emotion.

15 Addresses of interesting and effective sites.

16 Site outline or names of pages and subpages.

17 E-commerce features.

Jargon buster

Call to action: What you want the visitor to do on your site – buy a product, register for a newsletter, obtain information about a particular product, request an appointment and so on.

Brilliant Web Design

Client Survey

Targeted audience demographic

Age: _____

Gender: _____

Occupation: _____

Income: _____

Location: _____

What do you expect/desire visitors to do on your site? For example, look up product information, obtain technical support or customer assistance, place orders, find out more about you or your company, register for something.

_____

_____

_____

What sort of tone do you want your site to convey? For example, fun, exciting, professional, innovative, empathetic?

_____

Please provide addresses of websites you find interesting and effective and describe anything you especially like or dislike about these sites.

_____

_____

_____

Please attach a site outline, if possible, or list the names of the pages or sections you want your site to include:

_____

_____

_____

Will visitors need to be able to purchase products or place orders on your site?

_____

Figure 2-3 Client survey: target audience

Did you know?

Check out competitors' websites, but do not allow them to strongly influence your design. In some industries, all the top players have websites with similar designs and colour schemes. When looking at the competition, think about what you can do to make your site stand out.

Brilliant Web Design

Client Survey

Name any forms that will be required, for example, to register for a newsletter, make a reservation, obtain a quote, or schedule an appointment.

_____

_____

Do you have a logo or other graphics you would like incorporated into the site design?

_____

Do you have a colour scheme that must be incorporated into the site design?

_____

List any interactive media (animations, streaming video or audio) you want to include on the site.

_____

_____

_____

Will you need assistance in developing and editing content?

_____

Will you need assistance in managing the site and updating content or will this be handled in-house?

_____

Figure 2-4 Client survey: a site's contents

For your information

If you lack the artistic talent to develop graphics for the site, consider hiring a graphic artist to develop the logo and other graphic elements for you.

Conducting a client survey (cont.)

18 Forms required.

19 Logo or graphics to include.

20 Established colour scheme.

21 Interactive media (animations, streaming video or audio).

22 Content development.

23 Content updating preferences.

2

Timesaver tip

Develop a comprehensive list of contents to include on the site. Later, you can begin organising the content into pages.

Gathering existing assets ▶

Gather existing assets yourself or, if you are creating a site for a client, ask the client to provide existing assets, such as those shown in Figure 2-5.

1 Content from existing site.

2 Company logo.

3 Product photos.

! Important

Although using existing content can help speed up the process and trim the budget, avoid using second-rate content. Make sure the company logo and photos are of the highest quality.

🕐 Timesaver tip

Web developers rarely start from scratch. They usually have access to some existing content that can help drive the site design and simplify development.

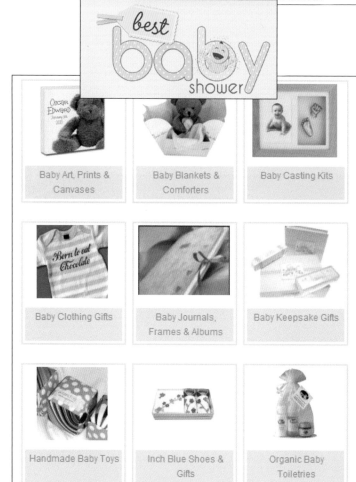

Figure 2-5 Existing assets to be gathered for site compilation

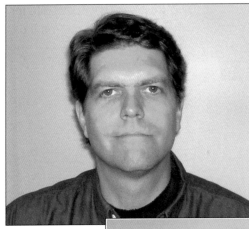

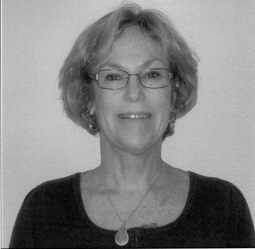

4 Management or personnel photos.

5 Management or personnel biographies.

For your information

If you are developing a site for a company or organisation, encourage them to include photos and biographies for a Who We Are page, as shown in Figure 2.6. People generally like to know who they are doing business with.

Sally Rogers, President, is responsible for the day-to-day management of all corporate activities related to Sallco's operations. Sally also takes credit for assembling the incredibly talented and dedicated team that continues to develop innovative, high-quality products and services and does everything possible to ensure Sallco distributors and customers can tap the full potential of Sallco's collaborative technologies in their organizations. Prior to launching Sallco, Sally served as Senior Marketing Manager for Collaborative Systems International, Safebet Logic, Telltale & Associates, and Bingford Computing, and as Marketing Liaison of Callalink and Lowmain Computers. Sally holds a degree from Cambridge Marketing College and currently serves on the Board of Directors for the Spearhead Community Association. She enjoys golf, tennis, and spending time with her three children and the family dog.

Figure 2-6 Existing assets: photos and biographies

Gathering existing assets (cont.)

6 Brochures and other publications.

7 Video clips.

8 Audio clips.

For your information ⓘ

If you are developing a site for a client and are in charge of developing the content, consider taking on more of a role as editor. The client, who knows the organisation and its customers or clients better than you do, is in a much better position to develop engaging content.

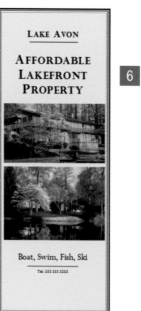

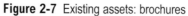

Figure 2-7 Existing assets: brochures

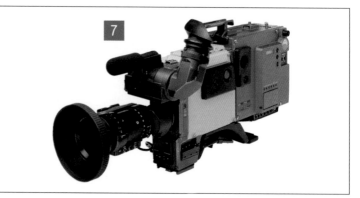

Figure 2-8 Existing assets: video

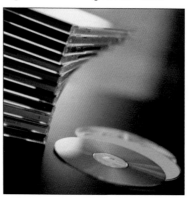

Figure 2-9 Existing assets: audio

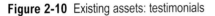

All of ACM's products have been topnotch, as well as affordable.
I had no trouble returning products. ACM provided a full refund that even
covered shipping!
With ACM's instructions and a little help from customer support, I was up
and running in minutes.

9

Figure 2-10 Existing assets: testimonials

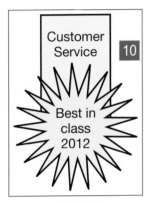

Customer Service **10**

Best in class 2012

Figure 2-11 Existing assets: awards

Gathering existing assets (cont.)

9 Customer testimonials (with permissions).

10 Credentials, certifications, awards.

11 Contact information.

2

! Important

Prior to posting information from or about anyone on the site, including testimonials, obtain written permission to do so. If you edit the content, present the person with the edited version to obtain approval. Never assume something is OK to share.

Setting measurable goals

Common website goals include:

1 Increase site traffic by 50%.

2 Increase sales by 25%.

3 Reduce calls to technical or customer support by 30%.

4 Raise approval rating by 10 points.

A site's purpose is rather vague. It provides some focus for the site, but it is too general to be of use in deciding whether the site is serving its purpose. To get more specific, set realistic, measurable goals, such as the goal for website traffic in Figure 2-12.

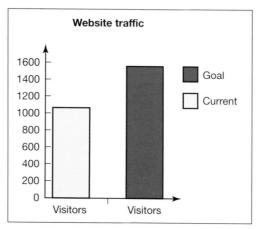

Figure 2-12 Set measurable goals

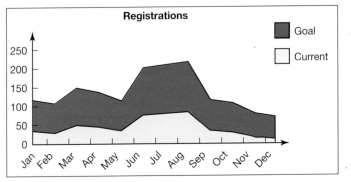

Figure 2-13 Registrations can be another website goal

See also

Website analytics can help you measure site traffic and give you a behind-the-scenes look at what people are doing on your site. See Chapter 13, 'Attracting traffic with search engine optimisation', for details.

5 Generate 40 new leads per month.

6 Register 50 newsletter subscribers per month.

7 Register 10 new affiliates per week (see Figure 2-13).

8 Improve close rate on sales by 15%.

Choosing the right site type

Common website types include:

1. Landing page to highlight a specific product, service or cause, as in Figure 2.14.

2. E-commerce site for selling goods and services and processing orders, as in Figure 2-15.

For your information

Just as a site can have more than one purpose or multiple goals, a site can consist of more than one site type. Many sites, for example, function as both a static website and a blog. Other sites may include a shopping area and an area where customers can obtain technical support.

Back in the old days of web design, almost all sites were static, with the primary goal of providing information to visitors. Now, the web is populated with a wide assortment of sites designed to achieve specific goals. To determine the best site type, examine your site's purpose and goals and find the best match.

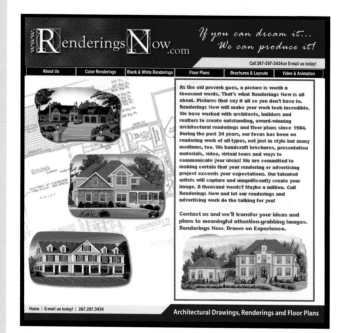

Figure 2-14 Example of a landing page

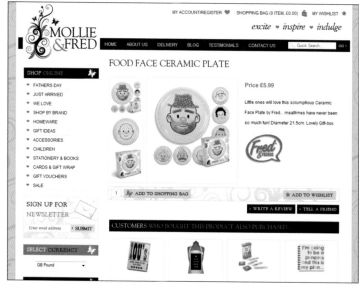

Figure 2-15 Example of an e-commerce site

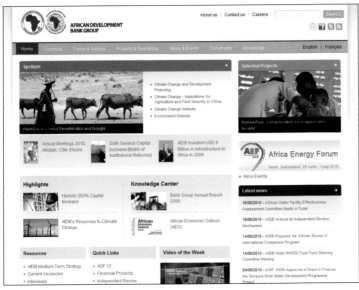

Figure 2-16 Example of a company website

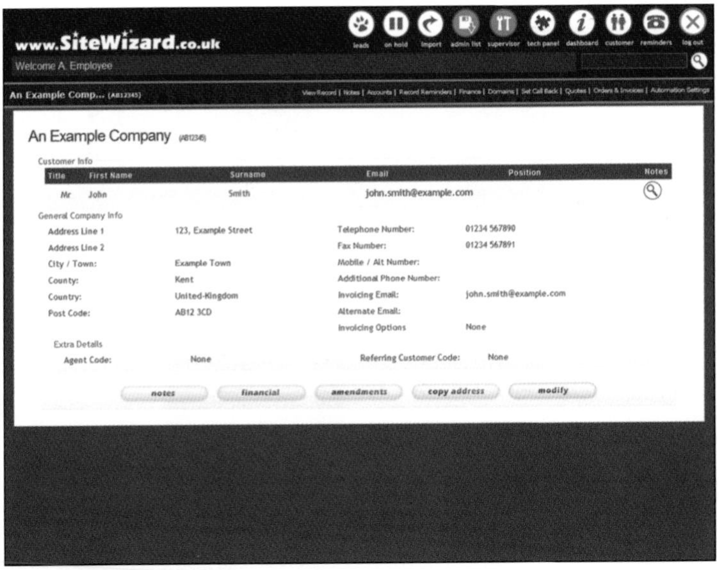

Figure 2-17 Example of an intranet

Choosing the right site type (cont.)

3 Company website for proving information about a company and the goods and services it provides, as in Figure 2-16.

4 Intranet for sharing information, documents and resources, as in Figure 2-17.

For your information

Try to develop a feel for why people will visit the site. Are they looking for information about the organization or an individual or about a product? Are they arriving with a problem they need help with? Getting a feel for the user can often tell you the type of site required.

Choosing the right site type (cont.)

5 Blog to establish thought leadership and engage others in discussions, as in Figure 2-18.

6 Community site for networking, information distribution, and event scheduling, as in Figure 2-19.

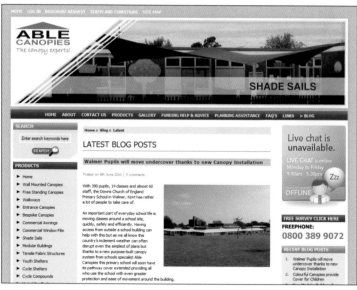

Figure 2-18 Example of a blog

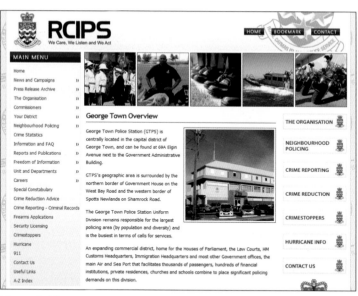

Figure 2-19 Example of a community site

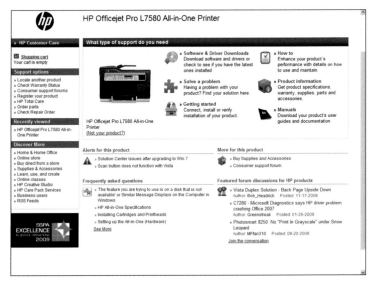

Figure 2-20 Example of a technical support site

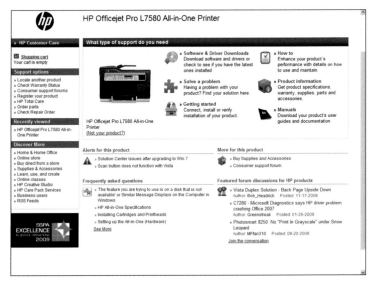

Figure 2-21 Example of a discussion site

7 Customer or technical support site, where people can find answers to their questions, as in Figure 2-20.

8 Discussion site, where people can help one another, as in Figure 2-21.

?

Did you know?

A discussion board has potential benefits and drawbacks. It enables peers to help one another, which can reduce the number of requests you need to address, but you do need to have someone in charge of monitoring the discussions. You may be able to recruit an eager, loyal, knowledgeable and trustworthy customer to do it for you.

Assembling your tools

Introduction

All web designers have a set of favourite tools for designing, creating, managing and troubleshooting the sites they create. These tools help designers create better sites more efficiently than if they had to code everything by hand. Eventually, you will assemble your own preferred gear. Until then, consider using some of the tools we recommend in this chapter, many of which are free.

Here, we provide suggestions on all the tools you need to design your site, create individual pages, manage the content, develop an attractive colour scheme, add multimedia components, generate forms and test your site to ensure it looks and functions properly in various web browsers.

What you'll do

Choose a blogging platform for site design

Choose a content management system (CMS)

Customise a blog or CMS design with templates

Accessorise a blog or CMS with plugins

Choose a web page authoring program

Choose a graphics program

Choose a multimedia development tools

Obtain an FTP program

Explore more web design tools

Choosing a blogging platform for site design ▶

Whether you are designing a static website or a dynamic blog, you can use a blogging platform as the core tool in designing, creating and managing the site. WordPress is a great choice. Due to its popularity, you can find plenty of predesigned templates, plugins and online support for creating a great site, and you can choose to include or omit a blogging component.

Checking out WordPress

1 Log in to manage your site online (Figure 3-1).

2 From the dashboard (Figure 3-2), you can manage all aspects of your site.

3 Create pages.

4 Create posts.

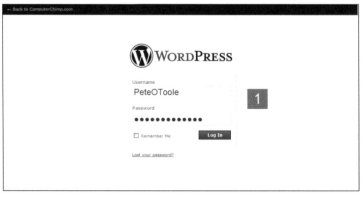

Figure 3-1 Log in with user name and password

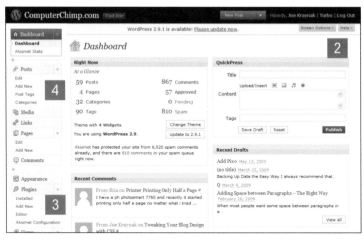
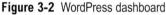

Figure 3-2 WordPress dashboard

Jargon buster 💡

Page: A static web page apart from the blog.
Blog posts: Entries listed on one page of the blog (usually the home page) in reverse chronological order – newest post first.

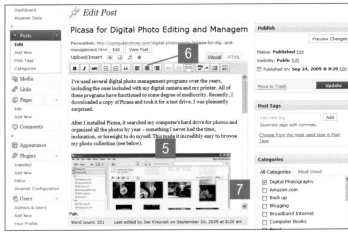

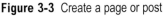

Figure 3-3 Create a page or post

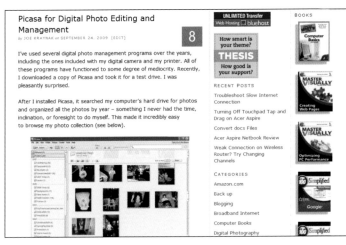

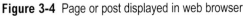

Figure 3-4 Page or post displayed in web browser

For your information

Another great blogging platform is TypePad. For a free trial, visit *www.typepad.com*.

Choosing a blogging platform for site design (cont.)

5 Insert content (Figure 3-3).

6 Format text.

7 Insert images.

8 The blogging platform displays the formatted content (Figure 3-4).

For your information

You can try WordPress for free and you do not even need to sign up for a hosting service. Go to WordPress.org and register for a free WordPress blog.

See also

You can customise the design by choosing a different template and editing the template's styles. See 'Customising a blog or CMS design with templates', later in thiis chapter.

Choosing a content management system

Checking out Joomla!

1. Log in to manage your site online (Figure 3-5).

2. From the control panel, you can manage all aspects of your site (Figure 3-6).

3. Assign the site a name via Global Configuration (Figure 3-7).

For your information

Joomla! is a powerful website creation and management tool that would require an entire book of its own to cover in detail. To get started, check out the *Absolute Beginner's Guide to Joomla!* at *docs. joomla.org/Beginners*.

A CMS is very similar to a blogging platform but is typically more powerful and complex and hence more difficult to learn. One of the more popular CMSs is Joomla!.

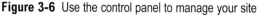

Figure 3-5 Log in to Joomla!

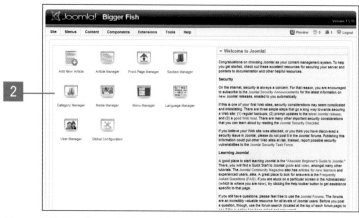

Figure 3-6 Use the control panel to manage your site

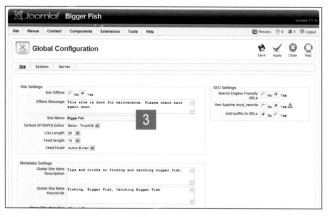

Figure 3-7 Use Global Configuration to assign the site a name

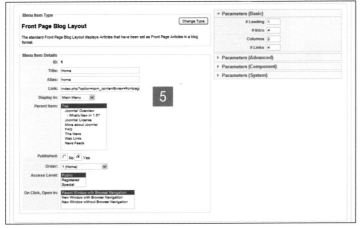

Figure 3-8 Add articles

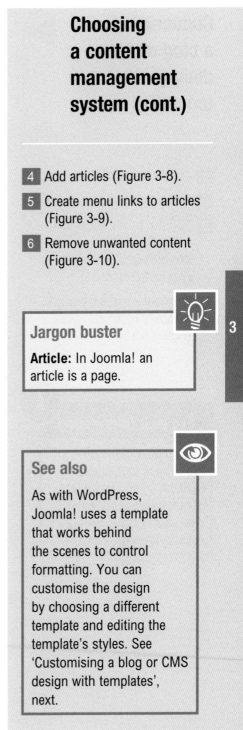

Figure 3-9 You can create links to articles

Figure 3-10 Get rid of unwanted content

4 Add articles (Figure 3-8).

5 Create menu links to articles (Figure 3-9).

6 Remove unwanted content (Figure 3-10).

Jargon buster

Article: In Joomla! an article is a page.

See also

As with WordPress, Joomla! uses a template that works behind the scenes to control formatting. You can customise the design by choosing a different template and editing the template's styles. See 'Customising a blog or CMS design with templates', next.

Customising a blog or CMS design with templates

What's cool about blogs and CMS is that the content and design remain separate. CSS stylesheets work behind the scenes to control the structure and formatting of each page. Because of this, you can completely alter a site's design at any time, simply by choosing a different template or tweaking the template's stylesheet.

1 Access the templates screen.

2 Select the desired template.

3 You can install additional templates from the WordPress dashboard (Figure 3-11).

4 The new template changes the site's look and layout (Figure 3-12).

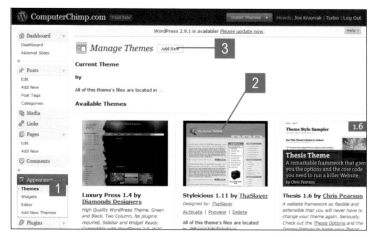
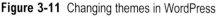

Figure 3-11 Changing themes in WordPress

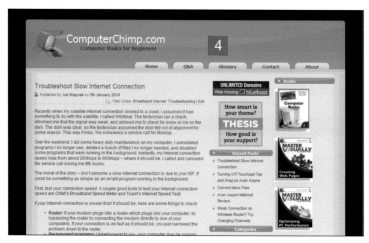

Figure 3-12 New theme applied to site

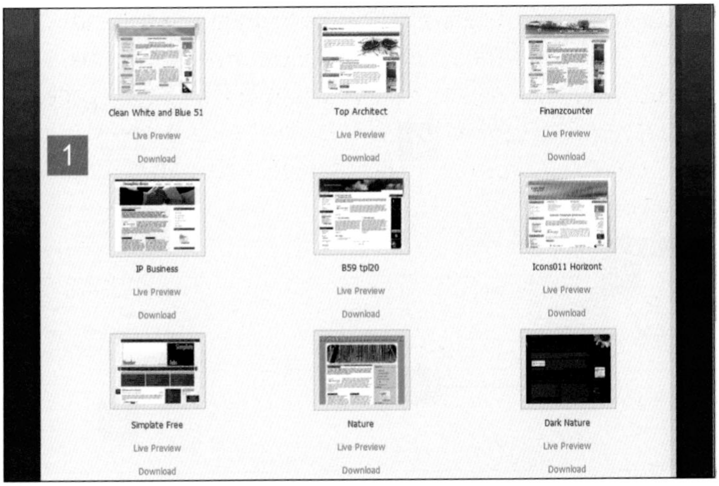

Figure 3-13 There are plenty of Joomla! templates to choose from

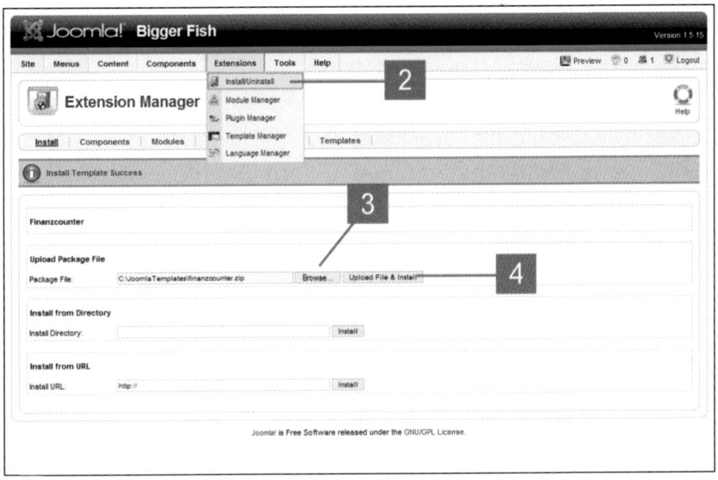

Figure 3-14 Install a Joomla! template

Customising a blog or CMS design with templates (cont.)

Installing a Joomla! template

1. Search the web for Joomla! templates and download one you like. See Figure 3-13.
2. From the Joomla! control panel, click Extensions, Install/Uninstall (Figure 3-14).
3. Browse for the Joomla template file you downloaded.
4. Click Upload File & Install.

3

Customising a blog or CMS design with templates (cont.)

Editing a theme

1. Access the screen for editing themes (Figure 3-15).
2. Choose the stylesheet you want to edit.
3. Make the desired changes.
4. Save your changes.

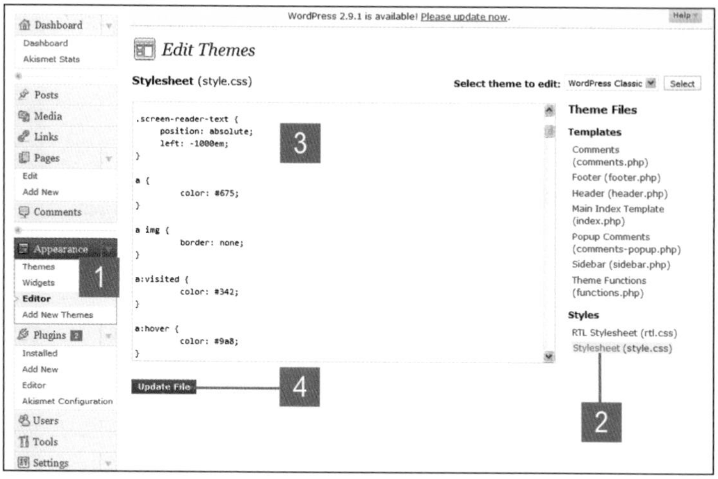

Figure 3-15 Edit a theme to customise the design

For your information

For details about editing HTML or CSS, check out *Brilliant HTML & CSS* by James A. Brannan (Prentice Hall, 2009).

Did you know?

Prior to editing a file, copy and save its contents to your computer so that you can restore the original if problems occur.

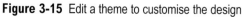

Every blogging platform and CMS has all the features and tools required to design, build and manage a site, but you can add even more with plugins. See Figure 3-16.

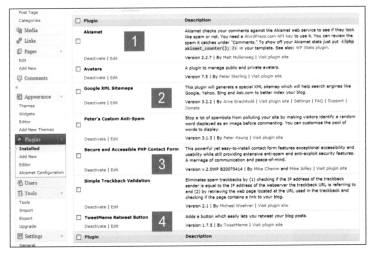

Figure 3-16 Sample plugins

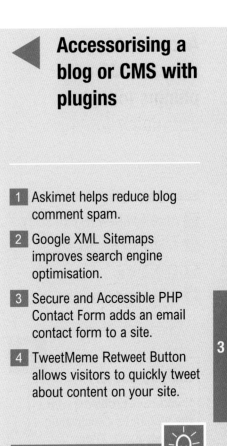

Accessorising a blog or CMS with plugins

1 Askimet helps reduce blog comment spam.

2 Google XML Sitemaps improves search engine optimisation.

3 Secure and Accessible PHP Contact Form adds an email contact form to a site.

4 TweetMeme Retweet Button allows visitors to quickly tweet about content on your site.

Jargon buster

Plugin: A component that adds a feature or capability to a software package.

Accessorising a blog or CMS with plugins (cont.)

Installing plugins in WordPress

1 Click Add New (Figure 3-17).

2 Search for the plugin.

3 Click Install.

4 Click Install Now.

?

Did you know?

If you have problems with the plugin, try deactivating and deleting it. Then, reinstall it manually by downloading the plugin to your computer and then uploading it to your blog's wp-content/plugins directory. You can then activate it from the dashboard.

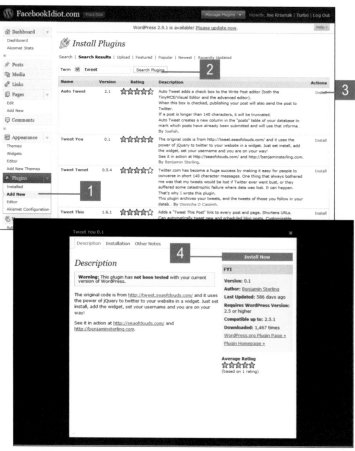

Figure 3-17 Installing plugins in WordPress

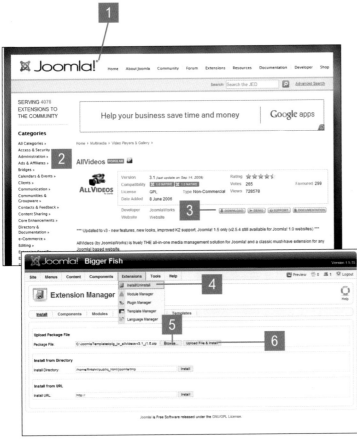

Figure 3-18 Installing extensions in Joomla!

Installing extensions in Joomla!

1. Go to extensions.joomla.com – see Figure 3-18.

2. Browse or search the categories for the extension you want to use.

3. Download the extension to your computer.

4. From the Joomla! control panel, click Extensions, Install/ Uninstall.

5. Browse for the Joomla! plugin file you downloaded.

6. Click Upload File & Install.

Choosing a web page authoring program

With a web page authoring program, you create pages locally (on your computer) and then upload them to the web server. You can choose between two types of web page authoring programs: professional strength (easier) or more basic (for coding by hand).

1 WYSIWYG interface makes formatting as easy as in a word-processing application. See Figure 3-19.

2 Click a tab to view the source.

For your information

Several professional-strength web page authoring programs are available, including Dreamweaver, Microsoft Expressions and Nvu. We recommend KompoZer (*http://kompozer.net*), a free program based on Nvu that's a simple but powerful alternative to Dreamweaver.

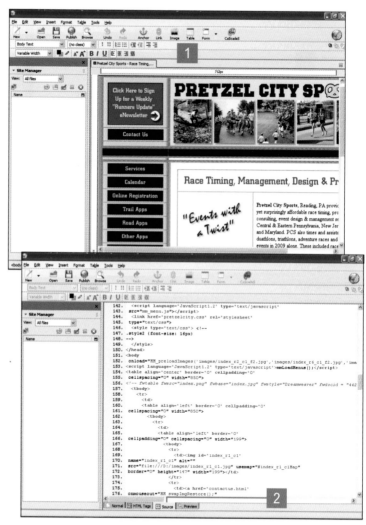

Figure 3-19 Professional website builder

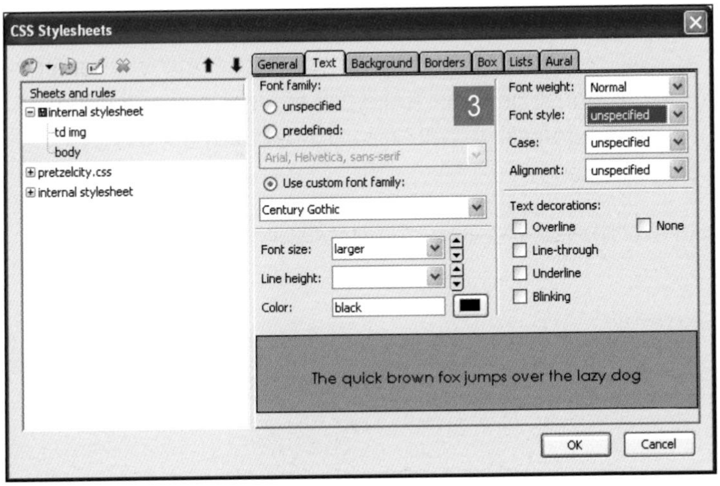

Figure 3-20 Creating CSS rules

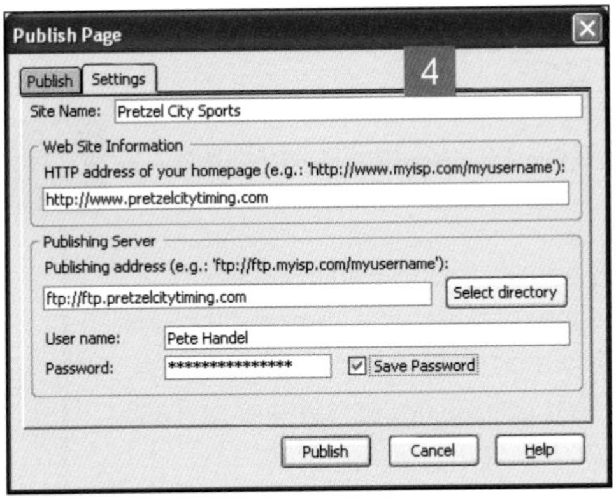

Figure 3-21 Publishing pages

Choosing a web page authoring program (cont.)

3 You can create CSS rules for specific objects. See Figure 3-20.

4 You can publish pages by uploading them to your hosting service via FTP. See Figure 3-21.

See also

For more about uploading with FTP, see 'Obtaining an FTP program', later in this chapter.

3

Choosing a web page authoring program (cont.)

HTML/CSS editor

1. A basic HTML/CSS editor, as in Figure 3-22, is strictly for working on individual pages.
2. You edit everything manually – no WYSIWYG.

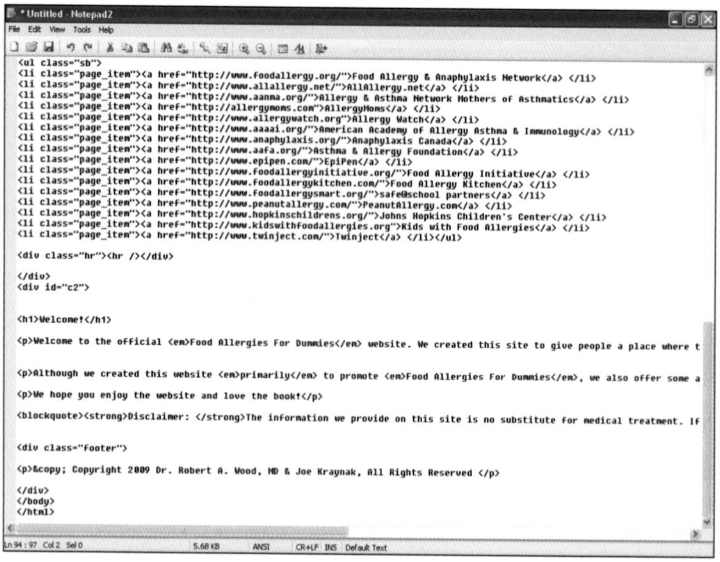

Figure 3-22 Editing individual pages in HTML

For your information

Many HTML editors number the lines of code, colour codes syntax and check for coding errors.

Timesaver tip

You can use any text editor, including Notepad, to edit HTML and CSS files, but better programs include Notepad2 (*http://sourceforge.net/projects/notepad2*), a souped-up Notepad that colour codes syntax, or Taco HTML editor (*http://tacosw.com*) for the Mac.

Jargon buster

CSS: Allows you to create rules to control the formatting of specific objects, including headings, text and images. By editing a CSS rule, you change the formatting of all objects tagged to follow that rule.

Most sites include graphics – digital photographs, graphic headers or banners, background images, lines, buttons and so forth. Even if you do not create the graphics yourself, you should have a program that enables you to improve the quality of images and adjust their size. See Figure 3-23.

Required features:

- resize graphics
- crop images
- adjust brightness and contrast
- convert to jpg, gif or png format.

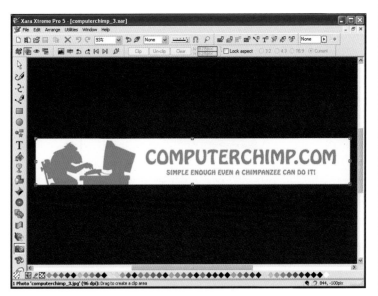

Figure 3-23 It's all in the graphics

◀ **Choosing a graphics program**

ⓘ

For your information

Almost all graphics programs include the basic features listed here and require little or no artistic talent. If you're artistic and want to create images from scratch, choose a higher-end product.

3

Choosing a graphics program (cont.)

Graphics programs

1. Adobe Photoshop (*www.adobe.com*) is the choice for professional graphic artists and designers. See Figure 3-24.

2. Xara (*www.xara.com*) offers a selection of excellent graphics programs for your needs and budget. See Figure 3-25.

3. CorelDraw Graphics Suite (*www.corel.com*) includes drawing and photo editing features. See Figure 3-26.

For your information

Visit the sites for free trial versions of the various products and take each of them for a test drive before purchasing one.

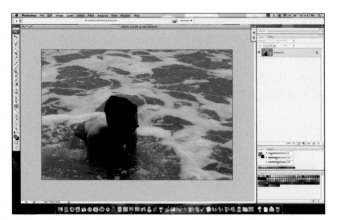

Figure 3-24 Adobe Photoshop

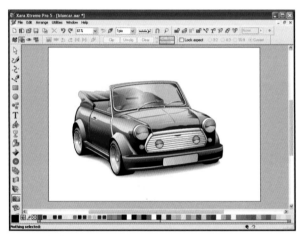

Figure 3-25 Xara

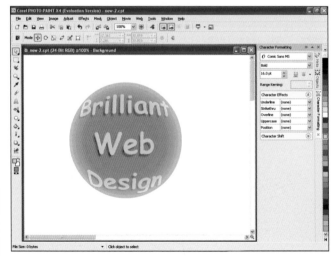

Figure 3-26 Corel

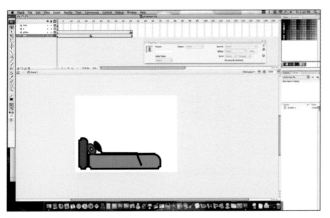

Figure 3-27 Adobe Flash

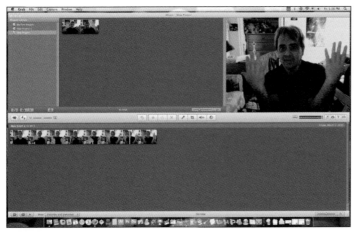

Figure 3-28 Apple QuickTime

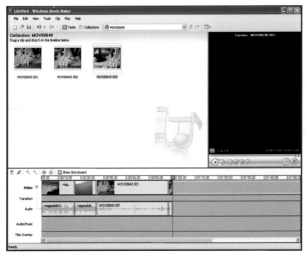

Figure 3-29 Windows Movie Maker

◀ **Choosing multimedia development tools**

If you plan on enhancing your site with audio, video and animation, gather some additional tools.

1 Adobe Flash (*www.adobe.com*) enables you to add sound, animation and interactive effects to web pages as small Flash files. See Figure 3-27.

2 Apple QuickTime (*www.apple. com/quicktime*) and iMovie (*www.apple.com/imovie*) are excellent for editing audio and video and exporting them for web applications. See Figure 3-28.

3 Windows Movie Maker (included with XP, Vista and Windows 7) is an affordable tool for editing and sharing video. See Figure 3-29.

3

ⓘ

For your information

Adobe Flash enables you to create interactive animations that load quickly and play right inside the browser window. Adobe Shockwave is for more complex multimedia applications that exceed a browser's capability.

Obtaining an FTP program

An FTP program enables you to upload files directly to your hosting service's web server. Most hosting services provide an FTP program that you can access after you log in, but having a program that runs on your computer is usually faster and more convenient.

Recommended FTP programs:

1. FireFTP (*http://fireftp.mozdev.org*) is a free plugin for the Firefox web browser. See Figure 3-30.

2. FileZilla (*http://filezilla-project.org*) is another free, easy-to-use FTP program. See Figure 3-31.

3. Fetch (*http://fetchsoftworks.com*) is an excellent FTP program for the Mac. See Figure 3-32.

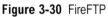

Jargon buster

FTP: Stands for *file transfer protocol* – the language used to transfer files between two computers over the internet.

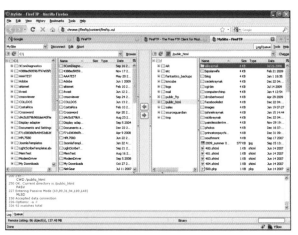

Figure 3-30 FireFTP

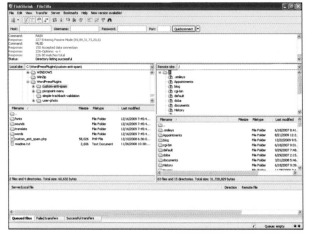

Figure 3-31 FileZilla

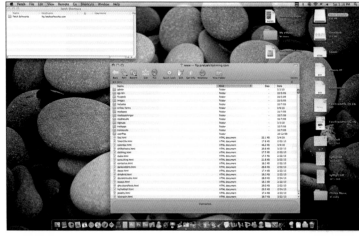

Figure 3-32 Fetch

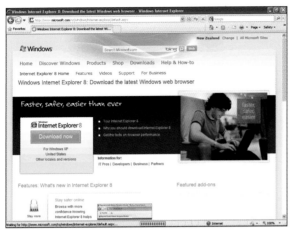

Figure 3-33 Internet Explorer

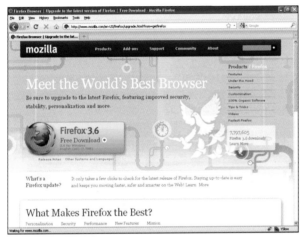

Figure 3-34 Firefox

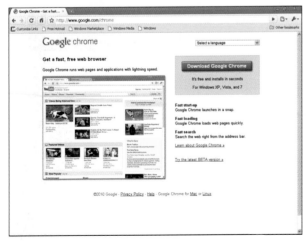

Figure 3-35 Google Chrome

In addition to the standard web design tools, consider adding some tools to your collection to help with testing, troubleshooting and enhancing your site. Most of these recommended tools are free.

Recommended web browsers

1. Microsoft Internet Explorer (*www.microsoft.com/ windows/ie*) – Figure 3-33.

2. Firefox (*www.firefox.com*) – Figure 3.34.

3. Google Chrome (*www.google. com/chrome*) – Figure 3-35.

3

Timesaver tip

Internet Explorer and Firefox account for over 80% of the market, so at least test your site using the most current versions of those two browsers. Google Chrome has a respectable following.

Exploring more web design tools (cont.)

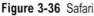

4 Safari (*www.apple.com/safari*) – Figure 3-36.

5 Opera (*www.opera.com*) – Figure 3-37.

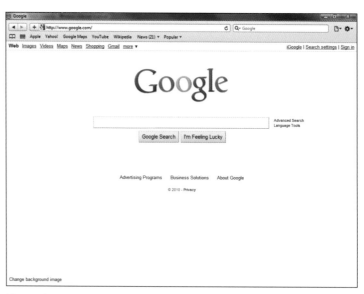

Figure 3-36 Safari

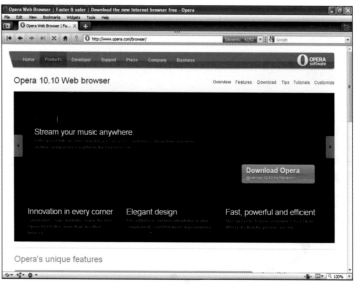

Figure 3-37 Opera

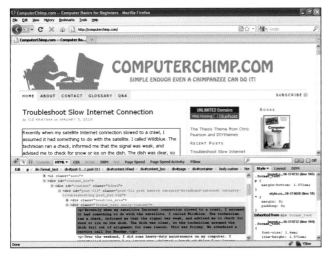

Figure 3-38 Firebug for troubleshooting CMS and HTML

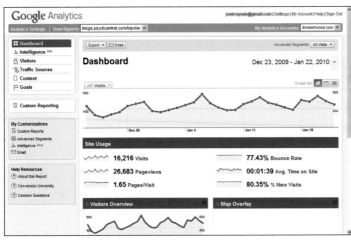

Figure 3-39 BannerFans for designing attractive banners

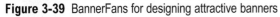

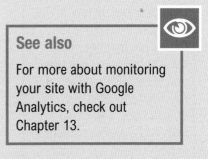

Figure 3-40 Google Analytics for tracking site traffic

Exploring more web design tools (cont.)

Recommended tools

1 Firebug (*htpp://getfirebug.com*) is a Mozilla Firefox plugin for inspecting CSS and HTML and troubleshooting a site – see Figure 3-38.

2 BannerFans (*http://bannerfans. com*) is a free online tool for designing attractive graphic headers – see Figure 3-39.

3 Google Analytics (*www.google. com/analytics*) is a powerful tool for monitoring site traffic – Figure 3-40.

See also

For more about monitoring your site with Google Analytics, check out Chapter 13.

Exploring more web design tools (cont.)

4 ColorSchemer (*www. colorschemer.com*) is a great tool for identifying complementary colour combinations for a site – Figure 3-41.

5 phpFormGenerator (*www. phpformgen.sourceforge.net*) is a great tool for building forms to collect data – Figure 3-42.

For your information

ColorSchemer is one of the few tools we recommend that is not free but, if you need help finding colours that work well together, it is indispensable. As shown here, it can also help you develop a colour scheme using the colours from an existing photo or illustration.

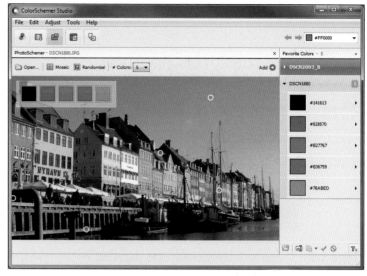

Figure 3-41 ColorSchema

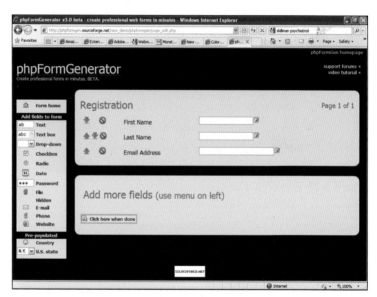

Figure 3-42 phpFormGenerator

Designing your website structure and layout

Introduction

A website must be based on a design. Many sites are just a collection of web pages tied together by the fact that any of them can be reached from the menu system. That's fine; perhaps that's all that is needed. There are some sites that have pages that a person viewing the site cannot access at all – that's bad practice. To be precise, these particular pages may show up in searches on Google, for instance, but from the menu of a site the visitor might not know how to get there or perhaps even that they exist.

Website design follows two paths: the organisation of the content and the layout (and connectivity) of the pages. Each of these areas requires a certain approach. Content is king. That phrase is used too often, but nonetheless it's vital to a website. People come to a site to read about something, learn something, see something, even hear something – all forms of content. So thinking of your site's content should stay a priority. The structure of the site is meant to support the content.

The structure of the site is the physical layout of the pages and, of course, the layout of any single page. There are a number of elements that in nearly all cases should appear on every page: the navigation facility, the footer, the logo or other identifier of the site and so on.

What you'll do

Explore content structure

Explore page and site structure

Learn about link strategy

Learn about wireframing

Explore different layouts

Consider white space vs. a heavy design

Use website templates

Content

What is your site meant to show? What information should it provide to visitors? What type of visitors is important – the general public, potential clients or some other segment? These questions are meant to direct your planning of the content on the site.

For example, if you are trying to sell the latest and greatest gadget for the kitchen, then your content should mention the gadget, of course, but also have some keywords in it, such as kitchen, cooking, food preparation or whatever makes sense. When it gets down to keywords we enter the world of search engine optimisation (SEO). That's a field unto itself. SEO practices are meant to get your web pages high up on searches.

Here we suggest thinking of the organisation of your content. Organised and accessible content helps in SEO, with the aim being how to help visitors navigate through your site to get to the information they seek.

Plan how your content should be accessed. Figure 4-1 shows a simple schematic for a website that offers information on its products.

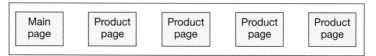

Figure 4-1 A simple product information site

Often there is an abundance of content and a more complex scheme is necessary to present it. Figure 4-2 shows a content layout with content that is categorised. This is a common configuration for content on a website.

On any website the menu or navigation system should be available on every page. This is especially helpful on a busy site such as the one shown in Figure 4-2.

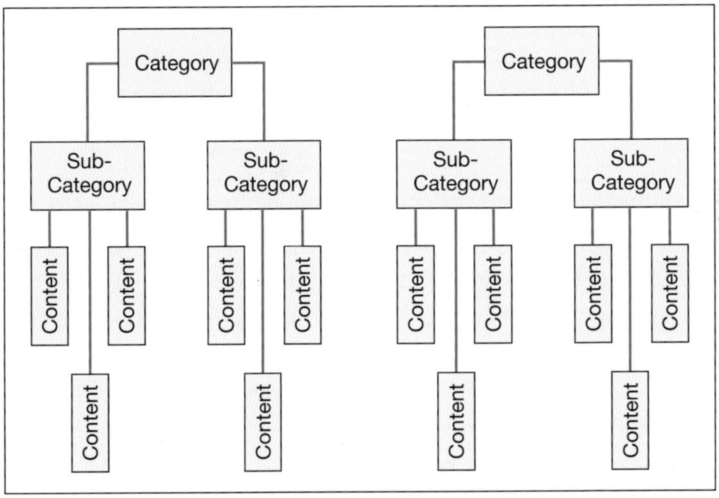

```
         Category                    Category

Sub-        Sub-           Sub-          Sub-
Category    Category       Category      Category

Content Content  Content Content  Content Content  Content Content

Content       Content         Content        Content
```

Figure 4-2 Content organisation based on categories

A great deal of content on the internet is presented as articles. Articles come in different lengths, of course. So although an article can be on one long page, it can be broken up into a succession of pages, as shown in Figure 4-3. If you use this method, make sure that all the article pages are linked to each other.

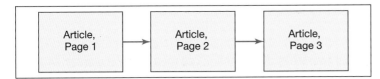

Figure 4-3 Breaking up an article to appear on successive pages

For your information

Categorising information is a great way to help people navigate through your website. By having links based on categories, a visitor is immediately taken to subsets of content of interest.

Did you know?

There is another reason for breaking an article onto successive pages. This provides more page views of the site and also more ways for a person to get into the site via search engines.

4

Website structure

The structure of your site must be planned out before putting the site together. The structure is designed to complement the design and types of content. Every website has a main page – the page that appears when the URL is entered into a browser address bar. Past that are any number of pages. True, there are single-page sites, but then there are sites with thousands of pages. Managing this type of structure is key to a successful site.

Traditionally, landing pages, although just web pages, were specialised typically by outside influences such as advertising having a 'call to action' to visit that particular page and sign up, order something, etc. That still holds, but it is best to think of any page on your site as a landing page since a person may 'land' on your site from any available page. Figure 4-4 shows this methodology.

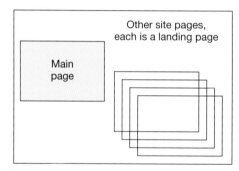

Figure 4-4 Any page is an entry point into your site

Many sites have areas that are restricted from the public. The typical two areas of restriction are members-only areas and an area reserved for the administrators of the site. These areas are password protected. If a person not yet logged in should enter a page in a restricted area, code in the page will redirect them to a login page. Only after a successful login will the person be allowed to go where there login level allows them to. Figure 4-5 shows an example of this type of website structure.

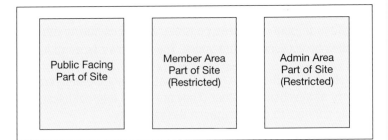

Figure 4-5 Public and restricted sections of a website

In addition to the visible web pages may be external files that are referenced into the web pages. These typically are CSS and JavaScript files. Although both CSS and JavaScript can be written directly into a web page, it is often advantageous to reference external files so that they can be used from multiple pages. Figure 4-6 shows how this is set up. The external files are referenced.

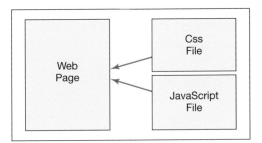

Figure 4-6 External CSS and JavaScript files are referenced

4

Link strategy

Links (also known as hyperlinks) are the key to making navigation through a website possible, as well as having other websites be accessible from yours. There are two types of links:

1. Internal links: these are the links that connect the different parts of a website together. They are called internal because they connect to other pages in the same site.

2. External links: these are links that lead from your site to other sites. Thinking this through it comes to mind that a link that leads from your website to another is providing the other website with another way for people to access that site. Linking across sites is a popular practice and is an important part of an SEO strategy.

Links can be textual or graphic. In either event they are created using the HTML anchor tag (<a). Inside the opening and closing anchor tags is text for a textual link. When a graphic is used, the image tag (<img) is set within the anchor tag. Figure 4-7 shows a page with textual and graphic links. Clicking on a graphic will lead to another page in the site in the same manner that clicking on the text will.

The HTML code for the link types is:

```
Text: <a href="animals.html">Animals</a>
Graphic: <a href="animals.html"><img
src="images/animals/babyleppy.jpg"
alt="animals"></a>
```

Either of the above links leads to the animals.html page.

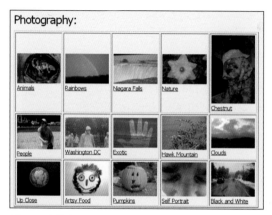

Figure 4-7 Textual and graphic links

Wireframing occurs on the page level. It is the act of designing the basic blocks of a page. A wireframe is not a completed page – it shows where page elements should go. Wireframing is usually the first step in designing a page.

A wireframe can be just a handful of placed boxes or may show a bit more detail. As you work on a wireframe you may have versions, each a bit more defined than the last. The next three figures show the progression of a wireframe in designing the main page of a website.

Figure 4-8 is a basic wireframe. In fact, it's a bit more than a basic wireframe since some colour was added. A true basic wireframe would not contain colour. This wireframe includes colour to help the areas stand out a bit better.

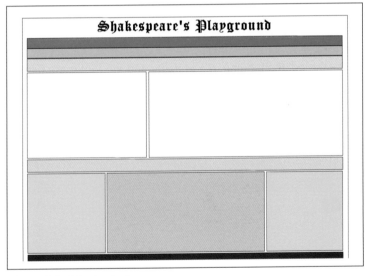

Figure 4-8 A basic wireframe

The boxes in a wireframe are placeholders for the different elements on a page. Continuing with this wireframe, the purpose of each boxed area is indicated, here in Figure 4-9.

Wireframing (cont.)

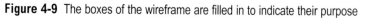

Figure 4-9 The boxes of the wireframe are filled in to indicate their purpose

In Figure 4-9, sections such as the tag line area, the menu, the main section and the footer are shown. The wireframe shown in Figure 4-10 is more filled in than a wireframe typically would be. Graphics, the tag line, menu items and the footer are filled in. At this stage, the wireframe is enhanced to the point of being the start of the page design – with elements actually filled in.

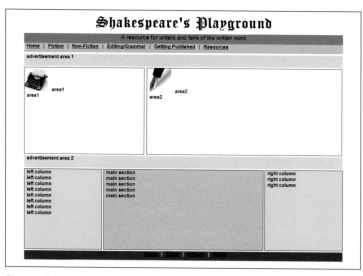

Figure 4-10 The page evolves past the wireframe stage

So what should your website look like? The structure must support the content, but aside from that there is much freedom on the design. A common classification of websites is how many columns they occupy. Even within a page a variety of columnar applications can be applied. This is easy to see in Figure 4-10 where the page being designed has two columns in the upper section, followed by an area of three columns.

Figure 4-11 shows a striking web page made from two columns. The columns clearly do not have to be even. In fact, it is good practice to apply a rough ratio of 1/3 to 2/3. This means one of the two columns takes up one-third of the available space.

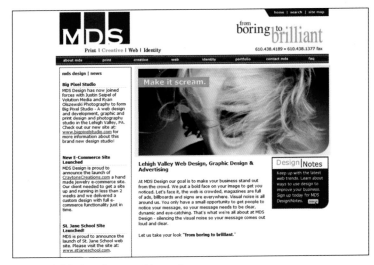

Figure 4-11 A web page of two columns

Layouts (cont.)

Figure 4-12 show a web page that does not distinctly break the page into four columns. However, the columnar effect of the graphics gives the appearance of it being a four-column page.

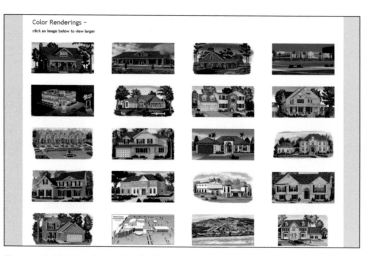

Figure 4-12 Graphics give the four-column appearance

Design is art. There is no exact set of rules to follow except to bear in mind generally accepted design methods. That said, the purpose of the site will surely drive the type of design to use.

Figures 4-13 and 4-14 show a striking difference in approach. Figure 4-13 shows a deep contrast between the coloured boxes and the black background. This conveys a feeling of excitement.

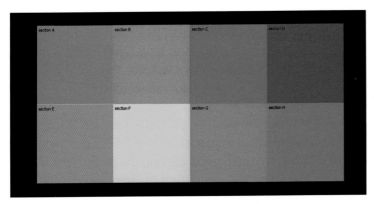

Figure 4-13 Coloured boxes on a black background

The targeted audience behind the site in Figure 4-14 is an older crowd. It's a site where life stories can be entered and shared. As such the approach is of a gentler nature – easy on the eyes and the depth of information on a page. It is a sparse site, designed that way for its purpose and audience.

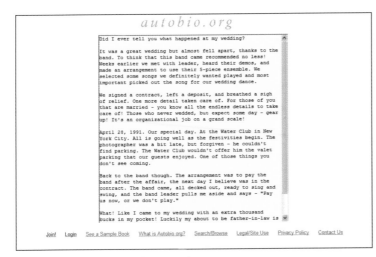

Figure 4-14 An easy-on-the-eyes site

Using website templates

Many predesigned templates are available for free or at a reasonable cost. Searching the internet with a phrase such as 'free web templates' will turn up search results leading to many sites. These templates are designed by artists and come with, typically, a main page, a CSS file and some images. Besides being ready-to-go templates, reviewing the HTML and CSS is a good exercise to become familiar with how these interesting templates are created.

There is often some licensing structure when you use these templates. The common thing is to leave a link on the bottom of the page back to the designer's website. Past that the idea is to alter the template to match your requirements.

Website templates are available that are structured to work with popular CMS platforms such as WordPress and Joomla!. Visiting *http://wordpress.org* and clicking the Extend link and then Themes showcases dozens of templates you can download and use.

Adding colour

Introduction

Some of the biggest decisions you make when designing a website relate to the colour scheme. In addition to making everything on the site appear attractive and readable, colours provide a way to give your site personality and possibly evoke certain emotions from your audience.

Selecting the wrong colours can make text difficult to read, immediately drive visitors from your site and perhaps send the wrong message, on an emotional level, about what your site is all about. Choosing the right colours can make visitors feel more at home, make your site appear more attractive and make content more accessible.

In this chapter, you will learn about colours in theory and in practice, so you can choose a suitable colour scheme and implement it on your site.

What you'll do

Consider colour associations

Mix primary colours

Identify complementary colours

Create neutral colours

Identify analogous colours

Alter colour with saturation

Change colour values

Cheat with an existing colour scheme

Design a colour scheme

Translate colours into codes

Considering colour associations

Jargon buster

Colour association: The emotional, psychological or cultural connection a person has with different colours.

Important

Colour associations are not the sole factor in choosing website colours. You may develop a colour scheme around an existing logo or graphics you want to use on your site, or a style that helps brand your product. Consider colour associations, but do not make them the sole determining factor in choosing colours for your site.

Colour is an excellent tool for adding personality to your site, evoking an emotional response from visitors and communicating certain themes without the use of words.

When choosing colours for your site, understanding how colours function and the effects they tend to have on people viewing your site can help you make better choices.

Colour associations

Colour associations enable you to use colour to express or evoke certain emotions. In Western cultures, for example, red tends to be associated with love and passion, while blue sets a more peaceful and soothing tone. Be aware of these associations when you begin developing a colour scheme for your site.

Black: depending on the context in which it is used, black can set a tone of mystery, death and evil, or class, elegance, high quality and truth (when juxtaposed with white, see Figure 5-1).

White: this typically represents purity, light and perfection, but it can also be used simply as a background, in which case it is a fairly neutral colour, void of emotion.

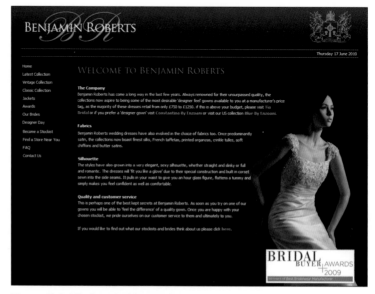

Figure 5-1 Black and white used to convey elegance and purity

Red: bright and deep reds are hot, fast, lusty, sensual and elegant. Because blood is red, this colour can also be used to set a tone of fear or courage (in a patriotic way).

Orange: bright, sunny and citrus-y, orange tends to evoke a sense of fun. It is a great colour for sites designed for children. Orange is also commonly used in coupons, ads and price tags to convey a sense of value or mark merchandise as a good deal.

Yellow: this is one step up from orange as a bright, sunny, fun colour. Due to its almost universal association with the sun, it tends to lift people's spirits and make them feel warm and happy. Consider Figure 5-2.

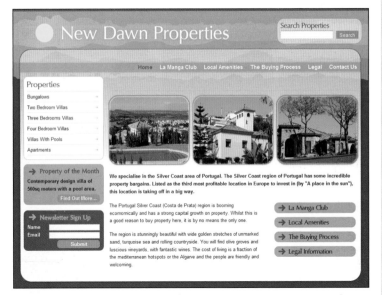

Figure 5-2 Red, orange and/or yellow convey warmth

For your information

Different shades of colour can convey different emotions. While deep reds may express love, passion or even anger, brownish, earthy reds can be much more soothing and even used as traditional autumn colours.

5

Considering colour associations (cont.)

See also

You can combine different colours for contrast, special effects, and even to evoke more than one emotion. See 'Designing a colour scheme', later in this chapter, to explore options for combining colours.

Green: this is the colour of grass, foliage and all things nature. Spring green symbolises hope, rebirth and growth. However, green can also symbolise money or wealth, sickness (as when someone turns a pale green) or envy (as in 'green with envy').

Blue: with respect to emotions, blue is the flip side of red. While red is hot, blue is cool and soothing, although it can also be a bit on the depressing side (as when somebody is 'feeling blue'). Blue also evokes a sense of trustworthiness and security – consider Figure 5-3. A blue sky background can convey a sense of hope and freedom.

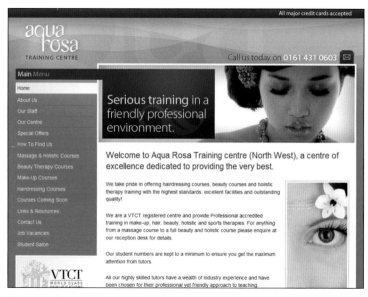

Figure 5-3 Blue is cool and soothing

Purple: purple, especially deep purple, traditionally has conveyed a sense of royalty and richness. However, context can significantly alter the emotions this colour conveys. In certain contexts, purple is associated with courage (the Purple Heart). Brighter shades of purple suggest fun.

Going hot or cold with colour temperatures

One of the primary associations of certain colours is related to temperature – cool and warm.

Cool colours: these are in the spectrum from green to blue to some darker shades of purple. They feel cooler because they remind people of fresh green forests, cool blue skies, oceans and ice. These colours tend to have a calming influence in terms of both emotion and design. See Figure 5-4.

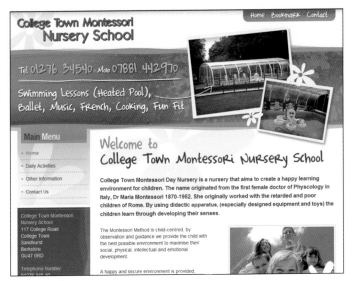

Figure 5-4 Cool colours produce a calming effect

5

Considering colour associations (cont.)

Warm colours: these colours are in the spectrum from violet to red (hot) to orange, yellow and even neon green. They also contain browns, pinks and burgundy. They feel warmer because they remind people of fire, sun, heat and speed. See Figure 5-5.

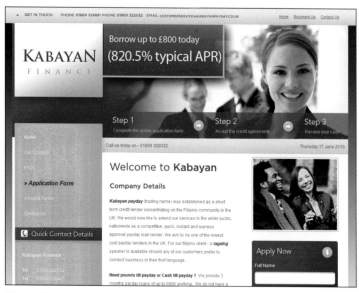

Figure 5-5 Warm colours can be used to heat things up

RGB (red, green, blue)

In web design, you use the RGB colour model, *an additive colour model*, because web pages are displayed onscreen. With RGB, the three primary colours are mixed in different proportions to create all available colours, including yellow, cyan and magenta, as shown in Figure 5-6.

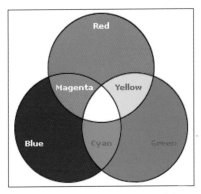

Figure 5-6 The RGB colour model

◀ **Mixing primary colours**

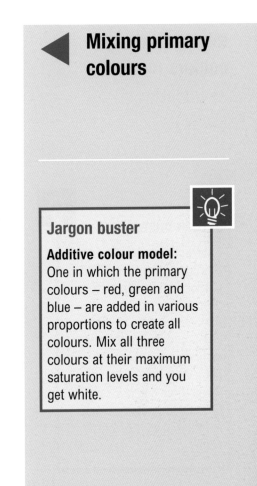

Jargon buster

Additive colour model: One in which the primary colours – red, green and blue – are added in various proportions to create all colours. Mix all three colours at their maximum saturation levels and you get white.

5

Mixing primary colours (cont.)

Jargon buster

Subtractive colour model: Starts with white and adds primary colours in various proportions to create all the colours. Mix all three colours at their maximum saturation levels and you get a dark grey. Because these three colours cannot produce true black, black is required as the 'fourth' colour.

CMYK (cyan, magenta, yellow, black)

In print, you use the CMYK colour model, a *subtractive colour model*, because you print on a white page. With CMYK, the three primary colours are mixed in different proportions to create all available colours, including blue, green and red.

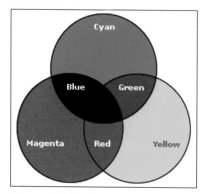

Figure 5-7 The CMYK colour model

For your information

The additive colour model is typically used for computers and other digital displays. The subtractive colour model is standard for print applications because, in print, you normally start with the white of the paper and then add primary colours to create colours on the page.

The colour wheel

Graphic artists use a colour wheel to mix the primary colours to create secondary and tertiary colours.

Figure 5-8 shows the RGB model, in which red, yellow and blue are the primary colours.

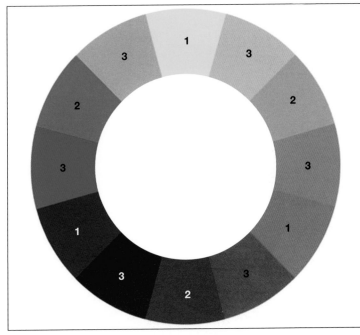

Figure 5-8 Mixing colours on the RGB colour wheel

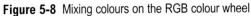

Jargon buster

1. **Primary colours:** The main colours in any colour model – red, green and blue in the RGB model, and cyan, magenta, yellow and black in the CMYK model.

2. **Secondary colours:** Created by mixing two neighbouring primary colours in equal proportion. For example, mixing yellow and blue produces green. Mixing blue and red produces purple.

3. **Tertiary colours:** Created by mixing a primary colour with a neighbouring secondary colour. For example, mixing blue with purple produces violet. Mixing yellow and green produces chartreuse.

5

Mixing primary colours (cont.)

Figure 5-9 shows the CMYK model, in which cyan, magenta and yellow are the primary colours. K stands for key black, a full combination of all three colours.

1 Primary colours.

2 Secondary colours.

3 Tertiary colours.

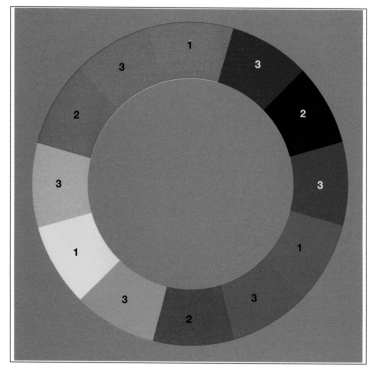

Figure 5-9 Mixing colours on the CMYK colour wheel

Use the colour wheel to identify complementary colours – those opposite one another on the colour wheel, as in Figure 5-10. Pairs of complementary colours include yellow and purple, red and green, and blue and orange.

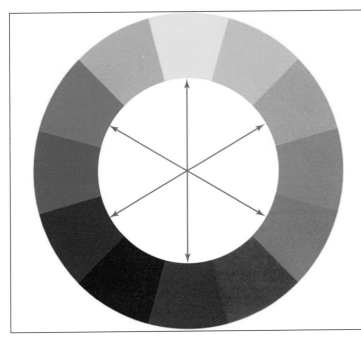

Figure 5-10 Complementary colours on the RGB colour wheel

Jargon buster

Complementary colours: Those that are opposite one another on a colour wheel. Complementary colours tend to look good when placed on the same page.

Important

Although complementary colours tend to look good together, avoid using them in a foreground/background relationship. This creates a phenomenon known as *simultaneous contrast*. Each colour makes the other look more vibrant, which is overstimulating.

5

Identifying complementary colours (cont.)

For obvious reasons, avoid using complementary colours in a foreground/background relationship, as in Figure 5-11.

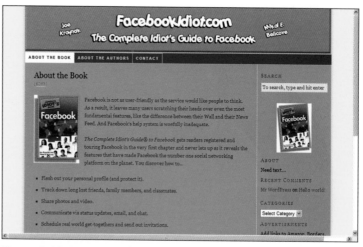

Figure 5-11 Poor use of complementary colours in a foreground/background relationship

Every colour has only one complementary colour, but by mixing the two colours you can create numerous neutral colours for added variation in your design.

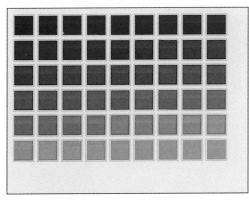

Figure 5-12 Complementaries: blue and orange and their neutrals

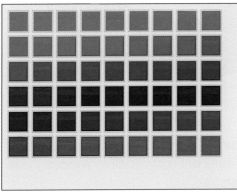

Figure 5-13 Complementaries: red and green and their neutrals

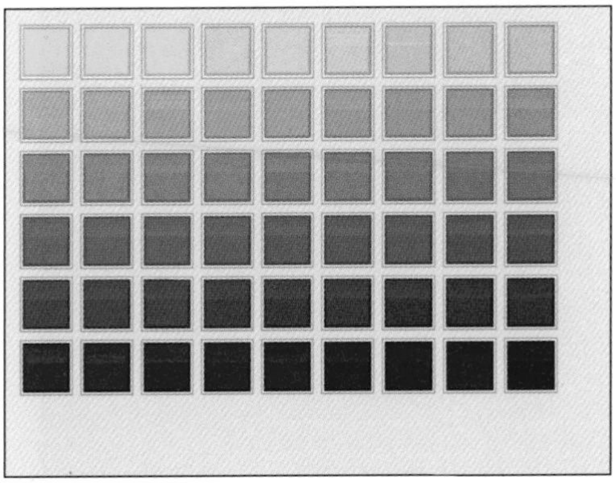

Figure 5-14 Complementaries: yellow and purple and their neutrals

◄ **Creating neutral colours**

1 Mix blue with orange to create neutrals, as in Figure 5-12.

2 Mix red and green to create neutrals, as in Figure 5-13.

3 Mix yellow and purple to create neutrals, as in Figure 5-14.

Jargon buster

Neutral colours: Neither warm nor cool. Typically, they include black, white, grey and various shades of brown.

For your information

Mixing any two complementary colours in equal proportion produces black. When you mix complementary colours, you are essentially creating different shades of the two colours, all of which look good with one another.

5

Identifying analogous colours

Analogous colours are next to one another on the colour wheel. For example, yellow is analogous to yellow-green and yellow-orange. See Figure 5-15.

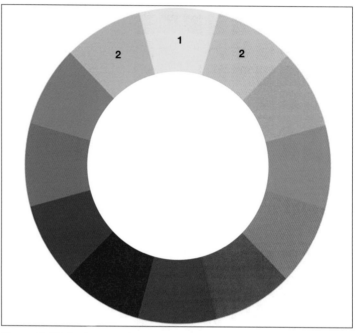

Figure 5-15 Analogous colours

Jargon buster

Analogous colours: Those that appear next to one another on the colour wheel. They tend to look good together and provide a sense of calm and unity.

Important

Avoid using analogous colours in situations that require contrast. For example, using analogous colours in a pie chart may make it difficult to discern the divisions between each slice of pie.

Using analogous colours in a design is usually a safe strategy, as long as you create sufficient contrast where necessary. See Figure 5-16 for an example.

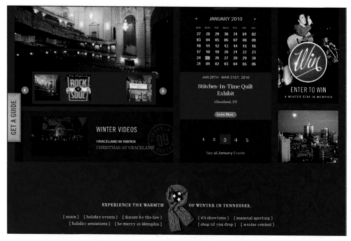

Figure 5-16 Website design using analogous colours

When you purchase paint for your home, you usually buy a gallon of white paint. The person at the store then adds one or more pure colours to make the paint the colour you want. The more pure colour is added, the more saturated the colour becomes and the more intense the colour.

In the same way, you can make colours more or less intense by increasing or decreasing their saturation. Figure 5-17 shows low, medium and high saturation.

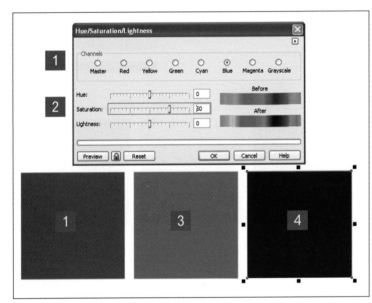

Figure 5-17 Medium, low and high saturation

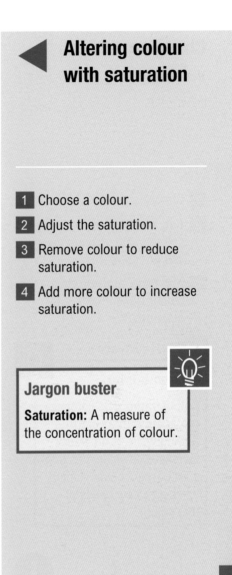

Altering colour with saturation

1 Choose a colour.

2 Adjust the saturation.

3 Remove colour to reduce saturation.

4 Add more colour to increase saturation.

Jargon buster

Saturation: A measure of the concentration of colour.

Changing colour values ▶

1 Choose a colour.

2 Add white to increase the colour value, making the colour lighter.

3 Add black to decrease the colour value, making the colour darker.

You can increase a colour's value to make it lighter or decrease the value to make the colour darker. In some graphics applications, you start with the desired colour and saturation and are then able to adjust the shade (lightness).

Figure 5-18 shows an application in which you choose the colour/saturation and then adjust the shade.

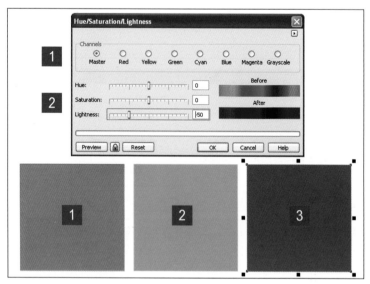

Figure 5-18 Medium, high and low colour values

Some graphics applications, such as the one in Figure 5-19, provide a colour wheel or selector that enables you to adjust the saturation and colour value at the same time.

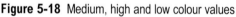

Figure 5-19 Application for choosing the colour/saturation and shade using one control

One way to develop a colour scheme is to start with a photograph, logo or image you want to use as the focus of your site. Use colours from the image to create your colour scheme.

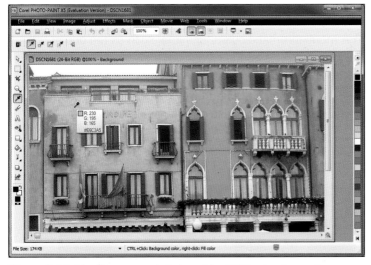

Figure 5-20 Mousing over a photo to get the RGB value for a colour

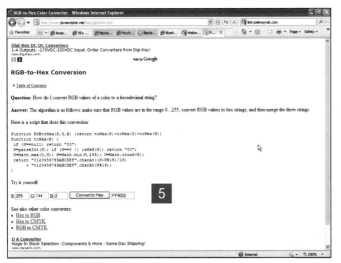

Figure 5-21 Using an RGB to hex converter to get the colour's hex value

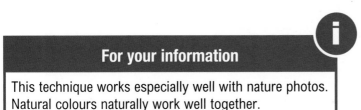

For your information

This technique works especially well with nature photos. Natural colours naturally work well together.

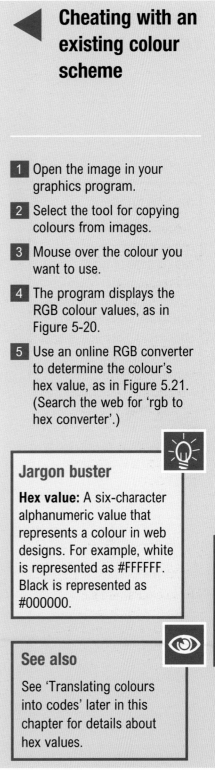

◄ **Cheating with an existing colour scheme**

1 Open the image in your graphics program.

2 Select the tool for copying colours from images.

3 Mouse over the colour you want to use.

4 The program displays the RGB colour values, as in Figure 5-20.

5 Use an online RGB converter to determine the colour's hex value, as in Figure 5.21. (Search the web for 'rgb to hex converter'.)

Jargon buster

Hex value: A six-character alphanumeric value that represents a colour in web designs. For example, white is represented as #FFFFFF. Black is represented as #000000.

See also

See 'Translating colours into codes' later in this chapter for details about hex values.

Designing a colour scheme

Using the colour wheel, you can confidently develop attractive custom colour schemes.

- An achromatic colour scheme, like the one shown in Figure 5-22 is the most basic, for instance a newspaper.
- A monochromatic colour scheme, such as the one in Figure 5-23, uses one colour but adds variation with tints and shades, resulting in a consistent and soothing design. Without much contrast, however, it can be challenging to use colour to emphasise specific areas of the site.

> **Jargon buster**
>
> **Achromatic:** Means without colour or black and white with shades of grey.
> **Monochromatic:** Means one colour, in addition to black and white. Variation can be added with tints and shades of that one colour.

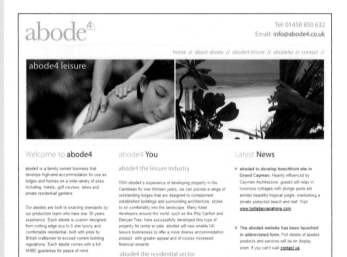

Figure 5-22 Achromatic design

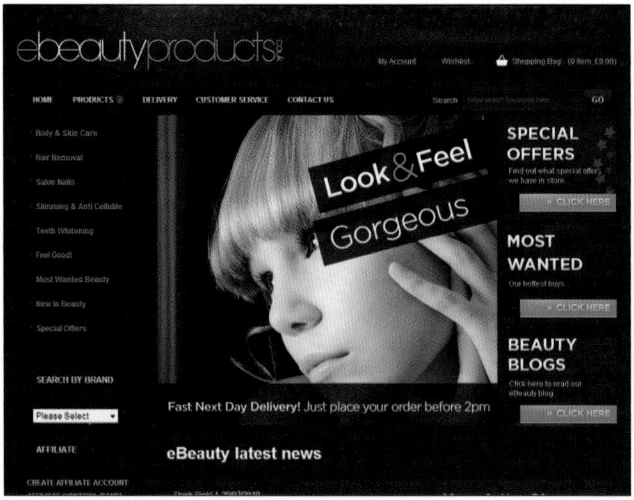

Figure 5-23 Monochromatic design

- An analogous colour scheme, such as the design in Figure 5-24, uses two similar colours to add more variation. One colour serves as the dominant, while the other enriches the design.

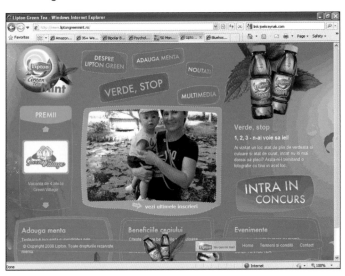

Figure 5-24 Analogous design

- Complementary colour schemes, such as the design in Figure 5-25, offer the greatest contrast for adding emphasis to specific areas or elements of the site. Use one colour as the dominant one, while using the other for accents.

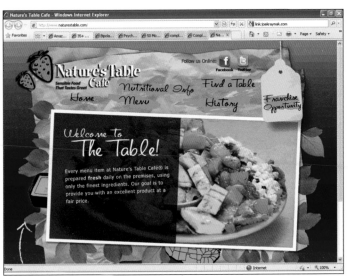

Figure 5-25 Complementary design

For your information

Consider using the cooler colour as the dominant one and the warmer colour as the accent. To add more contrast and emphasis, de-saturate the cooler colour.

5

Designing a colour scheme (cont.)

■ To add more variation, try using a split complementary colour scheme by choosing a dominant colour and the two colours adjacent to its complementary colour, as in Figure 5-26.

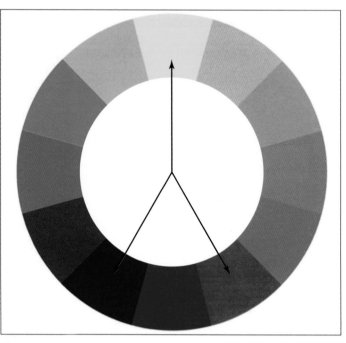

Figure 5-26 Split complementary colour scheme

- A triadic colour scheme (see Figure 5-27) does not offer as much contrast as a complementary one, but it is richer and more balanced.

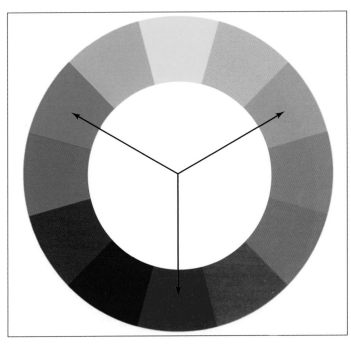

Figure 5-27 Triadic scheme

5

Designing a colour scheme (cont.)

For your information

Split complementary schemes use the two colours next to the base colour's complement.

Triadic schemes use three colours equally spaced on the colour wheel.

Tetradic schemes use four colours consisting of two pairs of complementary colours that are analogous to one another.

■ A tetradic (double complementary) colour scheme – Figure 5-28 – is the richest of all, with four colours, but establishing harmony and balance among the colours can be difficult.

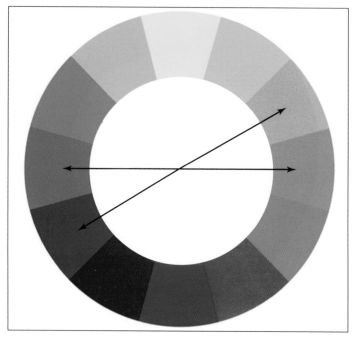

Figure 5-28 Tetradic scheme

Did you know?

To establish balance with a tetradic colour scheme, try choosing one colour as the dominant colour and using the other three colours to accent the design and add emphasis. Avoid using all four colours in equal amounts.

High-end graphics programs, such as Adobe Photoshop, may include tools to help you develop attractive colour schemes. You can also use colour scheme design tools online, such as Color Scheme Designer (*http://colorschemedesigner.com*) or purchase a program specifically for developing attractive colour schemes, such as Color Schemer (*www.colorschemer.com*).

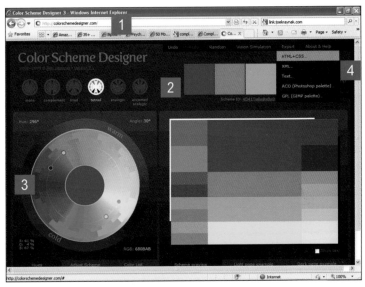

Figure 5-29 Color Scheme Designer

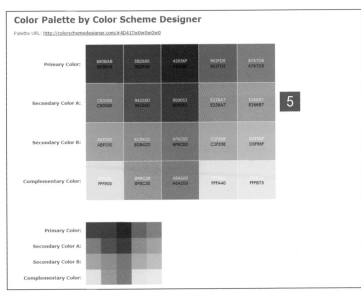

Figure 5-30 Color Scheme Designer palette with hex codes

Designing a colour scheme (cont.)

1 Go to *http:// colorschemedesigner.com* – see Figure 5-29.

2 Click a colour scheme type.

3 Drag the circles to select the desired colour(s).

4 Click Export, HTML+CSS.

5 Color Scheme Designer displays the colour palette complete with hex codes for the colours, as in Figure 5-30.

5

Translating colours into codes

You can colour any object on a web page, including the background, headings, body text and borders. To specify a colour, you add the colour attribute and then specify the colour. For primary colours, you can use the colour's name, such as {colour: blue;}. Otherwise, you must know the colour's hex value.

When using a colour scheme application or tool, it usually provides you with the hex values for every colour in the scheme. If you don't have the hex value but you do know the RGB values, you can use a converter to determine the hex value.

1 Go to *www.javascripter.net/faq/rgbtohex.htm*, as in Figure 5-31.

2 Enter the RGB values of the colour.

3 Click Convert to Hex.

4 Take note of the colour's hex value.

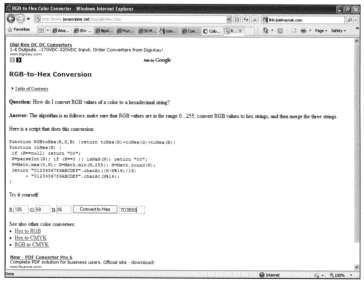

Figure 5-31 RGB to hex converter

For your information

A 24-bit true-colour monitor can display 16 million different colours. A 16-bit monitor can display more than 65,000 colours. Older monitors can display only 256 colours, 216 of which are considered 'web safe'. To produce additional colours, the monitor must mix colours, which can lead to unexpected results. The palette of web-safe colours is now considered old and not an issue when designing your colour scheme. For reference though, a list of web-safe colours can be found at *www.w3schools.com/html/html_colours.asp*.

Designing the text elements

6

Introduction

Text is key to a website. Putting aside all the bells and whistles, reading content is the main web activity. The fanciest sites on the web are of not much value if the text is obscured and inaccessible.

Text and fonts are the two distinctive categories in textual presentation. Fonts essentially are designed alphabets. There are hundreds of fonts available, yet only a handful are useful on the web. The catch is that for a font to display the way it should, it needs to be installed on the person's computer so that their browser can use it. That's why many website designers stick to a certain set of font families – so that they know the fonts will appear correctly to the user. The trick for using fancy fonts is to turn them into graphics. In this way they are presented as an image and will look exactly as they should regardless of loaded local fonts. There are advantages and disadvantages to this, as you will learn here.

There are many 'treatments' that can be applied to text and fonts, such as bolding, underlining, spacing, colours and more. All these attributes are explained in this chapter.

What you'll do

Learn the font types and font families

Understand how CSS settings are used to change text appearance

Apply font type, size, weight, style and variations

Apply colour, indent, alignment and other textual alterations

Use text as graphics

Font types and font families

If you look closely at the type in various publications, both online and off, you'll notice that sometimes letters have little extra lines, such as the letter 'I' having lines across the top and bottom. These lines are known as serifs. Fonts that use them are serif fonts.

The fonts that leave these off are known as sans serif (without serifs). Computers come with a handful of fonts, of each type. Times New Roman (or just Times) is a serif font. Arial and Verdana are sans serif. Compare the first two lines in Figure 6-1. The first is in a serif font, the latter is sans serif.

> A rose is still a rose by any other name
>
> **A rose is still a rose by any other name**
>
> `A rose is still a rose by any other name`

Figure 6-1 Comparing font types

The third line in Figure 6-1 is the Courier font. This is a monospace-style font, which means that each letter takes up the same amount of space. This font is used to simulate typewriters of the past. It is not used often.

The fonts in Figure 6-1 are styled using div tags and CSS. The HTML is this:

```
<div id="container">
<br /><br />
<div id="one">
A rose is still a rose by any other
name
</div>
<br /><br />
<div id="two">
A rose is still a rose by any other
name
</div>
<br /><br />
```

```
<div id="three">
A rose is still a rose by any other
name
</div>
```

The CSS comes from an external file. The CSS looks like this:

```
#one {
 font-family: times, "times new roman",
serif;
 font-size:20px;
 }
#two {
 font-family: arial, verdana, sans-
serif;
 font-size:18px;
 }
#three {
 font-family: courier, "courier new",
serif;
 font-size:18px;
 }
```

The fonts are indicated by the font-family CSS property (font-family) and each family is followed by possible exact fonts (ex. arial). Finally, each family list ends with a general 'serif' or 'sans-serif'. This allows the browser to display an appropriate general sans or sans-serif font if all of the named ones are unavailable – which is rare.

As a general rule use a serif font for longer portions of text. The serifs actually help guide the eyes while reading. Sans-serif fonts are best used for headlines, banners and headings. The size of the font may also drive what type of font to use.

Did you know?

Generally, sans-serif fonts are used for headings and serif fonts are used for longer sections of text. However, creative applications of fonts can bend these usual practices.

Font size

The CSS font-size property allows you to set the size using various types of measuring – pixels, percentage and more. In particular you can indicate font size using any of the following:

- fixed keywords of xx-small, x-small, small, medium, large, x-large or xx-large
- a relative value of smaller or larger
- a length set in pixels, ems, points, inches or centimetres
- a percentage.

The default size is medium if no other sizing is indicated. Figure 6-2 shows various font sizes. The text is altered using keywords, pixels, percentages and so forth.

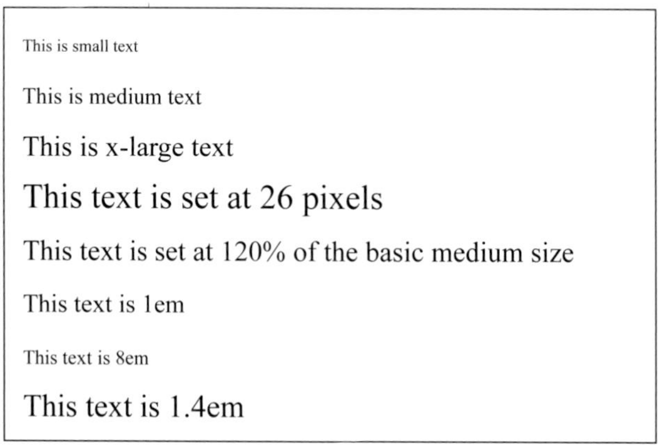

This is small text

This is medium text

This is x-large text

This text is set at 26 pixels

This text is set at 120% of the basic medium size

This text is 1em

This text is 8em

This text is 1.4em

Figure 6-2 Various font sizes

Setting the font weight is the equivalent of turning bold on and off. CSS actually lets you specify nine variations of font boldness. In practice, though, these are not useful since the fonts themselves don't support them. Some day perhaps. For now, to indicate bold with CSS, use this:

```
font-weight:bold;
```

You can replace the word bold with the word normal if you do not want bold text; a non-bold appearance is the default anyway.

Italics are set with the font-style property, like this:

```
font-style:italic;
```

Italic text is not easy to read for long passages of text. Use italics in headings and occasionally to make a word or phrase stand out. The same holds for setting text in bold.

Figure 6-3 shows a good example of how a heading is treated with bold and italic (sans serif too!), while the body of the text has a standard font appearance.

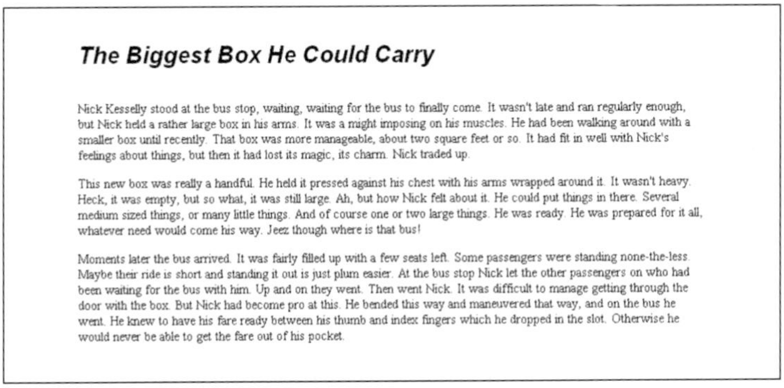

The Biggest Box He Could Carry

Nick Kesselly stood at the bus stop, waiting, waiting for the bus to finally come. It wasn't late and ran regularly enough, but Nick held a rather large box in his arms. It was a might imposing on his muscles. He had been walking around with a smaller box until recently. That box was more manageable, about two square feet or so. It had fit in well with Nick's feelings about things, but then it had lost its magic, its charm. Nick traded up.

This new box was really a handful. He held it pressed against his chest with his arms wrapped around it. It wasn't heavy. Heck, it was empty, but so what, it was still large. Ah, but how Nick felt about it. He could put things in there. Several medium sized things, or many little things. And of course one or two large things. He was ready. He was prepared for it all, whatever need would come his way. Jeez though where is that bus!

Moments later the bus arrived. It was fairly filled up with a few seats left. Some passengers were standing none-the-less. Maybe their ride is short and standing it out is just plum easier. At the bus stop Nick let the other passengers on who had been waiting for the bus with him. Up and on they went. Then went Nick. It was difficult to manage getting through the door with the box. But Nick had become pro at this. He bended this way and maneuvered that way, and on the bus he went. He knew to have his fare ready between his thumb and index fingers which he dropped in the slot. Otherwise he would never be able to get the fare out of his pocket.

Figure 6-3 Different font styling for the title

Font weight and italics

6

Did you know?

Another way to apply bold to text is to use the <strong> tag either in the CSS file or directly in the HTML.

Padding text

A design may dictate that text is not laid out all across the page. Text may be contained in sized areas. These areas may have borders. When text is contained in a boxed area (a div), it will butt against the edges. The appearance is not a good one – the text has no room to 'breathe'. Adding padding alleviates this problem by putting a designated amount of space around the text.

Figure 6-4 shows the same text contained in two divs. The bottom has been given a padding value of 7px. This means that on each side of the text, 7 pixels of space are placed between the text and the border of the box.

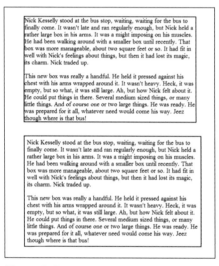

Figure 6-4 Padding is added to the bottom box

The CSS for the two divs is this:

```
#eighteen {
    width: 500px;
    border-style:solid;
border-width:thin;
    font-size:18px;
```

```
}
#nineteen {
    width: 500px;
    border-width:thin;
    border-style:solid;
        font-size:18px;
        padding:7px;
}
```

Referring to the CSS and then the figure you'll note that although the width of each div is 500 pixels, the bottom box looks wider. This is because of the padding. There are 7 pixels of padding on both the left and right sides of the text, making the boxes appear to differ in width by 14 pixels. By increasing the size of the top box to 514 pixels (`width:514px;`) the boxes line up, as shown in Figure 6-5.

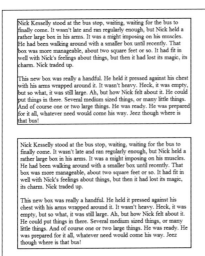

Figure 6-5 Compensating for the extra pixels from the padding

For your information

The space that padding takes up has to be considered in the general layout. Div sizing will need to be adjusted.

Text colour

Colour brings a website to life. Just as text can be enhanced with bold or italics, colour is another tool at your disposal. Consider Figure 6-6.

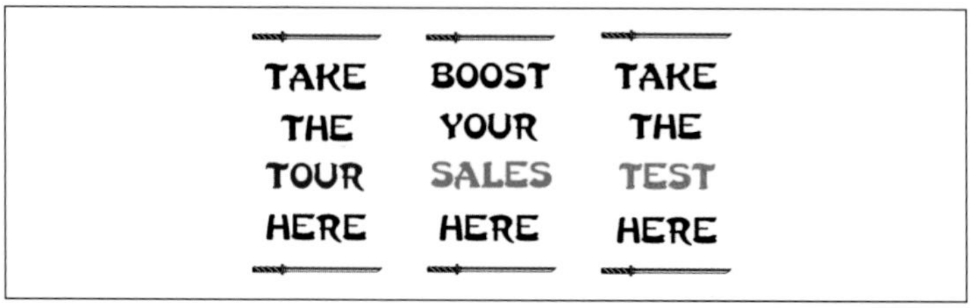

TAKE	BOOST	TAKE
THE	YOUR	THE
TOUR	SALES	TEST
HERE	HERE	HERE

Figure 6-6 Colour enhances text

The CSS property to change text colour is the quite simple 'colour', for example:

- color:blue;
- color:#00ff00;

The latter refers to setting a colour using the RGB (red-green-blue) system. You can read more about colour in Chapter 5.

Although it is common to set the colour for a div (and all text in the div receives the same colour treatment), the way to change colour on a letter-by-letter basis is to use the HTML span tag. Figure 6-7 shows how colour has been assigned to individual letters.

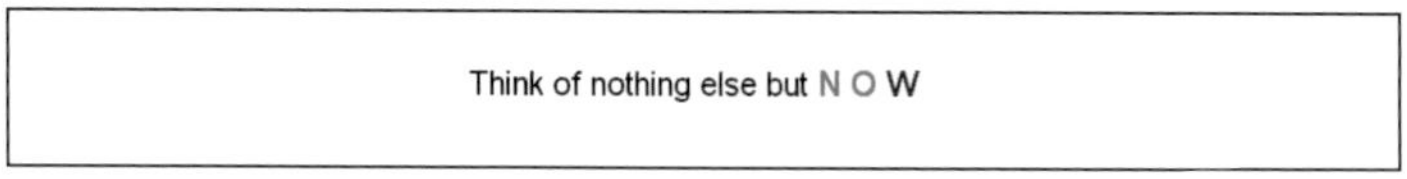

Think of nothing else but N O W

Figure 6-7 Applying colour to individual letters

Here is the HTML code that creates the text line in Figure 6-7:

```
Think of nothing else but <span
style="color:#00ff00;font-
weight:bold;font-size:24px;">N</
span> <span style="color:#ff0000;font-
weight:bold;font-size:24px;">O</
span> <span style="color:#0000ff;font-
weight:bold;font-size:24px;">W</span>
```

Word spacing is the setting of how much space exists between words. Letter spacing is the setting of how much exists between each letter in a word. Both of these settings are set with CSS and can be put to use for interesting effects.

With either, setting a value of 0 pixels is the default. In effect, you don't have to indicate this – the browser would render the word spacing at that value anyway. From there you can increase or decrease the number of pixels. Increasing the number of pixels puts more space between words and decreasing the pixels pushes words closer together. Decreasing means you have to use a negative value such –5px.

Figure 6-8 shows how word spacing has been applied to a line of text. The first line is at the normal setting. The second line is at 10 pixels and the third line is at –5 pixels. Note that the second line is stretched out and the third line is compressed. An effect of stretching out the words such as in the second line is useful in headings and titles. The compressed look is a more thorny proposition. Probably its use should be short and sparing – just for the occasion when you need something to shake up the design. The CSS settings for the second and third lines are:

- word-spacing:10px;
- word-spacing:-5px;

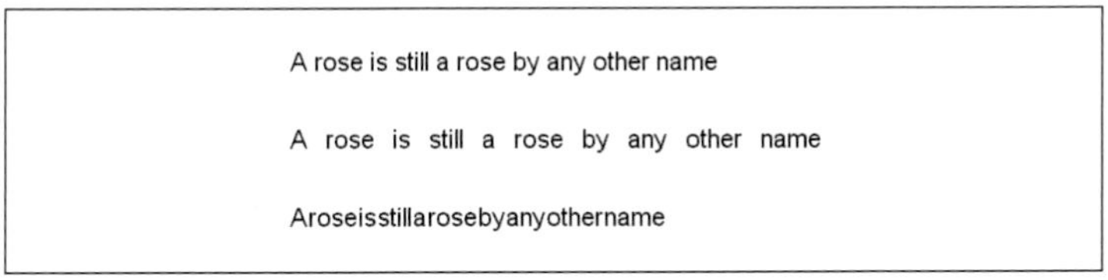

A rose is still a rose by any other name

A rose is still a rose by any other name

Aroseisstillarosebyanyothername

Figure 6-8 Altering word spacing

Word spacing and letter spacing (cont.)

Figure 6-9 shows the similar stretch and compress effects but applied to the spacing between letters. The second line has a setting of 5 pixels and the third line has a setting of –3 pixels. The first line is standard spacing. The CSS for the second and third lines are:

- letter-spacing:5px;
- letter-spacing:-3px;

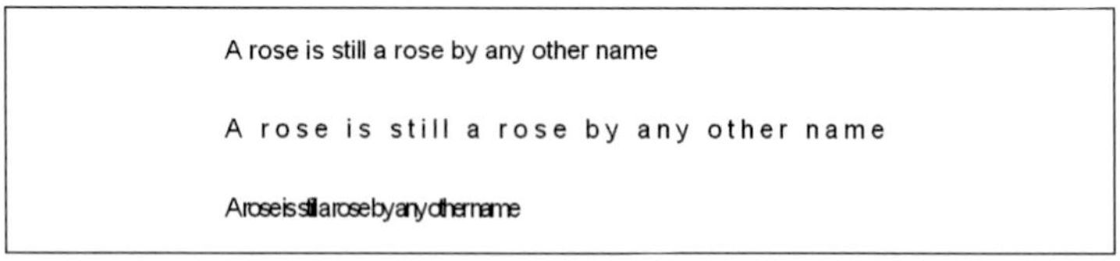

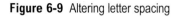

Figure 6-9 Altering letter spacing

Word spacing and letter spacing can at times seem quite similar, while at other times the distinction is clear. For example, in Figures 6-8 and 6-9, the second lines appear similar while the third, compressed lines are more distinctive relative with each other.

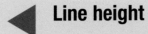
When text is presented in multiple lines, the amount of space between lines can be set with the line height property. Line height can be set in three ways:

- a number – the number is multiplied with the current font size to set the line height
- length – this allows a fixed value using pixels, centimetres, etc.
- percentage – a percent based on the current font size.

Figure 6-10 shows the same paragraph with three different line height settings. The first is in the standard setting – the line height matches the font size. The second paragraph is set at .7 (seven-tenths) of the font size – this pulls the lines closer together. The bottom paragraph is set at 140%. The CSS for the bottom two paragraphs looks like this:

- line-height: 0.7
- line-height: 140%;

> Nick Kesselly stood at the bus stop, waiting, waiting for the bus to finally come. It wasn't late and ran regularly enough, but Nick held a rather large box in his arms. It was a might imposing on his muscles. He had been walking around with a smaller box until recently. That box was more manageable, about two square feet or so. It had fit in well with Nick's feelings about things, but then it had lost its magic, its charm. Nick traded up.

> Nick Kesselly stood at the bus stop, waiting, waiting for the bus to finally come. It wasn't late and ran regularly enough, but Nick held a rather large box in his arms. It was a might imposing on his muscles. He had been walking around with a smaller box until recently. That box was more manageable, about two square feet or so. It had fit in well with Nick's feelings about things, but then it had lost its magic, its charm. Nick traded up.

> Nick Kesselly stood at the bus stop, waiting, waiting for the bus to finally come. It wasn't late and ran regularly enough, but Nick held a rather large box in his arms. It was a might imposing on his muscles. He had been walking around with a smaller box until recently. That box was more manageable, about two square feet or so. It had fit in well with Nick's feelings about things, but then it had lost its magic, its charm. Nick traded up.

Figure 6-10 Variations of the line height property

Text alignment

When there is a paragraph of text, you need to decide how to align the lines within the paragraph. Mostly the text is left aligned, with justified text being the second most common form. Justified text is when the lines fit perfectly all the way, left to right. In a way justified text is a mix of left and right aligned text.

Centred text is commonly used for headings. Paragraphs do not look right when the text is all centred. Right aligned text is a rather cool way of setting text and has a creative side to it.

Figure 6-11 shows all four alignments of the same paragraph. The easiest to read is undoubtedly the left aligned text. Note how the centred text looks odd.

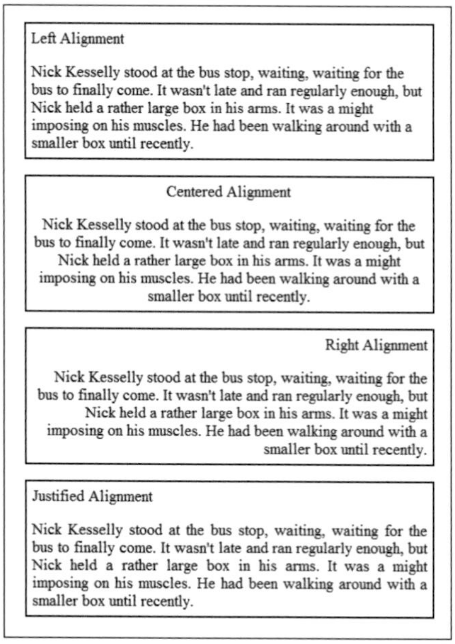

Left Alignment

Nick Kesselly stood at the bus stop, waiting, waiting for the bus to finally come. It wasn't late and ran regularly enough, but Nick held a rather large box in his arms. It was a might imposing on his muscles. He had been walking around with a smaller box until recently.

Centered Alignment

Nick Kesselly stood at the bus stop, waiting, waiting for the bus to finally come. It wasn't late and ran regularly enough, but Nick held a rather large box in his arms. It was a might imposing on his muscles. He had been walking around with a smaller box until recently.

Right Alignment

Nick Kesselly stood at the bus stop, waiting, waiting for the bus to finally come. It wasn't late and ran regularly enough, but Nick held a rather large box in his arms. It was a might imposing on his muscles. He had been walking around with a smaller box until recently.

Justified Alignment

Nick Kesselly stood at the bus stop, waiting, waiting for the bus to finally come. It wasn't late and ran regularly enough, but Nick held a rather large box in his arms. It was a might imposing on his muscles. He had been walking around with a smaller box until recently.

Figure 6-11 Four types of text alignment

The CSS of the four divs is here:

```
#thirtyone {
       font-size:20px;
   width: 500px;
   border-width:thin;
   border-style:solid;
      padding:7px;
   text-align:left;
}
#thirtytwo {
       font-size:20px;
   width: 500px;
   border-width:thin;
   border-style:solid;
      padding:7px;
   text-align:center;
}
#thirtythree {
       font-size:20px;
   width: 500px;
   border-width:thin;
   border-style:solid;
      padding:7px;
   text-align:right;
}
#thirtyfour {
       font-size:20px;
   width: 500px;
   border-width:thin;
   border-style:solid;
      padding:7px;
   text-align:justify;
}
```

Text alignment (cont.)

It is easy to ignore alignment and simply let all text be left aligned. However, a little thought can bring some new text design ideas into play. Figure 6-12 shows part of a site where the text is justified.

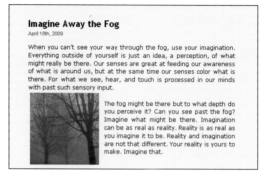

Figure 6-12 Justified text

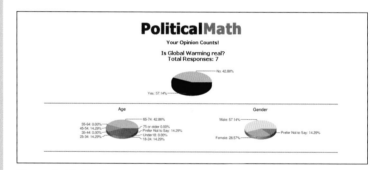

Figure 6-13 Mostly headings, centred

Figure 6-13 shows an example of a web page that has little text, mostly headers. So, of course, these are centred.

Early in this chapter we discussed using common fonts to ensure that viewers will see what they are meant to see in their web browsers. When the creative juices are jumping, however, the technique is to use graphics. That is, the graphics are letters or words, but created as a graphic with the aid of an art program. Thus you can create any text look you desire and it will appear correctly because the person is looking at a graphic.

Figure 6-14 shows an example. This is the heading from a web site for a church. The letters are set in a stained glass look. The words are readable and this graphic will appear the same to everyone.

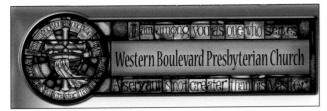

Figure 6-14 Text as a graphic

Figure 6-15 illustrates another example of text made as a graphic. The figure shows the top part of the website. Not all you see is a graphic – for example, the menu system is real text.

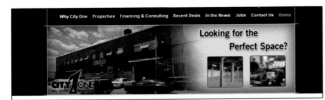

Figure 6-15 A mixture of text and image in a graphic

Text as graphics

6

Text as graphics (cont.)

Figure 6-16 isolates the part that is the graphic text. This portion of the text was made as a graphic so the shadow effect could be added to it.

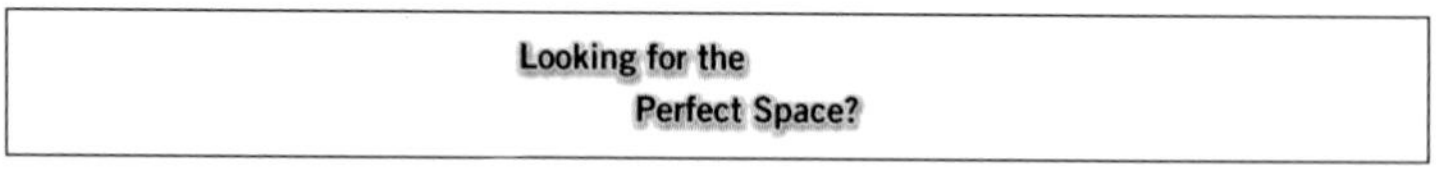

> **Looking for the**
> **Perfect Space?**

Figure 6-16 Using a graphic approach to be able to include the shadow effect

Did you know?

Text in Flash files suffers from the same limitation. The search engines cannot read the text out of a Flash file.

Now for the advantages and disadvantages of text replaced with graphics. In a nutshell: SEO. When search engine spiders come to index a site, they can't read the text in a graphic. Using the alt attribute in the image tag is clearly a good idea. However, if you have a sizeable amount of text in a graphic, not all of it can reasonably go into the alt attribute. Perhaps enough will, perhaps not. For this reason it is not always the case that design should have control over all that goes into a site.

Accenting your website with graphics

Introduction

The web is visual. Websites are varied in colour, images and everything else that the eye can take in. Flash presentations can be amazing to watch. Videos abound – from YouTube and other sources, even from your own website account should you put video files up.

This chapter is about traditional web graphics, not animations, Flash or movies. Traditional graphics are usually photographs saved as a JPG, PNG or GIF. There are reasons for using different file formats and we discuss these in this chapter. Graphics are used as logos, to show items on a page and for the background of a page. Branding involves using graphics for instant identification.

Also in this chapter we show how graphics are created, found, altered and applied. For example, we show different ways a background image can be used with the help of CSS.

What you'll do

Review how a logo instantly identifies an entity

Learn about different graphic types

Learn where to get graphics

Learn how graphics programs are used to alter images

Use CSS to work with page backgrounds

Images and branding

Logos and other identifiable visuals are part of a company's branding. This is a noticeable phenomenon on the internet. The most popular sites each have their own distinctive looks.

While it is true that branding involves more than just the graphics (for example, a certain font may be prevalent), some images instantly identify a site. Mostly the logo is one word or a set of words that is the name of the company, but it's more than just the name that establishes the identity: the logo is typically stylised with colours, a catchy design and so on.

Figures 7-1, 7-2 and 7-3 show logos from well-known websites which can almost be considered household names. Sometimes a company's name is so ingrained into our communications that the name comes to denote a common action. Google is a perfect example. When doing a search on the web someone might say 'I'm Googling'.

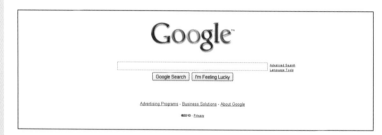

Figure 7-1 The ever recognisable Google

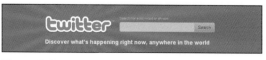

Figure 7-2 Twitter and the popular act of tweeting

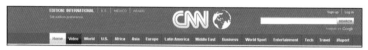

Figure 7-3 The well-known CNN logo

All of these logos are graphics. They appear as letters but of course are highly stylised. The point is that a logo is important. Brand identity is not the focus of this book, but for a chapter on graphics, logos cannot be left out. When designing your site, put thought into the logo – what it will be and where it will be placed. It may end up being the most recognisable part of the site.

There are numerous types of graphic file formats. Each has properties that make it useful, or not, depending on how the graphic is to be presented. When it comes to websites, besides the obvious appeal of the graphics, a consideration is the speed at which they will load on the page.

So, a rule of thumb is the smaller the file size, the faster the graphic will load. In line with this is the idea that the more graphics there are, the longer it takes the page to load. With high-speed connections this is not always a noticeable factor, but in the planning of a site it is a good thing to keep in mind.

Subjectively, the three most popular graphic file types for web pages are JPG, PNG and GIF. Jpegs, as they are often called, are the most common of all. The following table summarises the file types.

7

Years ago a lawsuit determined that the GIF format violates a patent. In essence, GIFs should not be used without permission. In reality, they are so prevalent that enforcing the patent is difficult.

File format	Comments
JPG	Smaller file sizes (relatively). A drawback is that the process of creating a JPG causes a loss of picture quality, although the extent of this loss can be quite minor. The file size decreases as more of the quality is dropped. Most designers will not skimp on quality and therefore will leave a JPG at its best possible definition.
PNG	The PNG format does not lose any quality. It is a newer format and was originally meant to replace the GIF type (below). The main difference between PNG and GIF is that a PNG image is not limited to 256 colour shades. However, a PNG cannot be animated.
GIF	GIF files are limited to 256 shades of colour. Basically this file type came into use some time ago when computer monitors could not show any more than the 256 colour variants. Even so, GIFs remain popular for images that do not need much colour variation, such as single colour or black and white images. GIFs can be animated – they can have frames that get cycled through and in this way show movement.

Graphic types (cont.)

Another way of classifying graphic files is by whether they are raster or vector based. Raster images are made of 'real' images such as photographs or scanned-in artwork. Graphic programs can also make raster images.

Raster images are sets of pixels. Indeed, a large raster image contains many pixels – and therefore creates a large file size. JPG, PNG and GIF are all raster based. Resizing raster images can ruin their quality, especially when enlarged, and they can gain jagged edges.

Vector images follow a different approach. Vectors are made with graphic programs and the files are saved essentially as mathematical formulas of how to recreate the graphic. Vector images can be resized without any undesired effect – the mathematical formulas simply recreate the image at the new size. A common vector use is for clip art.

Figure 7-4 shows a logo from a website. It is a raster image.

𝕾𝖍𝖆𝖐𝖊𝖘𝖕𝖊𝖆𝖗𝖊'𝖘 𝕻𝖑𝖆𝖞𝖌𝖗𝖔𝖚𝖓𝖉

Figure 7-4 A logo at its standard size

Figure 7-5 shows a portion of the logo resized to be larger. Notice how the letters have become jagged.

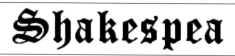

Figure 7-5 Making the logo larger creates an unwanted jagged effect

Because of the sizing issues with web graphics it's good to get a grasp on how they work – particularly with regards to pixels per inch (ppi). Think of digital cameras and their megapixel ratings. A camera with a 6 megapixel rating and one with a 10 megapixel rating take the same photograph. The 10 megapixel version will come out much larger. This is because the pixels per inch are higher; the number of pixels is greater. On your computer monitor you are probably seeing the images at 72 pixels per inch. This makes them look quite large, probably bigger than the whole image can be seen at once at 100% zoom. One image will be larger than the other. Either is way too big for a website. They need to be reduced in size, which you can do in a graphics program or by indicating their size using CSS.

Figure 7-6 shows a picture taken with a 10 megapixel camera. Figure 7-7 shows how the photograph appears in a web browser without any resizing or other sizing constraint. As you can see, the photograph is much larger than can be shown in the browser.

Graphic types (cont.)

? 7

Did you know?

Web browsers display images at 72 ppi.

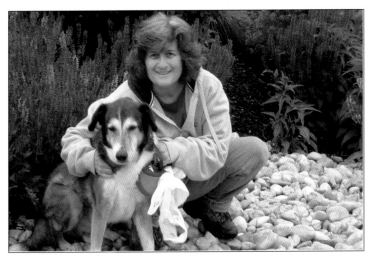

Figure 7-6 A photograph with a high pixels per inch count

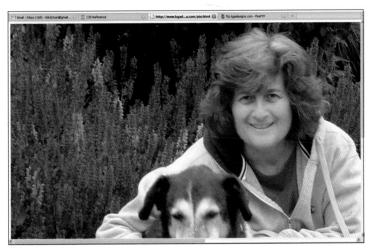

Figure 7-7 A photograph at its true size is much larger than the browser window

Where to get graphics

For your information

It is quite easy to copy images from any website by right-clicking on the image, however this is not a good idea. Someone went through the work of creating that image and assuming you can just take it and use it for yourself, without permission, is wrong.

If you have a decent camera, the best source for photographs is your creativity. Take pictures! With a graphics program you can later alter the image in any way necessary for the targeted website. Don't believe that your photographs are not worthy – they are. Perhaps some practice and learning about your camera is needed, but in fact most images you see on the web are photographs taken with a standard camera. Give it a try!

Next, the best source is online photo repositories. From these you purchase images and usually they are not expensive. A well-known site for this is Getty Images (*www.gettyimages.co.uk*), shown in Figure 7-8.

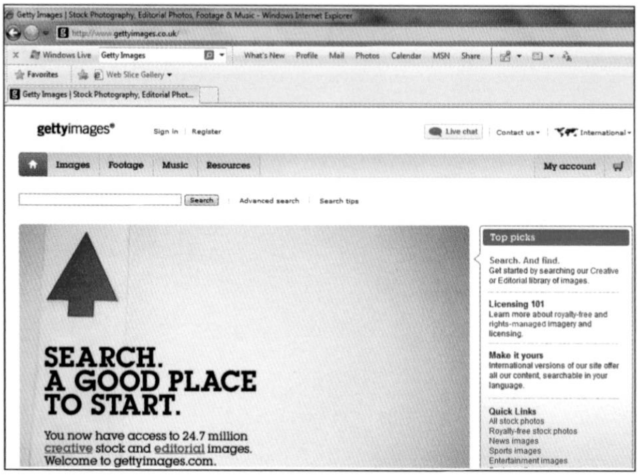

Figure 7-8 Getty Images, a site where you can purchase quality images

When purchasing images make sure you read the legalities concerning what you can use the images for. We strongly suggest reading the site's terms and conditions.

There are sites that provide free photographs. A popular one is Wikimedia Commons (*http://commons.wikimedia.org/wiki/Main_Page*), shown in Figure 7-9.

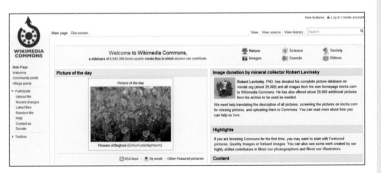

Figure 7-9 Wikimedia Commons

Working with graphics programs

Graphics on a website may be an altered version of an original image. There are many actions that can be applied to an image, such as:

- cropping
- altering colour and contrast
- applying filters (used for effects, some quite bizarre)
- rotating.

There are numerous graphics programs. Some run on the Windows operating system, others run on Apple computers, some have versions for both.

Adobe Photoshop is considered to be the top-notch graphics program. There are both Windows and Apple versions. Often Photoshop is bought as part of a package named Creative Suite. This package comes with Flash, Illustrator, Dreamweaver and other Adobe programs. There are various configurations of Creative Suite.

Adobe products are relatively expensive, but there are plenty of lower-cost alternatives. Educators and students may be eligible for reduced pricing – check the website for details (*www.adobe.com*).

There is a 'light' version of Photoshop called Photoshop Elements. This is an affordable alternative with many of the features of the full product. Figures 7-10 and 7-11 show an image before and after being altered using Photoshop Elements.

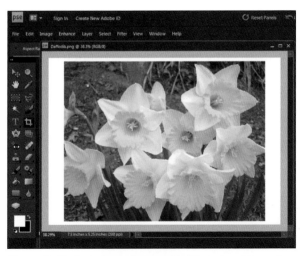

Figure 7-10 A photograph opened in Photoshop Elements

Figure 7-11 shows a way in which the image can be altered. In this example the colours have been changed – the yellow flowers are now orange. The background colour has been slightly altered as well.

PaintShop Photo Pro by Corel (*www.corel.com*) is a great, inexpensive photo-editing program. The program has a long history and a significant list of features. Otherwise, you can search the internet for free graphics programs – there are many available.

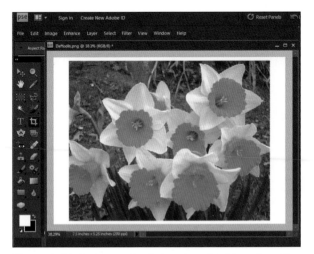

Figure 7-11 An image after being altered in Photoshop Elements

Working with graphics programs (cont.)

Graphics programs are most often used to open a photograph to edit it. However, they can be used to create new art. Figure 7-12 shows an image being created using the drawing tools in PaintShop Photo Pro version 7 (an older version). When the image is finished it can be saved in a native format, a JPG, or in a choice of many other file formats.

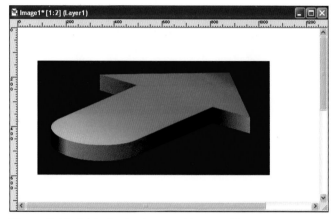

Figure 7-12 Original artwork created in a graphics program

Of course, not all graphics on the web are photographs. Figure 7-13 shows a scanned-in work of art that was saved as a JPG. The graphics program runs the scanner and the image is placed into the graphics program.

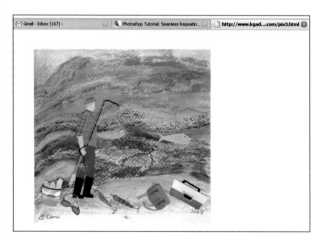

Figure 7-13 Artwork shown on a web page

In modern web programming, graphics are often presented from being referenced in the CSS file. Images are set using the background or background image property. Assuming the page is structured using div tags, the background image in the div is called from the corresponding CSS reference block. An example will help clear up any confusion about this.

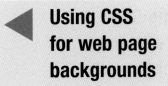
Figure 7-14 shows a web page with a repeating red ball image. The red ball is the referenced image for the container div. The CSS looks like this:

```
#container {
        margin:auto auto;
        background: url(redball.jpg);
}
```

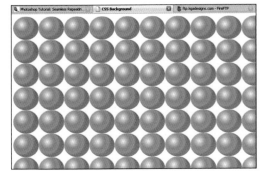

Figure 7-14 A repeating background

The red ball may be the desired graphic, but not dozens of them! So CSS to the rescue. By adding the no-repeat attribute, just a single red ball appears, as seen in Figure 7-15. The CSS now looks like this:

```
#container {
        margin:auto auto;
        background: url(redball.jpg)
        no-repeat;
}
```

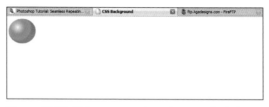

Figure 7-15 Using no-repeat produces a single image

What about positioning the image? There are a few ways to do this. You can use the keyword 'center' to place it midway across the page. Another technique is to use left and top positions. The upper left corner is 0,0. Changing these will move the image to the right and/or lower down. The values can be pixels or percentages. Here in Figure 7-16 the image is set at 100px, 100px. This means the image will move 100 pixels to the right and 100 pixels down, as seen in the figure. The CSS now looks like this:

```
#container {
        margin:auto auto;
        background: url(redball.jpg)
        100px 100px no-repeat;
}
```

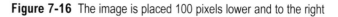

Figure 7-16 The image is placed 100 pixels lower and to the right

CSS provides the flexibility to manipulate the background image as needed. Many websites make use of a background, but one that is not obtrusive to the text and other elements on the page. This type of image generally is repeated but seamless. This means that although repeated throughout, such as in Figure 7-14, the image is constructed in such a way that, as it becomes adjacent, there are no discernable boundary lines. Seamless patterns can be created using graphic programs. A search on the web will produce results of how to make a seamless image with your software.

Figure 7-17 shows a seamless image created using PaintShop Pro.

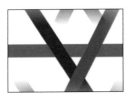

Figure 7-17 A single seamless image

Figure 7-18 shows how the page background looks with the seamless image. The CSS is set to repeat, but the divisions between the images are not to be seen.

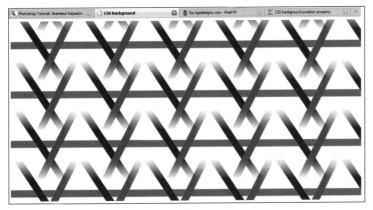

Figure 7-18 Using a repeating seamless pattern

Putting your design in motion

Introduction

Animated web page elements generate immediate interest. They are used in numerous instances, perhaps most often in advertising. There are many ways to put animation on a page, such as with Flash, videos or JavaScript-based carousels or slides.

Audio is another feature to put on a page. Although you won't see audio, you'll certainly notice it. Indeed, audio is a necessity for podcasts and videos. In this chapter we explore the different types of animations and audio you can put on your site.

What you'll do

Learn about Flash

See how an animated GIF file is created

Understand how video works on the web

Review how JavaScript can add animation

Learn to add audio

Flash

Flash is a unique web entity. Flash files are essentially movies but with a few twists. Besides showing 'action', Flash files can contain programming, with a language named ActionScript. ActionScript gives a Flash movie the ability to be interactive – for example, to wait for user input to perform an action. It's not necessary for a Flash movie to have ActionScript, but it makes Flash quite powerful.

Flash movies are created using the Flash product by Adobe. Flash uses a timeline and frames – similar to how actual movies are made. The raw design files have the .fla extension. They are then compiled into movies that are referenced from within a web page. The compiled files end with the .swf file extension. The compiled movies are set to repeat and therefore play endlessly on a web page. Figure 8-1 shows a movie being created within the Flash product.

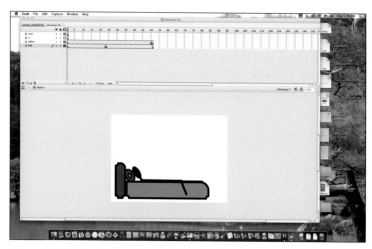

Figure 8-1 Using Flash to compose a movie

Flash is quite flexible and many designs can be created and implemented. There are websites that provide Flash templates for your use. One is Flash Village (*http://flashvillage.com*) and another is Flashmo (*www.flashmo.com*), shown in Figure 8-2.

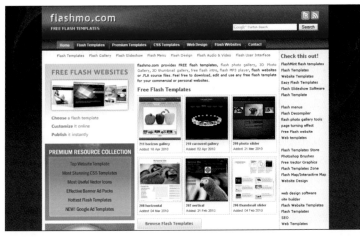

Figure 8-2 A popular Flash template site

Flash is used on a web page in one of two ways. There may be areas of a page that show a Flash movie or the whole page may be a running Flash file. Either way, the movie is played through the Flash viewer – a browser plugin that is usually already integrated into each browser on the market.

For your information

Flash files cannot be read by search engine spiders, so web pages that are completely Flash are not likely to be high up in search results. It is better to use Flash in sections of a web page.

Animated GIF files

GIF is an image file type that can be of a single image or can cycle through a series of images, thereby providing animation. Animated GIFs have to be assembled from a series of still images (such as JPGs). This is done either with specialised software or through an online service.

Figure 8-3 shows how frames are used in assembling the file. In this example, a globe is turning – a bit more so in each successive frame. When the file is finished and viewed, it will be in motion: the Earth spinning.

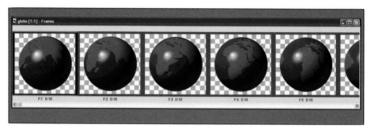

Figure 8-3 Assembling an animated GIF

Figure 8-4 shows the finished file. You do not see the frames and were this not on paper you would see it spinning.

On the internet you will find websites dedicated to making animated GIFs. You upload image files, make selections and the file is generated for you to download. For one such example, visit *http://gickr.com*.

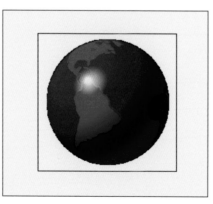

Figure 8-4 This image spins when viewed on a web page

Video files and ways of producing movies can be confusing. Video on the web went through some hoops to arrive at where it is today. As a result there is a number of video file types. On a web page a video has to be shown in some type of player, which adds to the confusion.

Some popular players are Windows Media Player, QuickTime and RealPlayer. Each plays one or more file types and that's where confusion can set in with your design efforts. Popular file types are WMV, MPG (MPEG), MOV and AVI. But which player should you use for which type of movie? For example, QuickTime is an Apple product and its associated type is MOV. So in order for a web page to play a MOV-based movie, the QuickTime player needs to be installed on the computer. QuickTime is usually not installed on Windows computers so a separate download of the player has to occur before the video can be seen. Windows Media Player is, of course, the standard player on Windows computers and can play many video types.

An interesting twist is that the Flash player is installed on most computers and if not it is easy to download. In a sense Flash movies are no different than standard videos even though they can do more than play movies (i.e. interaction).

Enter YouTube. YouTube is one of the biggest sites on the internet and in fact is owned by Google. YouTube alleviates the problems of matching files and players as it can take practically any video file type and make it playable on any web page or in any browser. Figure 8-5 shows the YouTube website.

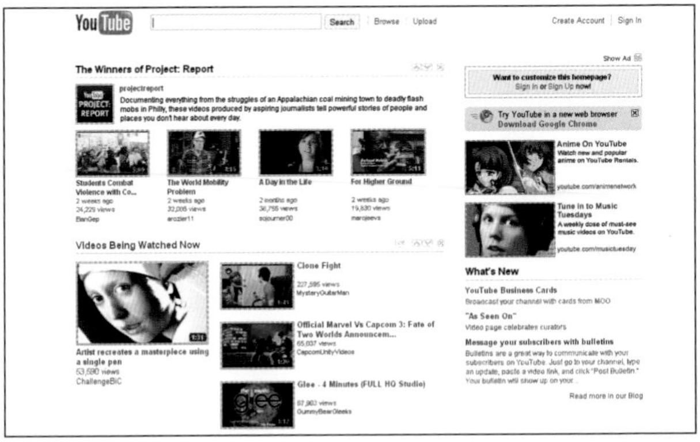

8

Figure 8-5 The YouTube website

Video on the web (cont.)

YouTube can take large files (up to 2 gigabytes) and handles a wide variety of file types. It lets you upload your video files and will process your video into a format that it uses. It then provides the HTML code to embed on your site so you can link to the video. YouTube provides a player as part of the callback to the website for the video and as such you don't need to worry about having a compatible player.

YouTube is a free membership site. You sign up for an account and then you can upload videos. Figure 8-6 shows the result of an uploaded video. You can add a title, description, tags, set privacy rules and categorise the video.

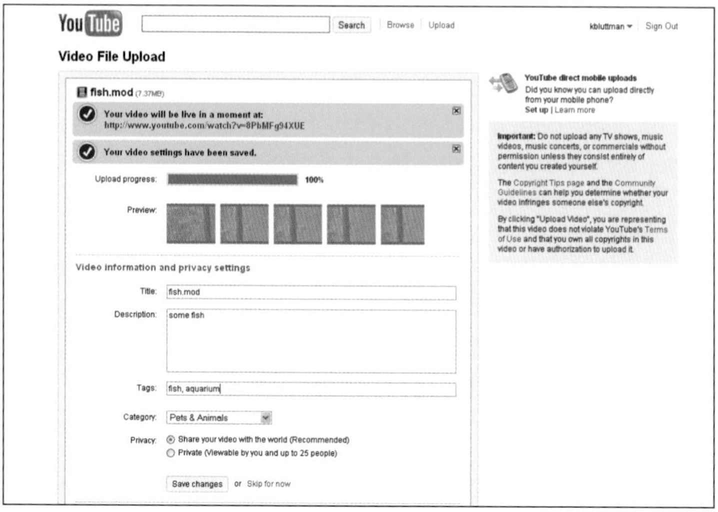

Figure 8-6 Uploading a video on YouTube

Once a video is uploaded and processed, YouTube provides a link back to the video on its site and also a section of HTML code that lets you embed the video link on a web page. Figure 8-7 shows how YouTube provides this code.

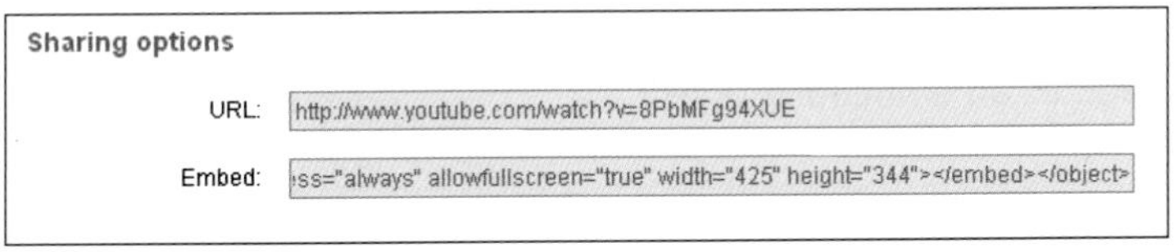

Sharing options	
URL:	http://www.youtube.com/watch?v=8PbMFg94XUE
Embed:	ss="always" allowfullscreen="true" width="425" height="344"></embed></object>

Figure 8-7 YouTube provides the URL to the video and also HTML code to embed on your site

YouTube lets a member create a channel. This loosely follows the idea of having a television channel all to yourself. All your videos can be grouped on your channel and people can subscribe to your channel.

Having a channel is a great marketing tool for companies. Information on new products, people, etc. can be disseminated using video. Figure 8-8 shows Ken's channel page.

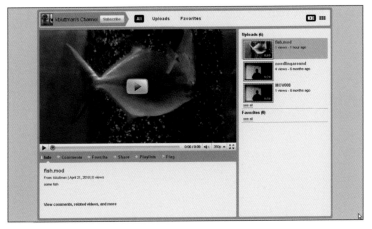

Figure 8-8 A YouTube channel

For your information

All uploaded video must be original or at least not infringe any copyright.

8

Video on the web (cont.)

Figure 8-9 shows how a YouTube video appears on a web page as an embedded object.

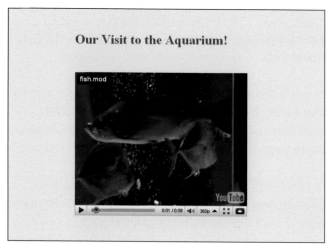

Figure 8-9 A YouTube video on a web page

JavaScript is a powerful language that can create many effects in the browser. It has the ability to manipulate individual parts of a page and the types of manipulation are plentiful. For example, JavaScript can hide or show parts of a page, move objects around on a page and can be used to create sophisticated utilities such as slide shows.

Figure 8-10 shows a slideshow on a web page. It is built with JavaScript and while it can't be shown here on paper, this utility has the ability to control the speed of the slide transitions and can add custom text to go with each picture.

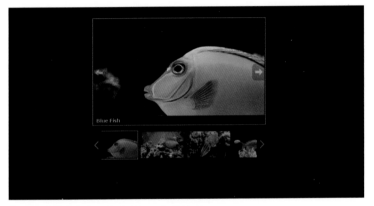

Figure 8-10 A JavaScript-based slide show

The latest trend is to use specialised JavaScript libraries that have many functions already built into them. This relieves the drudgery of having to create your own utilities. JavaScript is powerful, but that power comes at a price – it can be difficult to program.

A JavaScript library is referenced from the page, similar to the way a CSS file is. One of the most popular libraries is JQuery. Figure 8-11 shows another slide show, this one built with JQuery.

JavaScript animation

8

JavaScript animation (cont.)

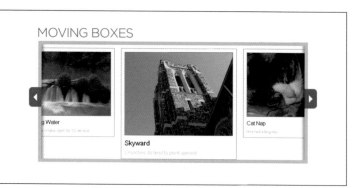

Figure 8-11 A slide show assembled using the JQuery library

Here is a guide to the various popular libraries:

JQuery	*http://jquery.com/*
YUI (Yahoo User Interface)	*http://developer.yahoo.com/yui/*
Prototype	*www.prototypejs.org/*
Scriptaculous	*http://script.aculo.us/*

Becoming familiar with how these libraries work will let you add many cool visuals to your site. The great thing is you don't have to learn JavaScript, just how to implement the libraries. All of them are supported by plenty of documentation and a large user community.

Although video has an audio component, there are times when only audio is needed. There are some websites that play audio upon loading the page and there may be no way to turn it off. This is bad practice as a visitor has no choice but to listen or navigate away from the site.

Best practice for supplying audio is to have an audio player on the page that allows a visitor to start, pause and stop the sound. Audio players work in the same way as video players, but they don't have to be of a given size. The most popular audio players are built in Flash. The player is uploaded to your website and embedding code is put into the page to show the player. The actual audio files are referenced either in the embed code or via an external file that resides on the web server. And, of course, the audio files themselves have to be there!

A search on the internet for 'flash audio players' will return results to a great variety of players. Some play a single audio file, others can handle playlists. Some have simple start, pause and stop buttons, others may have buttons to cycle through the playlist, adjust volume and even adjust the look of the player. Some interesting players to look at can be found at these sites:

- *www.flashmp3player.org/*
- *www.flabell.com/flash/Simple-Flash-Mp3-Player-37*
- *www.varal.org/media/niftyplayer/*

Audio

8

Implementing a content management system

Introduction

A content management system (CMS) is one that focuses on easy content entry and management. That serves as a basic description. In practice, a CMS can usually do more, such as allowing users to join to contribute their content and/or comment on existing content, uploading graphics and serving as a type of membership site.

Although a CMS can be custom designed and programmed, there are available free, open-source platforms that most designers use. The leading two are WordPress and Joomla!. WordPress began as a blogging platform, but its flexibility and support in the way of plugins enables it to do many things. Joomla! also has an extensive number of plugins.

Each product requires you to install it, have a database and learn how to use the administration section (where the site owner is able to handle the tasks of the website). Each product uses templates for the design. There are hundreds to choose from; some free, some not. Creating templates for these products seems to be a joy for designers as the structure of the platforms makes it an easy task.

In this chapter we'll introduce a few platforms but stick with WordPress for examples of what can be done.

What you'll do

Understand the basics of a content management system

Review your needs and pick the appropriate platform

Get an overview of the installation process

See how posts, pages and plugins are used

Get an overview of template customisation

Content management basics

▶

Content is king – an often used expression but still a basic tenet of having a successful website. The purpose of a CMS is to make it easy to input, edit, delete and otherwise manage the content. The site owner or administrator logs into the site and adds new comments in the form of a blog post or a page. Visitors to the site will see this new content and may be able to add their own comments, depending on whether permission has been set up for them to do so.

A CMS is usually built upon a common interest or subject – cooking, politics, sports, etc. These types of systems are for enjoyment, discussion and opinions. Figure 9-1 shows a page from a blog. The CMS is the WordPress platform.

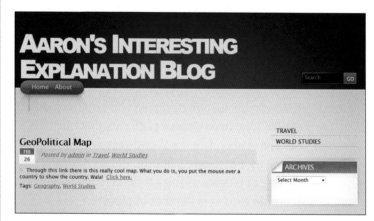

Figure 9-1 A blog entry

Another use could be as a company marketing tool. The content on such a site could be used to introduce new products or to give instructions. There could be an FAQ page, help pages, ways to contact the company and so on.

Some CMSs are meant to get members to sign up to use features or at least to be part of the social network aspect of the site. Figure 9-2 shows a site that is centred around a sports interest and encourages people to become members.

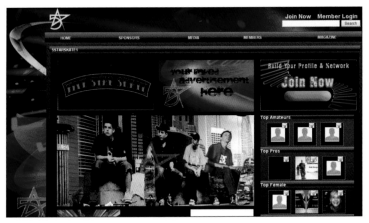

Figure 9-2 A CMS can be focused on having members

The platforms of WordPress, Joomla!, Drupal and others
are integrated systems that are installed and then can be
customised. The ability to customise these systems is a
speciality of web developers. Specifically, some customisation
requires special programming needs, but other changes
site owners may be able to do on their own using the tools
provided in the administration section. Figure 9-3 shows the
admin section for a WordPress site.

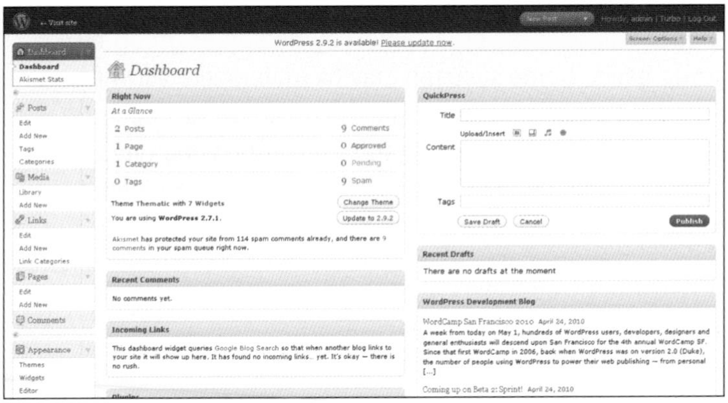

Figure 9-3 The WordPress administration section

When a site has permission for comments to be added to
posts, often spam will make its way in as comments. This can
be a big problem. It can turn people away, clog your system
and reduce your page rankings with the search engines. To
combat this a system should offer a way to fend off spam

9

Content management basics (cont.)

comments. WordPress has the Akismet feature. It captures spam comments and prevents them from being posted. The site owner can review them or if not they are just deleted after a certain amount of time. Figure 9-4 shows a summary of spam caught by Akismet for a given period of time.

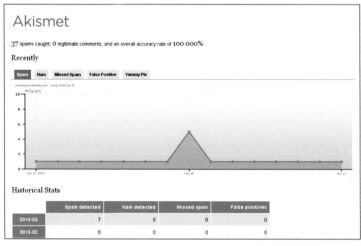

Figure 9-4 Akismet captures WordPress spam

Besides the standard editing features comes the ability to control input access on a person-by-person or group-by-group basis. Some systems may be quite open, allowing anyone to enter content. At the other end of the spectrum, some sites are set up to not allow this. Choosing one over the other depends on the purpose of the site. Do you intend to encourage discussion?

Selecting the correct CMS is not difficult once you have a focused list of what you need it to do. Things to consider are:

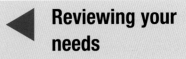
- Is the content mostly or completely originated and/or entered by the site owner/administrator?

- Is the site meant to only display content or also to encourage user discussions?

- Should there be a membership component so people can join and provide their content?

- Should the system provide social networking features (such as ability to share information and send messages)?

- How easy is it to install the software on the website?

This is just a small list of questions. You may have specific needs for which one system may be the best. Research the systems to see what is most useful for you. There is no 'got it all' system – each has its own strengths and weaknesses.

The various platforms have many common functions but also differences – see the table below.

Content management system	Comments
WordPress www.wordpress.org	Can be used for simple blogging or a fully fledged multiple-page site. Posts are the content entries and ability for people to add comments is controllable. Adding pages is what allows the platform to be used fully for a comprehensive site.
Joomla! www.joomla.org	Has nine built-in user groups with varying permissions, from no access to full administrative rights. Has built-in features such as a banner manager and the ability to easily create polls/surveys.

9

Reviewing your needs (cont.)

Content management system	Comments
Drupal *www.drupal.org*	Uses a threaded comment model for content. Also there is a book model. Users can personalise the look of the site. Version control is applied to content updates so a history of changes is available.
Pligg *www.pligg.com*	Works as a social networking-based CMS. Users can join groups that are of common interest. User-posted content can be rated by other users.

The few systems shown in the table are just some of the better known ones; it is not an all-inclusive list. Research the internet to find more. One thing to review is the available addins/plugins/modules. Many developers have contributed functionality to make a given CMS perform a task that is not built in. A few more systems to review are:

Silverstripe	*www.silverstripe.com*
Radiant	*www.radiantcms.org*
ModX	*www.modxcms.com*

Consider how the CMS will be installed. This can be a tedious and confusing process if you are not familiar with databases or adept at using FTP. Some ISPs (internet service providers) now offer automated installations as part of their control panel functions. However, this automation is not available for all CMS applications, usually only WordPress.

On the assumption that your ISP does not provide an automated installation, here are the steps you need to follow to install WordPress.

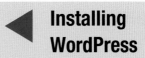

1. Create a database. You need a web hosting account that provides a MySQL database (nearly all accounts do provide them). When you create the database, make note of the database name (something you chose to make the database), the user name, the user password and the database address. The database address might be an IP address, a URL or simply 'localhost'. This depends on how your ISP sets it up.

2. Visit *www.wordpress.org* and download the software. You are first downloading to your computer. Figure 9-5 shows the WordPress website and as you can see there is a button to initiate a download.

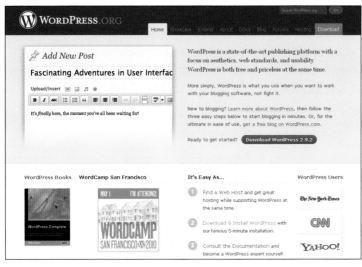

Figure 9-5 The WordPress website

3. A single compressed file is downloaded into a directory of your choice. Extract the contents from the compressed file. WordPress comprises three directories: wp-admin, wp-content and wp-includes. There are several other files, shown in Figure 9-6. Notice that one of them is called wp-config-sample.

Installing WordPress (cont.)

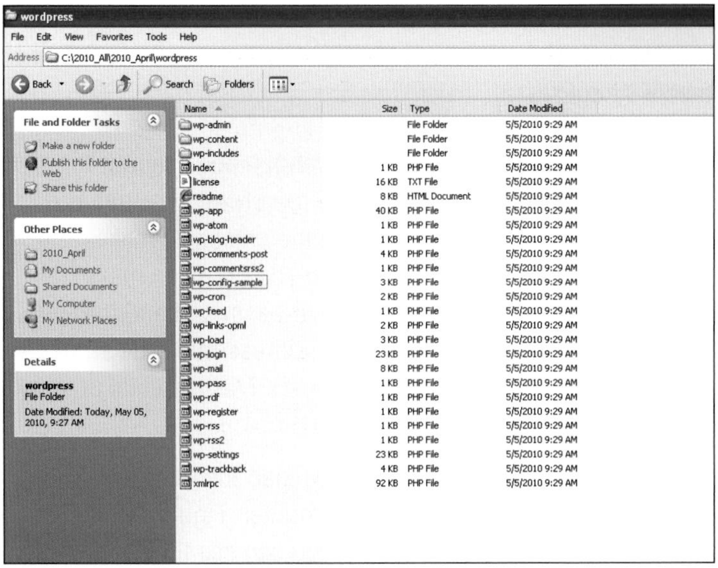

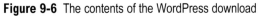

Figure 9-6 The contents of the WordPress download

4. Rename the wp-config-sample.php file as wp-config.php. Open the file in a text editor such as Notepad. In the file are placeholders where you enter the database name, user name, user password and database address. Save the file and close it.

5. FTP all the directories and files to your web server. They can go into the root of the website or into a subfolder.

6. Complete the installation by running the wp-install file within a web browser. Open a browser and navigate to the URL and possible subfolder to which you FTPd the files. Then append /wp-admin/install.php to the URL and run it. For example, if you installed WordPress in the root directory, you should visit: *http://example.com/wp-admin/install.php*.

7. Follow the instructions shown in the browser. If you encounter any problems, visit the WordPress site for help (*www.wordpress.org*). During this process you will be given the password to log into the admin section. Jot it down and DON'T LOSE IT!

When the WordPress installation is complete you will have a basic template at the URL you used. You can keep this template or find others that are more attractive.

Each CMS has its own nomenclature, particularly with regard to what a section of content is called. In Joomla! you create 'articles'. In WordPress you create a 'post'. To do this you go to the admin section and make use of the WYSIWYG editor. See Figure 9-10.

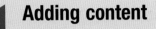
Figure 9-10 Creating a new post

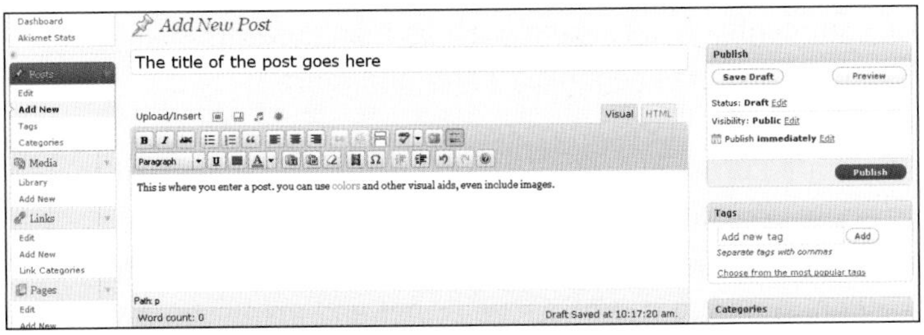

A post is given tags and is categorised. This makes it easy for people to find the post when visiting the site. Posts can be edited or deleted at any time. When a post is visible on the site, visitors may leave comments provided the permission setting to do so is set.

If/when you change to a new theme, no content is lost. The content simply appears in the way that the new theme has it set up with CSS.

Besides posts (which are bits of content that appear on the main page or on the single page), you can create new pages. These become dedicated separate pages and are accessed from links in the sidebar on each page. The ability to add pages is one of the best features for putting WordPress to use as a CMS.

9

Expanding features with plugins

▶

Plugins provide extended functionality. Being an open-source product, WordPress invites developers to create plugins and upload them to the WordPress site. From there site owners can download and install plugins. Plugins provide many types of features and can be found by a search or by category. The categories can be of a WordPress entity such as posts or comments, or for needs such as manipulating images, integrating with Facebook, Twitter and more.

There are currently around 10,000 plugins. This only goes to show how popular the extensibility of WordPress is. Once a plugin is installed it is controllable from the admin section. A plugin can be active or not and many come with additional options. Plugins can be edited in the same way that WordPress files are. Figure 9-11 shows a plugin Ken wrote that provides random quotes about music.

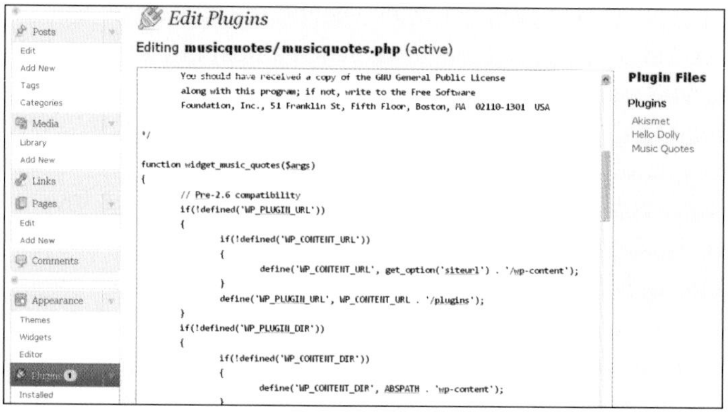

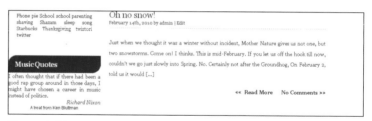

Figure 9-11 A plugin shown in the editing pane

The programming seen in Figure 9-11 may be incomprehensible to you, but if so it is not important since you do not have to know the programming to use a plugin, only for creating one. On the site itself this particular plugin shows up in the sidebar on the left, as in Figure 9-12.

Figure 9-12 A plugin that displays music quotes

Designing and processing forms

Introduction

Forms are the mainstay of how users interact with websites. Seen on most sites, forms take in user input and process it. The type of information that is entered as well as how it is processed is unique to the website. In between these two tasks is form validation.

Validation is used to ensure that the values entered into a form adhere to the type of data that is expected. For example, names, addresses, phone numbers, etc. are validated to ensure that something was entered – at least for the entries that are required (entry is not automatically required). Other types of validation ensure that a selection was made from a mutually exclusive list or from a multiple option list.

Finally, forms are 'submitted' – that is, a form is not processed until (usually) the user clicks the Submit button to send the form for processing. The processing of a form occurs on whichever page the 'action' attribute in the form tag sends the form data to. Forms also have other attributes, a common one being the 'method', which indicates in what manner the data is moved along to the next page.

Forms are comprised of a variety of input types – entry boxes, select lists and more. A very important part of forms is labels. Labels do not accept input; they are used to identify the entries. For example, if you are presented with an entry box that has no labelling, it is not clear what you are supposed to enter. However, if the entry box is preceded by a label that says 'Enter first name', then it is clear what to enter in the box.

Forms can be as simple as a single entry (think of a search box) or more in depth and lengthy, taking many inputs; it all depends on the need.

Processing form data is done with any number of programmable approaches, usually involving the use of a web programming language such as PHP or ASP.Net. Form processing is beyond the scope of this book, but at least knowing how the process works is useful, especially given that you have to identify in the form tag where the processing takes place.

All forms begin with the HTML form tag <form. The word 'form' does not comprise the full tag appearance – along with 'form' must come at least the 'action'. Here is a typical form tag:

```
<form name="new_employee"
action="submit_employee.php"
method="post">
```

i

For your information

The method can be 'post' or 'get'. When submitted using post, the information is sent to the processing page behind the scenes. When get is used, the form data is sent as name-value pairs appended to the processing page URL, for example submit_employee.php?firstname=Ken&lastname=Bluttman. There is no hard and fast rule for using post over get or vice versa. However, post should be used for any sensitive data, such as a password. Post is used far more often than get.

1 Provide an action that the form will take when submitted.

2 Provide a method.

10

Using text boxes

Text boxes (also known as entry boxes) appear as blank areas in which user input is entered – see Figure 10-1. Optional attributes can limit the size of the box and how many characters can be entered into the box. For example, a text box entry might look like this:

```
<input type="text" id="firstname"
name="firstname" size="40"
maxlength="40" />
```

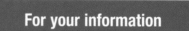

Figure 10-1 A typical web form

1. Start a text box entry by using the <input tag.

2. Give the text box a name and/ or an id. Using both is a good idea since some validation uses id, other uses name and the processing might use either.

3. Optionally, give a size or a maxlength. You can use one without the other.

4. Make sure you close the tag with either a /> or ></input>.

? Did you know?

It's a good idea to limit the amount of data that can be entered into a text box. For example, a value of 40 is more than adequate for a first name.

For your information

Text boxes accept single-line entry. To provide a multiple-line entry box you use the <textarea tag. With this tag you supply the number of rows and columns the box should be.

Tick boxes are used when more than one selection can be made, for example you can tick that you have visited France *and* Spain. Tick boxes appear as squares. Radio buttons are used for *mutual exclusivity*, which means only *one* selection can be made. For example, you can be only male *or* female. Radio buttons appear as circles that you click to select one. Figure 10-2 shows a form with both.

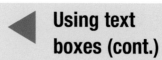
○ **A:** Yoga Nidra, Prana Vidya, 4-day Silence, AHYMS-A: 7/17- 8/1 (15 nights)

○ **B:** Yoga Nidra, Prana Vidya, Spirituality Wknd, 6-day Silence: 7/17- 8/1 (15 nights)

○ **C:** Prana Vidya, Spirituality Wknd, 6-day Silence: 7/19 - 8/1(13 nights)

○ **D:** Prana Vidya, 4-day Silence, AHYMS-A: 7/19 - 8/1 (13 nights)

○ **E:** 10-day Silence, AHMS-A: 7/18- 8/1 (14 nights)

○ **F:** 5-day Silence, AHMS-A: 7/23 - 8/1(9 nights)

- Or -

○ **Personalized Retreat:** Select check-in and check-out dates and the events you wish to attend. The accomodation fee is £80.00 per night:

Check In: July 17 ▾   Check Out: July 18 ▾

☐ **Yoga Nidra**

  ◉ Remove Selection

  ○ Weekend (w/o nights), 7/18: 9 AM - 6 PM & 7/19: 9 AM - 5 PM, by 6/1: £65, after 6/1: £130

  ○ **Or, individual afternoons:**

    ☐ Saturday (Swami Veda only), 7/18: 3 PM – 6 PM, £22

    ☐ Sunday (Swami Veda only), 7/19: 3 PM – 5 PM, £22

☐ **Prana Vidya: Yoga Teacher Workshop**, 7/19-7/24. £164

☐ **Spirituality Weekend**

Figure 10-2 A form with both tick boxes and radio button inputs

10

▶

Tick boxes and radio buttons are both presented in HTML as 'input' types. The way that radio buttons are set up to accept only one option at a time is to name all the options with the same name, but with a different value. This HTML snippet shows how:

Thank you for calling:

```
<input type="radio" id="thankyou"
name="thankyou" value="Y">Yes</input>
   <input type="radio" id="thankyou"
name="thankyou" value="N">No</input>
```

The input type is 'radio'. The name in this example is 'thankyou'. This means that any radio inputs that are named 'thankyou' will operate together to ensure that only one can be selected at a time. The value attribute differentiates the choices – in this example one radio has a value of Y and the other has a value of N (for Yes and No). Yes and No are shown on the form and only one can be selected. Figure 10-3 shows the form.

Greeting		
Thank you for calling:	○ Yes	○ No
Use Dealership Name:	○ Yes	○ No
Used First Name Only:	○ Yes	○ No
Asked "How may I help you?":	○ Yes	○ No
Used proper tone and voice inflections:	○ Yes	○ No

Figure 10-3 Using radio buttons on a form

In this example five sets of radio inputs are used. Each set has a unique name. The name 'thankyou' is applied only to the top row. Each other row has another name that is used for the radio inputs. This allows a Yes or No selection to be made for each row.

Select lists, such as the one in Figure 10-4, are dropdowns from which you can choose a single item.

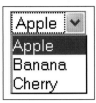

Figure 10-4 A select dropdown list

The HTML for a select is a bit different. Instead of using <input, the dropdown list is set up using the '<select' tag, with a number of <option tags. Each option tag contains a unique value:

```
<select name="fruit">
  <option value="apple">Apple</option>
  <option value="banana">Banana</option>
  <option value="cherry">Cherry</option>
</select>
```

Forms are submitted with a submit button, which uses the input tag:

```
<input type="submit" value="Click Me! />
```

The value of the submit button is what appears on the button, so a value of Click Me! produces a button that says Click Me!

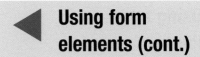

10

Using tables to line up forms

HTML tables give you control over how to line up items on a web page. There is much discussion about their use – that tables should not be used excessively, perhaps not at all. Using HTML div tags is the alternative and modern way to set up forms. However, using div tags for this purpose can take longer and be trickier to implement. As such, many web designers fall back on using tables to line up forms. Both methods are presented here. First is the table approach, shown here in Figure 10-5 as a simple login form.

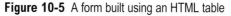

Figure 10-5 A form built using an HTML table

The form elements are placed inside table cells:

```
<form id="f" name="f"
action="checklogin.php" onsubmit="return
checkform(this)" method="post">
<table>
<tr>
 <td style="text-align:right">Enter
Login Name</td>
 <td><input type="text" id="loginname"
name="loginname" size="20" /></td>
</tr>
<tr>
    <td style="text-align:right">Enter
Password</td>
    <td><input type="password"
id="password" name="password" size="16"
/></td>
</tr>
<tr>
    <td colspan="2"> </td>
</tr>
<tr>
```

```
<td> </td><td><input
type="submit" value="Submit" /></td>
</tr>
</table>
</form>
```

In the login form in Figure 10-5, note how the labels (Enter Login Name, Enter Password) are right-aligned. This provides the visual appeal of having elements lining up. Looking through the various form figures so far in this chapter you will see how right-aligned labels provide a uniform look and appeal. The basic way to do this is to apply right alignment to the table cells that hold the labels using the style attribute and inline CSS, like this:

```
<td style="text-align:right">
```

1. Set up form elements in a table by placing the labels in the left cells.

2. Place the actual form inputs in the right cells.

3. Use styling to right-align the labels.

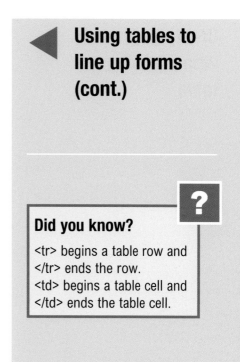

Using tables to line up forms (cont.)

?

Did you know?

<tr> begins a table row and </tr> ends the row.
<td> begins a table cell and </td> ends the table cell.

10

Creating a form without using a table

It's imperative that the labels in a form line up with the proper associated inputs. Tables provide the easy way to do this. Web designers will sometimes eschew this approach and set up a 'tableless' form, using div tags.

This form is created without tables, as in Figure 10-6.

Registration is required. It's easy and free!
Fill out the information below and away you go...

Your first name (1-20 characters):
Your last name (2-20 characters):
Your city (2-30 characters):

Your email address:
Enter your email address again:

A screen name, also is your login (6-16 characters):

Password (6-16 characters):

Submit

Figure 10-6 A tableless form

The underlying HTML contains two div tags. One holds the labels, the other holds the inputs. Their placement next to each other is handled using CSS (which is not shown here); however, see how in this HTML the divs are not mixed together. One div tag is named formlabels and the other is named forminputs:

```
<form id="f1" name="f1"
action="insertregistration.php"
method="post" onsubmit="return
checkform(this)">
<div id="formlabels">
   Your first name (1-20 characters):
<br />
   Your last name (2-20 characters):
<br />
   Your city (2-30 characters):<br />
   Your email address:<br />
   Enter your email address again:
<br /><br />
   A screen name, also is your login
```

```
(6-16 characters):<br /><br />
  Password (6-16 characters):<br />
<br />
</div>
<div id="forminputs">
  <input type="text" id="firstname"
name="firstname" value="" /><br />
  <input type="text" id="lastname"
name="lastname" value="" /><br />
  <input type="text" id="city"
name="city" value="" /><br />
  <input type="text" id="email"
name="email" value="" /><br />
  <input type="text" id="email2"
name="email2" value="" /><br /><br />
  <input type="text" id="loginn"
name="loginn" value="" /><br /><br />
  <input type="password" id="password"
name="password" /><br /><br />
  <input type="submit" value="Submit"
/><br /><br />
</div>
  </form>
```

10

Tabbed forms

▶

When there is a good amount of information to enter into a form, a variation is to create a tabbed form. With this approach a subjective number of tabs can be used, typically a function of the organisation of data being entered.

Figure 10-7 shows an example of a tabbed form. On each tab is a section of the form. The tabs were decided upon based on what data they are used to collect. Since the <form tag encloses all the tabs, all the various entries are considered part of a single form.

Please fill out this employment application.

| Name and Address | Work History | References |

Reference Name 1:
Reference Phone 1:

Reference Name 2:
Reference Phone 2:

Submit

Form 10-7 A form presented in tabs

This approach involves more than one form, but from the user viewpoint it is all part of a single large form, as the information being collected is all related. The technique involves having inputs on a page that when submitted cause another page to appear with more inputs. The new page contains a new form, not a continuation of the first one. What is important is that the information collected in each successive page is not lost. This is accomplished during the processing between pages. As each form/page is submitted, the form values can be:

- written to a database
- stored in session variables
- forwarded to the next page and incorporated as hidden fields
- any or all of the above.

A rather user-friendly technique is to provide forward and back buttons. Instead of a button saying Submit, it would say Next. This foward button operates in the same fashion as the Submit button, in fact it is the Submit button, just with the wording (the value attribute) saying Next instead of Submit. The Back button is handled differently. This is a special input type of button and has a JavaScript routine attached to return the user to the previous page (outside the scope of this book). It's especially helpful to fill up the form on the previous page with the previously entered values should the user click the Back button. This is possible because the values were stored with one or more of the above methods. Figure 10-8 shows a form section with a Back and a Next button.

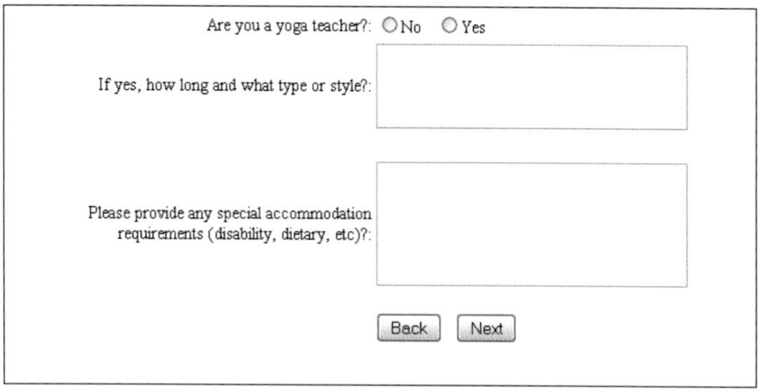

?

Did you know?

Hidden fields are a type of form input that hold a value and do not appear on the page. However, the value is 'visible' to the processing of the form. Hidden fields are used to carry along information necessary for the final form processing.

Figure 10-8 Using Next and Back buttons for multi-page forms

Validating form input

For your information

See *Brilliant JavaScript* by Ken Bluttman (Prentice Hall, 2009) to learn the details of validation.

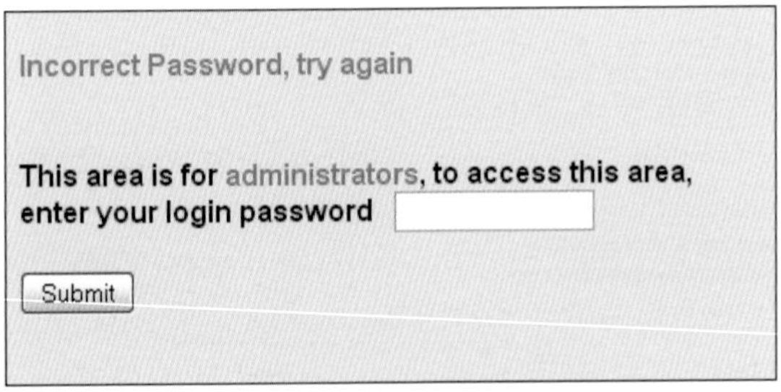

It's good practice to validate the entries made in a form. There is a variety of reasons:

1. Ensure the correct type of entry was made.

2. Ensure the entry followed a necessary structure.

3. Simply ensure that an entry was made.

4. Check for improper words or values.

For example, if you want a field to be required, you check that the entry box (or radio buttons, etc.) is not blank. Or if age is entered you should never see a value less than 1 or greater than perhaps 110.

Validation is performed in two ways. Either one is enough, although using both is best in case one misses something. The two types are JavaScript and custom testing during the form processing.

JavaScript is unique in that it occurs in the person's browser – local to the computer and not at the web server. JavaScript is great, powerful and flexible, but there is one catch: it can be turned off. That is why you should also have validation done during the processing of the form data. Remember, this is done with a web server language and, if something does not validate, the coding can redisplay the page with the form. Of course, some type of message is necessary so the person can understand something didn't go as planned. Figure 10-9 shows a form that was submitted and redisplayed with the appropriate error message.

Incorrect Password, try again

This area is for administrators, to access this area, enter your login password

Submit

Figure 10-9 Providing an alert that the entry was invalid

Form entry must be stored or acted upon – otherwise there is no point in collecting it.

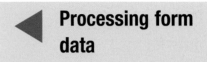

The Action attribute of the form tag indicates the page that will work with the entered data. The action may be as simple as storing the data or as sophisticated as the requirements call for. After a form is submitted the user must be presented with something – a thank you, a result or whatever is called for.

The called action page can be one that displays the result or message or can be an intermediate page that simply processes and then redirects at the end. In Figure 10-10, the submitted form on the lower left can have an action that calls the next visible page – the A path in the diagram. Or the action can call an unseen page, shown here as having the submitted form following the B path.

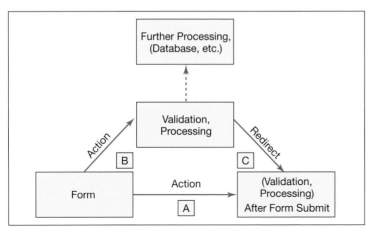

Figure 10-10 Form processing

Validation and processing can occur in either situation. In the direct path, A, the receiving page can validate and process and display the new page in a way that is based on what is submitted. This requires that the page is built with a web programming language, such as PHP. Following the B path is not much different; it depends on what makes sense for the actual application. If a path such as B is taken, then the processing page would end with a redirect to the next page the user should see – the one on the lower right.

10

Processing form data (cont.)

Any number of things can be accomplished when processing the form. Typical applications are registrations, sending emails, providing answers (a calculator type of application) or requesting information.

Designing for different platforms, browsers and screen resolutions

11

Introduction

Thanks to the web design standards, especially in CSS and HTML, you have a great deal of control over how your site appears and functions on a variety of computer systems.

However, due to variations in operating systems, monitors, screen resolutions, web browsers and even user-defined settings, you can never be completely certain that your site looks and performs the same on other people's systems as it does on yours. Pages that pop up quickly on your computer can take forever to load over a slower connection. A deep blue background on your screen may look black on someone else's computer. The fonts and type sizes you carefully chose may be completely different when viewed in another browser.

In some cases, the only way to respond to these variations is to accept them. For example, if a user chooses to disable graphics in his browser so pages load faster, that choice is out of your control. However, you can take steps to make your design more flexible and improve your site's performance for a majority of your visitors. In this chapter, we reveal techniques for making your site more universally accessible and visually appealing.

What you'll do

Accommodate different operating systems

Design for differences in monitors and screen resolutions

Design for different web browsers

Accommodate different user preferences

Account for slow internet connections

Deal with the mobile web

Accommodate users with disabilities

Accommodating different operating systems ▶

To accommodate differences among operating systems, do the following:

1 Use common, web-safe fonts, such as those in Figure 11-1. List alternative fonts in case the first choice is unavailable. This is done in the CSS.

2 Make sure the required media player is available for both Windows and Mac OS. See Figure 11-2.

3 Remain flexible – you can't control everything.

Timesaver tip

You can test your site in various operating system/browser combinations at BrowserShots (*http://browsershots.org*) or BrowserCam (*www.browsercam.com*).

See also

For more about fonts and font attributes, turn to Chapter 6 'Designing the text elements'.

Whether you are designing websites on a Windows-based PC or using Mac OS or Linux, consider the fact that people visiting your site may be using a different operating system. This could affect the appearance or function of your site.

Operating systems can differ in the following ways:

Font display: the available fonts and appearance of identical fonts can vary depending on the operating system.

Media players: availability of some players or versions of players may differ among operating systems.

Form objects: dropdown menus, scrolling lists and other form objects may appear differently in different operating systems.

Arial Black	Arial Narrow
Arial	Century Gothic
COPPERPLATE GOTHIC LIGHT	Courier New
Georgia	Gill Sans
Lucida Console	Lucida Sans Unicode
Palatino Linotype	Tahoma
Times New Roman	Trebuchet MS
Verdana	

Figure 11-1 Use web-safe fonts

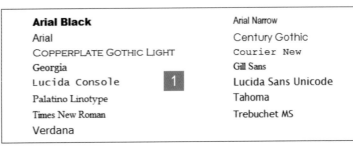

Figure 11.2 Media player available for different operating systems

For your information ⓘ

Windows claims about 92% of the market, while Mac OS claims about 5% and Linux about 1%. Mobile device interfaces, including iPhone, are quickly expanding their market share.

Screen sizes and resolutions vary more than ever with the introduction of wide-screen monitors and smaller netbook computers. In addition, visitors can resize their browser windows to whatever size they desire.

To accommodate possible differences in monitors and screen resolutions, make your design flexible and arrange content so that the most important items appear in the upper left portion of your pages, as in Figure 11-3.

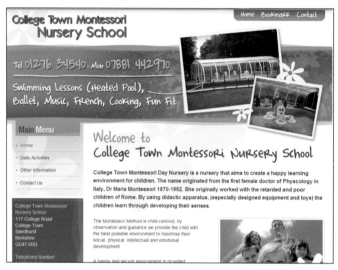

Figure 11-3 Position the most important elements in the upper left of the page

With a fixed-width layout, you specify the precise width of each column in pixels, as in Figure 11-4.

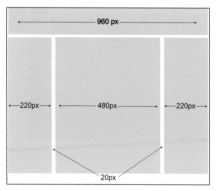

Figure 11-4 Schematic of a fixed-width layout

ⓘ
For your information

As of December 2009, market share for monitor resolutions on the web was broken down as follows:

1024 × 768 – 28%

1280 × 800 – 20%

1280 × 1024 – 11%

1440 × 900 – 9%

1680 × 1050 – 5.5%

1366 × 768 – 3.5%

800 × 600 – 3%

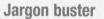

Jargon buster

Fixed-width layout: Keeps the page width the same regardless of the width of the display area, ensuring the page looks the same on all displays. Users with smaller screens may need to scroll left or right to view the entire page.

Designing for differences in monitors and screen resolutions (cont.)

Jargon buster

Fluid layout: Resizes columns and rewraps text to fit the width of the page inside the display area.

For your information

You can use fixed-width, fluid and elastic layouts in different areas on your site or even in different areas on the same page.

With a fluid layout, you specifiy column widths as percentages, as in Figure 11-5.

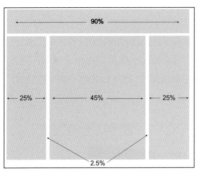

Figure 11-5 Schematic of a fluid layout

If you have a navigation bar on the left, consider assigning it a fixed width and setting the width property for the other column(s) to 'auto', as in Figure 11-6.

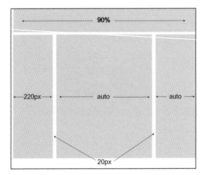

Figure 11-6 Schematic of a fluid layout with one column of fixed width

Important !

When creating an elastic layout, use the CSS max-width property to specify a maximum width of 100% for the body tag. This prevents the page width from exceeding the width of the browser window.

With an elastic layout, such as the one in Figures 11-7 and 11-8, you specify column widths in 'em' units, which adjusts the size of the column to the size of the text. If a user overrides your font setting to use a larger or smaller font, your column widths adjust accordingly.

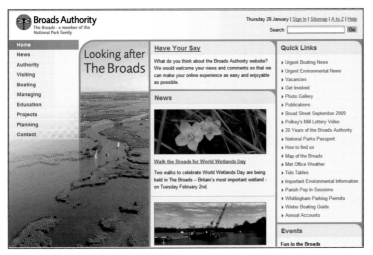

Figure 11-7 Elastic layout with small text

Jargon buster

Elastic layout: Resizes columns to accommodate any changes in text size, so line breaks and text wrapping remain unchanged. Elastic layouts tend to be the most flexible.

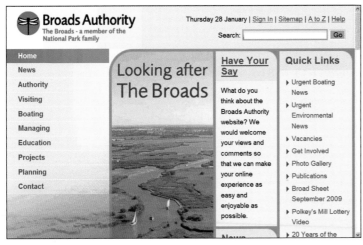

Figure 11-8 Elastic layout with large text

Designing for differences in monitors and screen resolutions (cont.)

To create an elastic layout, specify the initial font size in the <body> tag as a percentage (see Figure 11-9) and all other font sizes and measurements in the em unit, so that the browser can scale everything on the page, including column widths when the user zooms in or out.

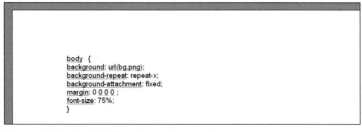

Figure 11-9 Set initial font size in the <body> tag to a percentage

Set column widths in ems (see Figure 11-10) so that they adjust to accommodate changes in text size.

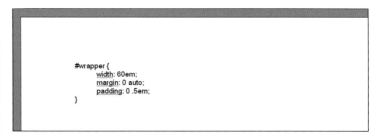

Figure 11-10 CSS column widths in ems

Most web browsers are standards compliant, so as long as you adhere to the current CSS and HTML standards, you don't need to worry too much about differences among browsers. However, you should always check your website's appearance and functionality in the top three web browsers: Internet Explorer, Firefox and Chrome. (Safari and Opera may also be considered in the upper tier.)

Proper HTML coding (Figure 11-11) and use of CSS (Figure 11-12) ensures the most universal support among standards-compliant browsers.

```
<html>
<body>

<h1>My First Heading</h1>

<p>My first paragraph.</p>

</body>
</html>
```

Figure 11-11 An example of proper HTML format

```
blockquote {
        width: 60%;
        margin: 0 auto;
        font-style: italic;
        border-left: 2px solid #2683AE;
        padding-left: 1em;
}
```

Figure 11-12 An example of sample CSS

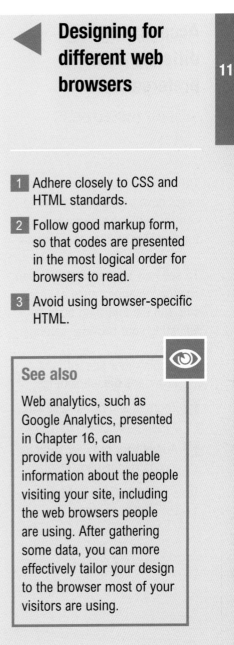

1 Adhere closely to CSS and HTML standards.

2 Follow good markup form, so that codes are presented in the most logical order for browsers to read.

3 Avoid using browser-specific HTML.

See also

Web analytics, such as Google Analytics, presented in Chapter 16, can provide you with valuable information about the people visiting your site, including the web browsers people are using. After gathering some data, you can more effectively tailor your design to the browser most of your visitors are using.

Accommodating different user preferences

Through their web browsers, users have a great deal of control over the appearance and functionality of sites they access.

To see how user preferences can change the appearance of your site, run the following tests by adjusting your browser settings:

1. Display your site with the browser's default settings.
2. Zoom in and out to test your site for changes in font size.
3. Adjust your browser settings to control the page display.

Take a look at Figures 11-13 to 11-15.

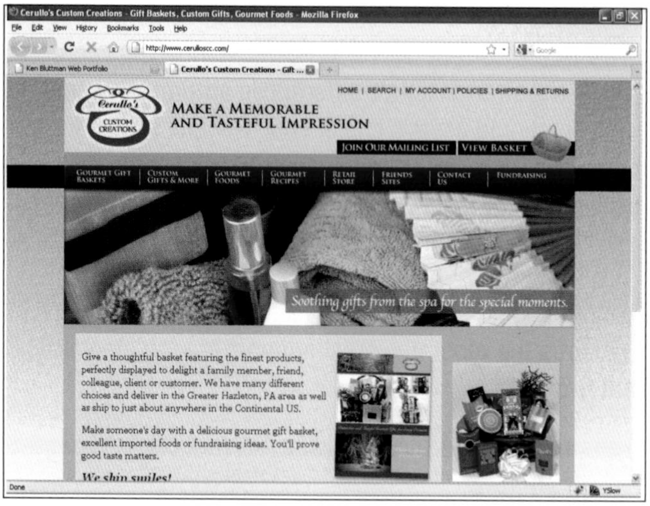

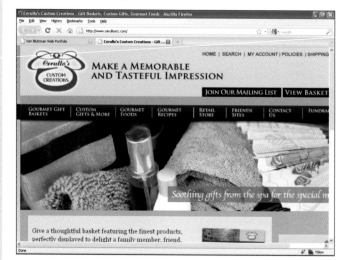

Figure 11-13 The original site

Figure 11-14 With zoomed-in text

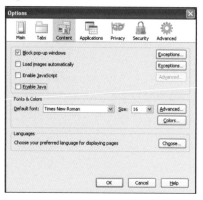

Figure 11-15 Mozilla Firefox options

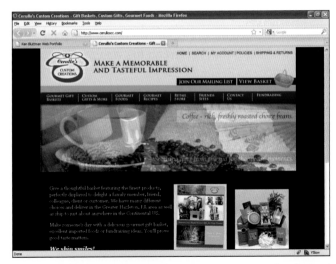

Figure 11-16 Background and foreground colours can be changed around

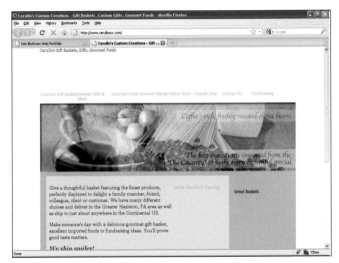

Figure 11-17 A site without images displayed

4 Try changing the foreground and background colours. If you use light text on a dark background, see how dark text on a white background looks. See Figure 11-16.

5 Turn off image display, as in Figure 11-17.

6 Disable Java and Javascript.

7 Turn off popup windows.

8 Try using your site without any objects that require added plugin functionality, such as Flash.

For your information

You may decide not to change anything on your site based on the results of your test, but be aware that changes in user preferences can significantly affect the appearance and perhaps even the functionality of your site.

Accounting for slow internet connections

Just because web pages appear instantly on your computer does not mean they will be so responsive on other people's computers, especially if they're surfing the web over a slow internet connection, as in Figure 11-18.

Unless you know your audience is comprised almost entirely of broadband internet users, do everything possible to streamline your pages so that they load more quickly.

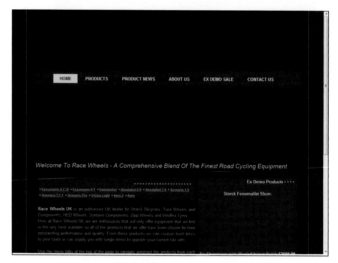

Figure 11-18 A partially loaded page can drive visitors away

See also

See Chapter 12, 'Designing for speed' for details on how to design your website for speed.

More and more internet users are accessing the web by way of mobile devices, including mobile phones, BlackBerries and iPhones, with tiny screens and limited navigation. A standard website may look terrible when displayed on such a tiny screen and may lack a great deal of functionality. Look at Figures 11-19 and 11-20 to see the difference when viewing a site on a mobile device.

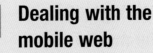

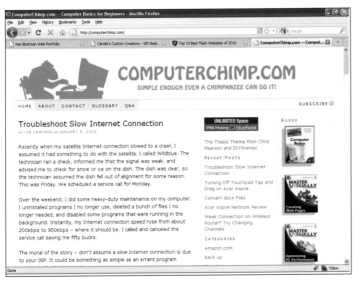

Figure 11-19 The standard website

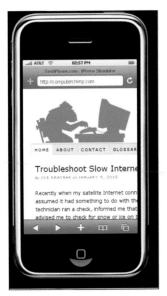

Figure 11-20 The same site displayed on a mobile device

Dealing with the mobile web (cont.)

1. Create an alternative website using XHTML-MP – see Figure 11-21.
2. Provide the content and functionality mobile users will want, as in Figure 11-22.

Important

When designing for the mobile web, streamline your design in content, appearance and functionality. Keep it simple.

When designing for the mobile web, consider the following factors:

Speed: mobile devices may have limited bandwidth.

Cost: users may pay per megabyte for downloading content. Hence, they may be reluctant to revisit a content-heavy site using their mobile device.

Screen sizes: these may vary, but they are all small, ranging in size from about 128px square to about 320 × 480px, and scrolling horizontally may be difficult.

```
<?xml version="1.0" encoding="UTF-8"?>
  <!DOCTYPE html PUBLIC "-//W3C//DTD XHTML 1.0 Transitional//EN"
        "http://www.w3.org/TR/xhtml1/DTD/xhtml1-transitional.dtd">
  <html xmlns="http://www.w3.org/1999/xhtml">

  (Your XHTML page contents goes here - we'll cover this next.)

  </html>
```

Figure 11-21 Sample XHTML-MP markup

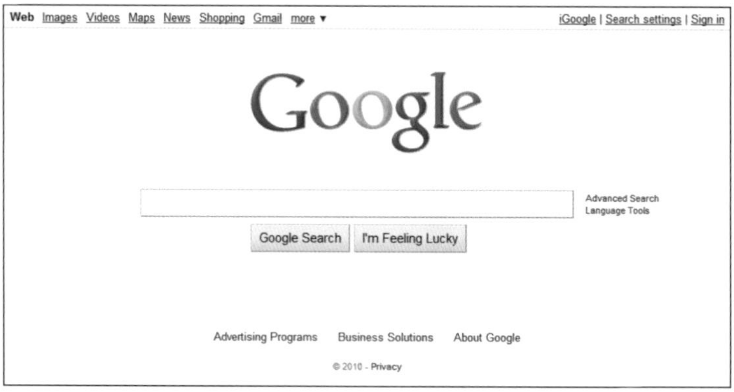

Figure 11-22 The resulting site shown in the web browser

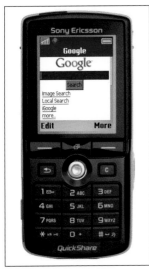

Figure 11-23 The resulting site shown on a mobile device

For your information

You could use a single domain for both your standard and mobile sites and implement user detection so that the server decides which pages to deliver to visitors based on their device and browser. However, this is quite complicated and beyond the scope of this book.

Also, locating both sites on the same server prevents mobile users from accessing your standard site for more information and increased functionality if they choose to do so.

3 Host the site on a subdomain, such as *m.yourdomain.com* or *mobile.yourdomain.com*. Figure 11-23 shows the site on a mobile device.

4 Validate your XHTML-MP markup at *validator.w3.org/mobile*.

5 Test your mobile website online in simulators for various phones.

Timesaver tip

At BrowserCam (*www.browsercam.com*) you can test your mobile website on a variety of mobile devices.

Accommodating users with disabilities ▶

You can accommodate users with disabilities by doing the following:

1. Specify font sizes as percentages, so browsers can zoom in on text.
2. Include alternative text for any and all images.
3. Provide transcripts for podcasts and other audio content.
4. Make your site easy to navigate with either a mouse or a keyboard.
5. Present content as simply and clearly as possible.

Users with disabilities should have equal access to the web, so your website should accommodate users with impaired hearing, vision, mobility or cognitive functioning:

Impaired vision: visitors with impaired or no vision may access your site using a special device, such as a screen reader, Braille reader or screen magnifier, or by using browser functions to zoom in or have the text read to them.

Impaired hearing: if your site includes any auditory components, such as video with sound, podcasts or music, those with impaired hearing may be unable to access that content.

Impaired mobility: users with impaired mobility may use something other than a mouse to navigate your site – perhaps a keyboard, foot pedal, joystick or sip-and-puff control.

Cognitive impairment: this includes attention deficit and limitations in reading comprehension and retention and problem solving.

Designing for speed

Introduction

People who surf the web have zero patience. If a page takes more than a couple of seconds to load, most users click the Back button and try the next link on the list. To keep people from losing patience with your site, optimise your site and all pages on it to load as quickly as possible.

In addition to increasing the speed of your site, optimisation strategies can conserve valuable system resources on your server. Smaller files conserve storage space, while pages that load more efficiently reduce CPU usage, especially on high-traffic sites.

In this chapter, we show you how to test pages to determine how long they take to load, identify issues that may be slowing down your site, and optimise your site and your web pages to load more quickly.

What you'll do

Test web page loading times

Identify bottlenecks

Reduce HTTP requests

Reduce image file sizes

Specify image dimensions

Use CSS sprites

Create an image map

Add an HTTP Expires header

Cache CMS-generated pages

Gzip components

Move CSS to beginning and JavaScript to end

Streamline CSS

Streamline JavaScript

Minimise DNS lookups

Testing web page loading times

1. Use your web browser to go to *http://tools.pingdom.com* – see Figure 12-1.

2. Click in the URL box and type the address of the page you want to test.

3. Click the Test now button.

4. Note the time required to load each page object.

5. Scroll down for a summary of the results, including the total time required to load the page, as shown in Figure 12-2.

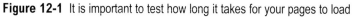

Figure 12-1 It is important to test how long it takes for your pages to load

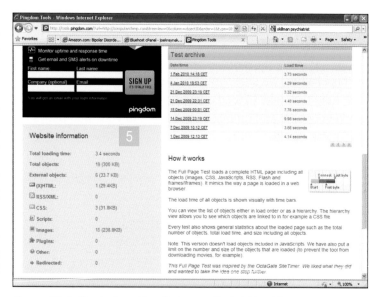

Figure 12-2 The test results will give you the total load time

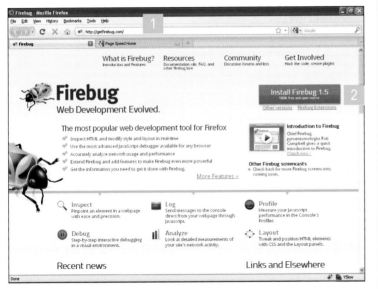

Figure 12-3 Install the Firebug plugin for Firefox

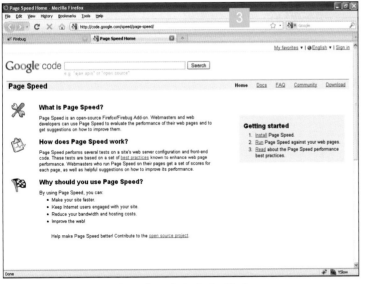

Figure 12-4 Install the Page Speed plugin for Firefox

1 Run Mozilla Firefox – see Figure 12-3.

2 Go to *http://getfirebug.com* and download and install the Firebug plugin for Firefox.

3 Go to *http://code.google.com/ speed/page-speed/* (see Figure 12-4) and install the Page Speed plugin for Firefox.

ⓘ

For your information

Google is not the only company that offers a page speed analyser for Firefox. Yahoo! offers a plugin called YSlow, which functions in much the same way. You can use either or both to test your pages, but they both require Mozilla Firefox and Firebug. You can find the YSlow plugin at *http://developer.yahoo.com/ yslow/*.

Identifying bottlenecks (cont.)

4 Open the page you want to test in the Firefox browser, as in Figure 12-5.

5 Click Tools, Firebug, Open Firebug.

6 Click the Page Speed tab.

7 Click Analyze Performance.

8 Note the possible bottlenecks marked with red warnings and yellow cautions, illustrated in Figure 12-6.

9 Click the plus sign next to an item for more information.

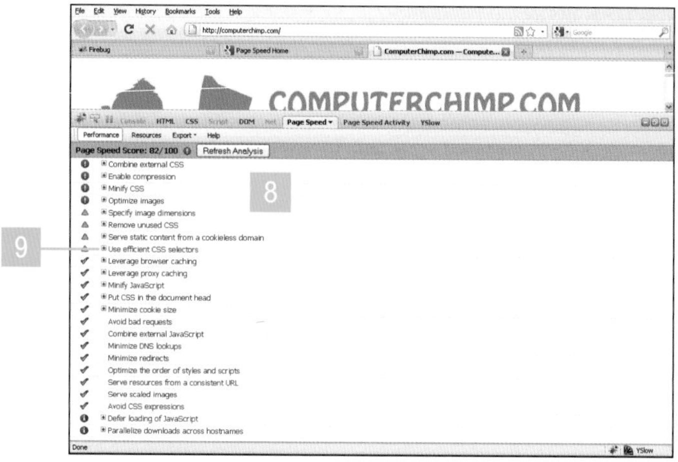

Timesaver tip

You can increase the size of the Firebug panel by dragging the top of the Firebug menu bar upwards.

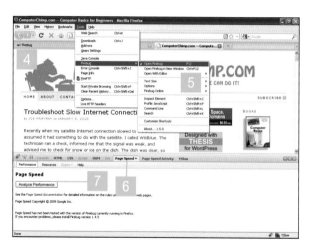

Figure 12-5 Use Page Speed to analyse performance and identify bottlenecks

Figure 12-6 Red warnings and yellow cautions indicate possible bottlenecks

For your information

Not all items marked with warnings or cautions are items you need to fix. For example, under Enable Compression, Page Speed may display a few items that are not being compressed even though Gzip compression is working well on your site.

Fix what you can, but don't become obsessed over items you are unable to fix.

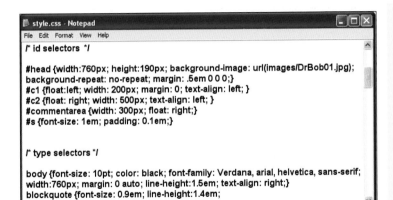

Figure 12-7 Combine all CSS into a single stylesheet

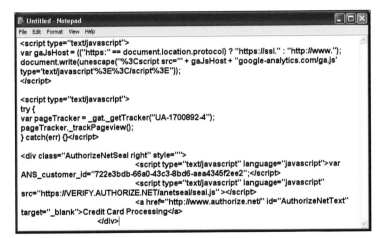

Figure 12-8 Combine all scripts into a single script

Reducing HTTP requests

1　Combine all CSS into a single stylesheet, when possible. See Figure 12-7 for an example.

2　Combine all scripts into a single script, when possible. See Figure 12-8.

12

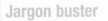

Jargon buster

HTTP request: A call from the browser to your web server for an object it requires to render a web page.

CSS sprites: A technique for combining multiple small background images into a single image and using CSS to reference the small images by location. This can significantly reduce the number of HTTP requests because the browser loads a single image.

Designing for speed 203

Reducing HTTP requests (cont.)

3 Combine background images using CSS sprites, as in Figure 12-9.

4 Use image maps, where possible, instead of numerous smaller images. See Figure 12-10.

See also

For more about CSS sprites, see 'Using CSS sprites' later in this chapter.

For more about using image maps, see 'Creating an image map' later in this chapter.

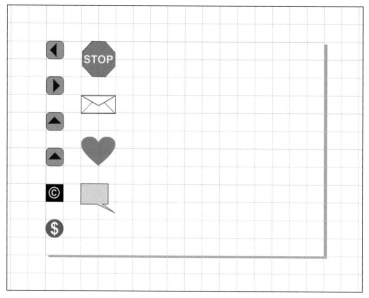

Figure 12-9 Combine background images with CSS sprites

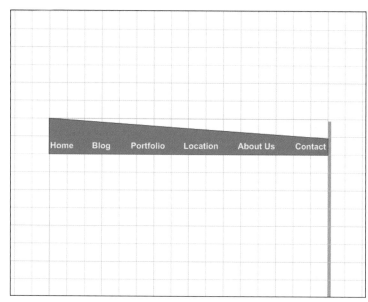

Figure 12-10 Make use of image maps

Reducing image file sizes

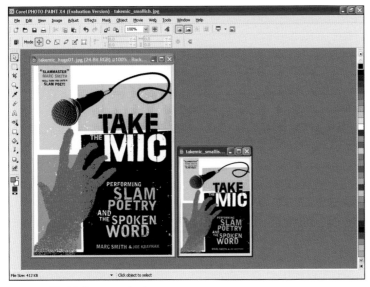

Figure 12-11 Image reduction

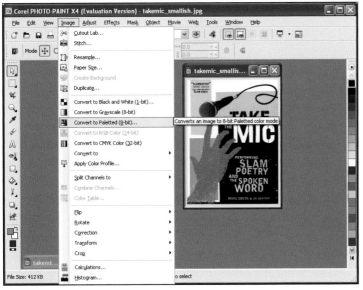

Figure 12-12 Colour reduction

1 Reduce the size (dimensions) of the image – see Figure 12-11.

2 Reduce the number of colours – see Figure 12-12.

12

For your information

The JPEG (JPG) format is usually best for photos and images with greater detail. GIF and PNG formats are better for images that use only a few well-defined colours, such as buttons and logos.

Reducing image file sizes (cont.)

3 Increase the compression percentage – see Figure 12-13.

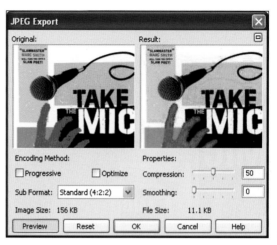

Figure 12-13 Increase compression percentage

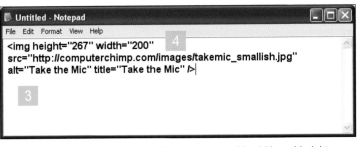

Figure 12-14 Note the image's dimensions

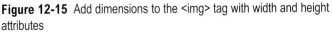

Figure 12-15 Add dimensions to the <img> tag with width and height attributes

Did you know?

If you are using the same image at different sizes, upload the largest version of the image you need and then scale the image for the smaller versions – setting smaller dimensions. If you are using the smaller version of an image exclusively, reduce the image size rather than merely scaling it down.

Specifying image dimensions

1 Open the image in a graphics program, such as the one shown in Figure 12-14.

2 Note the image's height and width in pixels.

3 Insert an <img> tag where you want the image to appear, as in Figure 12-15.

4 Specify the image's height and width attributes.

Timesaver tip

If you insert your images using a CMS or blogging platform, it automatically inserts height and width attributes for the image. However, if you change the image size later, make sure you edit the image attributes – the CMS or blogging platform may not adjust the attributes for you.

Using CSS sprites

1 Create your sprite, positioning the upper left corner of each image on the point where two gridlines intersect, as in Figure 12-16.

2 Identify the height and width of each image.

3 Calculate how far the image must move up and to the left for its upper left corner to be at point 0X,0Y.

4 Create a 1px-by-1px transparent gif image – see Figure 12-17.

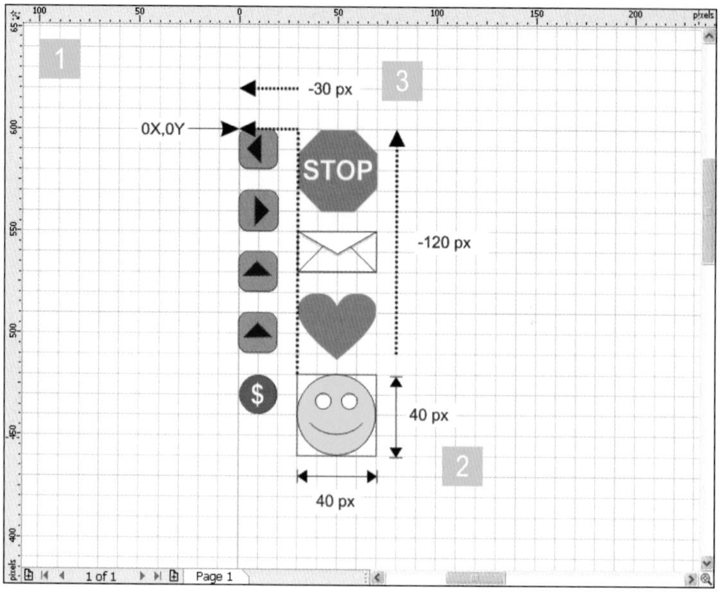

Figure 12-16 Create a CSS sprite by combining multiple images into a single image

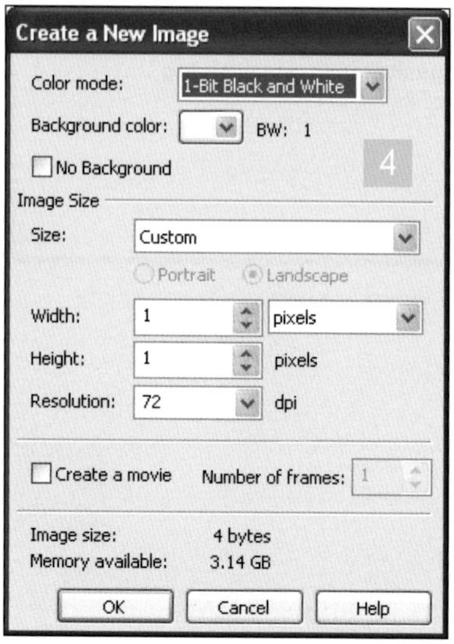

Figure 12-17 Create a transparent gif image 1px by 1px

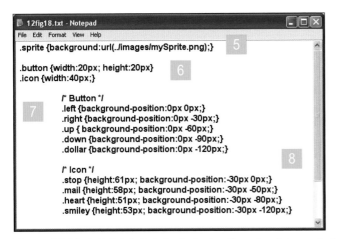

Figure 12-18 Add details to indicate the location of each image in the sprite

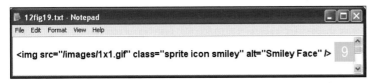

Figure 12-19 Define where you want images displayed on the page

Timesaver tip

SpriteMe (*http://spriteme.org*) offers a utility that can create sprites from existing background images on your site and generate the necessary CSS for you.

5 Create a CSS class called 'sprite' that loads the sprite, as in Figure 12-18.

6 Create a class for each category of images with a shared dimension – width or height.

7 Create a class for each image, including any necessary height or width attributes.

8 Use the background-position property to specify the number of pixels each image needs to shift up and to the left.

9 Use HTML <img> tags along with the CSS classes you have created to load images where you want them displayed on your page – see Figure 12-19.

Creating an image map

1 Identify coordinates on the image that define areas you want to be clickable – see Figure 12-20.

2 Insert <map> opening and closing tags where you want the image map to appear, including map name and id attributes – see Figure 12-21.

3 Add <area> tags to specify the areas of the image that will be clickable and the page each clickable area will open.

4 Insert an <img> tag after the closing map tag to insert the image and include a usemap attribute that references the map's id.

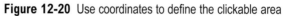

Figure 12-20 Use coordinates to define the clickable area

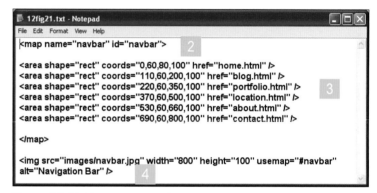

Figure 12-21 Use tags to specify clickable areas

Coordinates can define areas of different shapes:

x1, y1, x2, y2 for a rectangular area.

x, y, radius to specify a circular area with its centre at x, y.

x1, y1, x2, y2, x3, y3 ... to specify a polygon of any number of sides.

The Expires header tells web browsers how long to store objects in their cache before refreshing those objects. You typically set expiration dates for images, CSS files and scripts, so that browsers do not need to download these items again during recent return visits to the site.

A typical Expires header in a .htaccess file is shown in Figure 12-22.

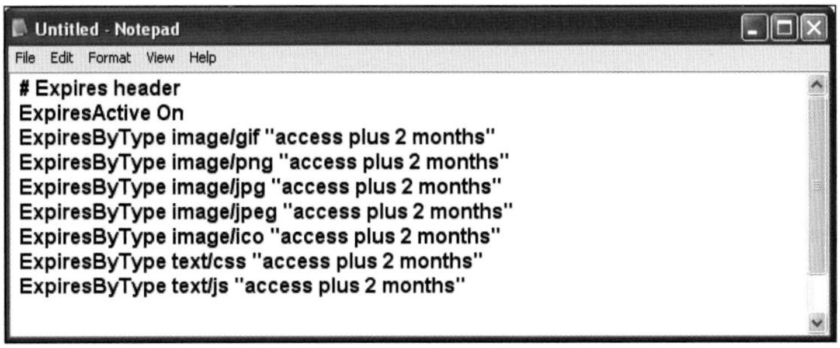

```
# Expires header
ExpiresActive On
ExpiresByType image/gif "access plus 2 months"
ExpiresByType image/png "access plus 2 months"
ExpiresByType image/jpg "access plus 2 months"
ExpiresByType image/jpeg "access plus 2 months"
ExpiresByType image/ico "access plus 2 months"
ExpiresByType text/css "access plus 2 months"
ExpiresByType text/js "access plus 2 months"
```

Figure 12-22 A typical Expires header in a .htaccess file

Adding an HTTP Expires header

1 Create or open the .htaccess file on your web server.

2 Add an Expires or Cache-Control header to specify the expiration of cached objects.

3 Save the .htaccess file.

Did you know?

The Expires or Cache-Control header varies depending on the server the web hosting service uses.

Timesaver tip

To view the HTTP headers, use the Live HTTP Headers plugin for Mozilla Firefox. This allows you to see whether your Expires header is being sent to browsers. You can download the plugin at *http://addons.mozilla.org*.

For your information

Set expiration dates for at least one month. You can set even longer dates for objects you are sure will not change for quite a while.

Did you know?

Your browser's options probably provide control over the cache. You could turn caching off or change the size of the cache to 0. Either of these actions will prevent caching.

Caching CMS-generated pages

When a visitor arrives at a site built on a blogging platform or content management system, database queries assemble the objects that comprise the page and then deliver it to the visitor's browser. This takes extra time.

A caching plugin stores a copy of the page after it has been assembled and serves up the static copy instead of having to build the page every time it is requested. This can speed up web page loading times considerably.

1 Install a caching plugin, as in Figure 12-23.

2 Enable caching.

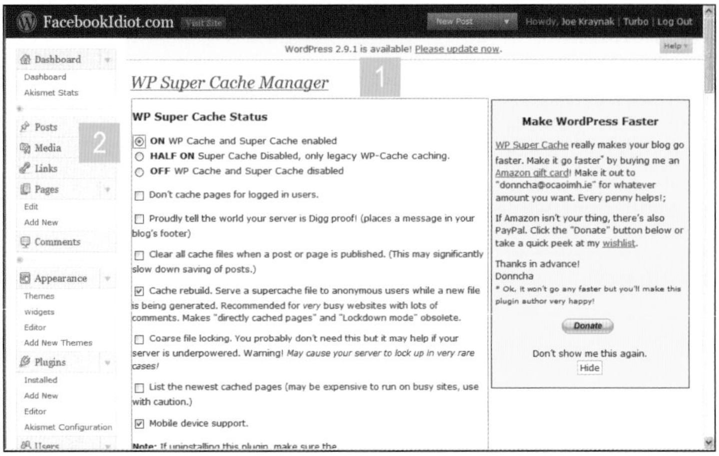

Timesaver tip

One of the best caching programs for WordPress is WP Super Cache, shown here.

Joomla! includes a System Cache Plugin. All you need to do is enable the plugin.

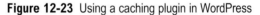

Figure 12-23 Using a caching plugin in WordPress

Did you know?

Whenever you're configuring your site, clear the cache and disable the caching plugin. Otherwise, some or all of your changes may not appear immediately on your site. In other words, you may be looking at older, cached versions of your pages.

Almost all web browsers support Gzip compression, which can significantly reduce the size of data transfers and response times. First, test your site to determine whether your web server is already sending compressed data.

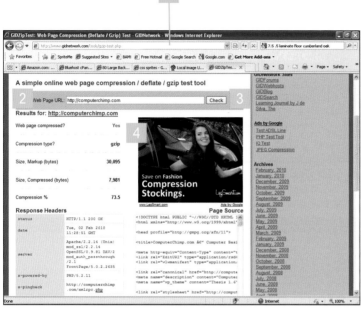

Figure 12-24 Testing for Gzip compression

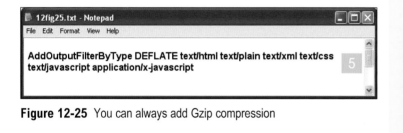

Figure 12-25 You can always add Gzip compression

Did you know?

Always back up the .htaccess file before editing it. Any errors in this file could render your site inaccessible. If this occurs, replace the edited file with your backup version.

Gzipping components

1 Point your web browser to *www.gidnetwork.com/tools/gzip-test.php*, shown in Figure 12-24.

2 Enter the address of the site you want to test for Gzip compression.

3 Click Check.

4 Note the result.

5 If your site shows it is not using Gzip compression, add the DEFLATE command to your .htaccess file, as shown in Figure 12-25.

For your information

Google Page Speed also tests for Gzip compression and displays a list of components not being compressed.

Moving CSS to beginning and JavaScript to end

1. Move any CSS to the beginning of your web pages, as in Figure 12-26.
2. Move any JavaScript to the end of your web pages, as in Figure 12-27.

For your information

By loading CSS first, the browser is able to render pages more quickly. Loading JavaScript enables visitors to view the page while the sometimes time-consuming JavaScript continues to load in the background.

```
<!DOCTYPE html PUBLIC "-//W3C//DTD XHTML 1.0
 Strict//EN" "http://www.w3.org/TR/xhtml1/DTD/xhtml1-strict.dtd">
<html xmlns="http://www.w3.org/1999/xhtml" dir="ltr" lang="en-US">

<head profile="http://gmpg.org/xfn/11">

<title>ComputerChimp.com — Computer Basics for Beginners</title>

<meta http-equiv="Content-Type" content="text/html; charset=UTF-8" />
<link rel="EditURI" type="application/rsd+xml" title="RSD"
 href="http://computerchimp.com/xmlrpc.php?rsd" />
<link rel="wlwmanifest" type="application/wlwmanifest+xml"
 href="http://computerchimp.com/wp-includes/wlwmanifest.xml" />

<link rel="canonical" href="http://computerchimp.com/" />
<meta name="description" content="Computer Basics for Beginners" />
<meta name="wp_theme" content="Thesis 1.6" />

<link rel="stylesheet" href="http://computerchimp.com/wp-
 content/themes/thesis_16/style.css?010410-174658" type="text/css" media="screen,
 projection" />
<link rel="stylesheet" href="http://computerchimp.com/wp-
 content/themes/thesis_16/custom/layout.css?010410-174732" type="text/css"
 media="screen, projection" />
<!--[if lte IE 7]><link rel="stylesheet" href="http://computerchimp.com/wp-
 content/themes/thesis_16/lib/css/ie.css?010410-174927" type="text/css"
 media="screen, projection" /><![endif]-->
<link rel="stylesheet" href="http://computerchimp.com/wp-
 content/themes/thesis_16/custom/custom.css?010410-174723" type="text/css"
 media="screen, projection" />

```

Figure 12-26 Position CSS at the beginning of web pages

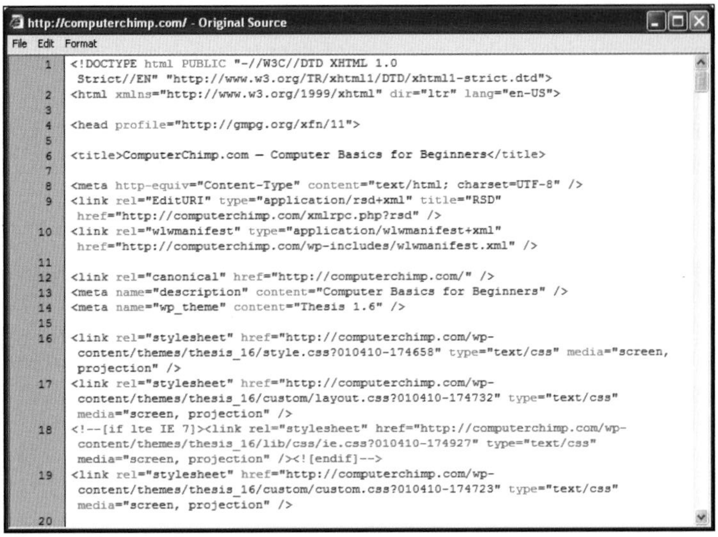

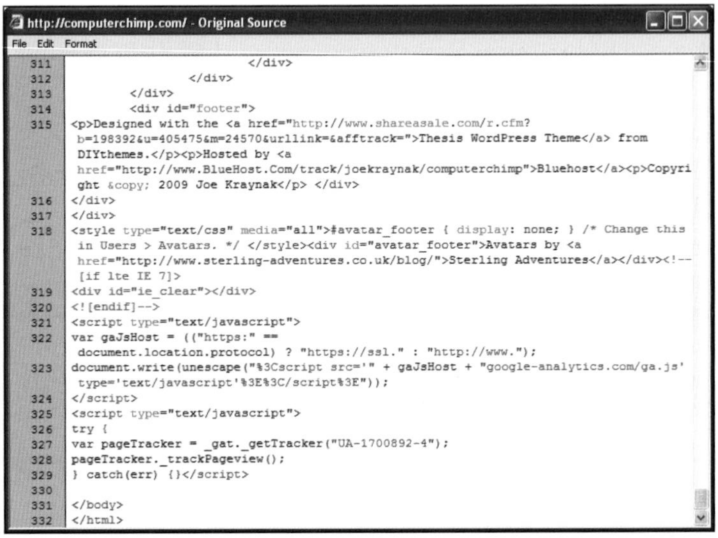


```
                        </div>
                </div>
        </div>
        <div id="footer">
<p>Designed with the <a href="http://www.shareasale.com/r.cfm?
 b=198392&u=405475&m=24570&urllink=&afftrack=">Thesis WordPress Theme</a> from
 DIYthemes.</p><p>Hosted by <a
 href="http://www.BlueHost.Com/track/joekraynak/computerchimp">Bluehost</a><p>Copyri
 ght &copy; 2009 Joe Kraynak</p> </div>
</div>
</div>
<style type="text/css" media="all">#avatar_footer { display: none; } /* Change this
 in Users > Avatars. */ </style><div id="avatar_footer">Avatars by <a
 href="http://www.sterling-adventures.co.uk/blog/">Sterling Adventures</a></div><!--
 [if lte IE 7]>
<div id="ie_clear"></div>
<![endif]-->
<script type="text/javascript">
var gaJsHost = (("https:" ==
 document.location.protocol) ? "https://ssl." : "http://www.");
document.write(unescape("%3Cscript src='" + gaJsHost + "google-analytics.com/ga.js'
 type='text/javascript'%3E%3C/script%3E"));
</script>
<script type="text/javascript">
try {
var pageTracker = _gat._getTracker("UA-1700892-4");
pageTracker._trackPageview();
} catch(err) {}</script>

</body>
</html>
```

Figure 12-27 Position JavaScript at the end of web pages

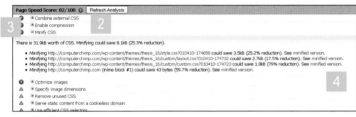

Figure 12-28 Create a backup copy of CSS files

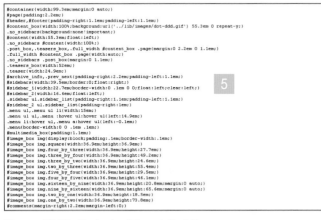

Figure 12-29 Minify the CSS file

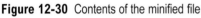

Figure 12-30 Contents of the minified file

See also

For more about Google Page Speed, see 'Identifying bottlenecks', earlier in this chapter.

Streamlining CSS

12

1. Create a backup copy of the CSS files that control the formatting on your site, as in Figure 12-28.

2. Run Google Page Speed, shown in Figure 12-29.

3. Click the plus sign next to Minify CSS.

4. Click the 'minified version' link for the CSS file you want to minify.

5. Replace the contents of the CSS file with the minified CSS for that file. See Figure 12-30.

Did you know?

Page Speed minifies (reduces the size of) the CSS file by removing all spaces and comments. Comments can be valuable in editing the CSS some time in the future, so we recommend performing this task only if you are comfortable editing CSS without the use of comments or are sure you will not need to edit the CSS later.

Streamlining CSS
(cont.)

6. Return to the Page Speed analysis results, shown in Figure 12-31.

7. Click the plus sign next to Remove unused CSS.

8. Use the results as your guide in removing CSS codes not in use on your site.

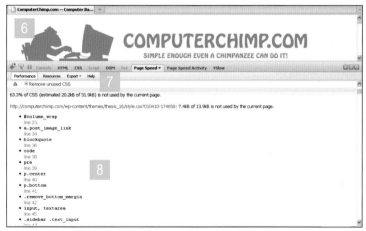

Figure 12-31 Identify and remove unused CSS styles

Did you know?

Be careful. Just because some CSS is not used on the page you tested, it may be used to format other pages on your site. Unused CSS may also be useful for formatting you are not using right now but may want to use in the future. Use the Page Speed results only as a guide for trimming CSS and always back up your CSS files before editing them.

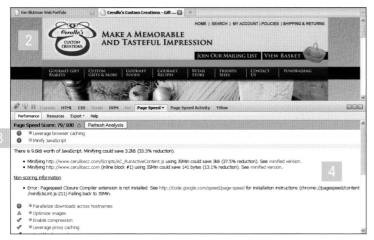

Figure 12-32 Page Speed reduces the size of the JavaScript

```
var isIE=(navigator.appVersion.indexOf("MSIE")!=-1)?true:false;var isWin=(navigator.appVersion.toLowerCase().indexOf("win")!=
(var version;var axo;var e;try{axo=new ActiveXObject("ShockwaveFlash.ShockwaveFlash.7");version=axo.GetVariable("$version");}
if(!version)
{try{axo=new ActiveXObject("ShockwaveFlash.ShockwaveFlash.6");version="WIN 6,0,21,0";axo.AllowScriptAccess="always";version=a
if(!version)
{try{axo=new ActiveXObject("ShockwaveFlash.ShockwaveFlash.3");version=axo.GetVariable("$version");}catch(e){}}
if(!version)
{try{axo=new ActiveXObject("ShockwaveFlash.ShockwaveFlash.3");version="WIN 3,0,18,0";}catch(e){}}
if(!version)
{try{axo=new ActiveXObject("ShockwaveFlash.ShockwaveFlash");version="WIN 2,0,0,11";}catch(e){version=-1;}}
return version;}
function GetSwfVer(){var flashVer=-1;if(navigator.plugins!=null&&navigator.plugins.length>0){if(navigator.plugins["Shockwave
if(versionRevision[0]=="d"){versionRevision=versionRevision.substring(1);}else if(versionRevision[0]=="r"){versionRevision=ve
var flashVer=versionMajor+"."+versionMinor+"."+versionRevision;}}
else if(navigator.userAgent.toLowerCase().indexOf("webtv/2.6")!=-1)flashVer=4;else if(navigator.userAgent.toLowerCase().index
return flashVer;}
function DetectFlashVer(reqMajorVer,reqMinorVer,reqRevision)
{versionStr=GetSwfVer();if(versionStr==-1){return false;}else if(versionStr!=0){if(isIE&&isWin&&!isOpera){tempArray=versionSt
var versionMajor=versionArray[0];var versionMinor=versionArray[1];var versionRevision=versionArray[2];if(versionMajor>parseF
return true;else if(versionMinor==parseFloat(reqMinorVer)){if(versionRevision>=parseFloat(reqRevision))
return true;}}
return false;}}
function AC_AddExtension(src,ext)
{if(src.indexOf('?')!=-1)
return src.replace(/\?/,ext+'?');else
return src+ext;}
function AC_Generateobj(objAttrs,params,embedAttrs)
{var str='';if(isIE&&isWin&&!isOpera)
{str+='<object ';for(var i in objAttrs)
{str+=i+'="'+objAttrs[i]+'" ';}
str+='>';for(var i in params)
{str+='<param name="'+i+'" value="'+params[i]+'" /> ';}
str+='</object>';}
else
{str+='<embed ';for(var i in embedAttrs)
```

Figure 12-33 The minified JavaScript

Streamlining JavaScript

1. Create a backup copy of the JavaScript used on your site.

2. Run Google Page Speed, as in Figure 12-32.

3. Click the plus sign next to Minify JavaScript.

4. Click the 'minified version" link for the JavaScript you want to minify.

5. Replace the original JavaScript with the minified JavaScript. See Figure 12-33.

See also

For more about Google Page Speed, see 'Identifying bottlenecks', earlier in this chapter.

Minimising DNS lookups

1 When possible, store files referenced in your web pages on your site's domain, as illustrated in Figure 12-34.

2 Reference local resources rather than referencing resources stored on other domains. See Figure 12-35.

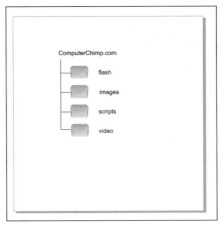

Figure 12-34 Stored files

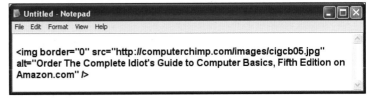

Figure 12-35 Reference local resources so that they load faster

Attracting traffic with search engine optimisation

Introduction

When you invest so much time, effort and expertise in designing a site, you want people to be able to find it. Most people discover websites through search engines, including Google, Yahoo! and Bing, which all use similar methods to find relevant content on the web and index it. By knowing what search engines look for, how they expect information to be presented and the tricks they typically penalise sites for trying, you can more effectively tailor your site and its contents to achieve higher search engine rankings.

In this chapter, we show you the basics of how search engines function, show you how to make your content more attractive to search engines and highlight SEO and web design practices you should avoid. By doing more of what really works and less of what does not work or is likely to result in penalties for your site, your site's search engine rankings will naturally rise.

What you'll do

Understand how search engines work

Use links strategically

Make your content search engine friendly

Add a robots.txt file

Add an XML sitemap

Add a meta description

Add meta keywords

Optimise images

Optimise video

Increase site popularity

Avoid bad SEO practices

Analyse and adjust your SEO

Understanding how search engines work

▶

Search engines are automated indexing machines. They search the web by following links, index the content they discover and deem relevant, then provide users with tools for searching the index. By understanding how search engines function, you gain a better understanding of the reasoning behind specific SEO techniques.

How search engines work

1 Web spiders (or crawlers) search the internet for links to relevant content – see Figure 13-1.

2 Spiders collect the URLs and corresponding documents and send them to the search engine's indexer.

3 When a user executes a search, the search engine displays links for index entries that most closely match the search entry in order of relevance.

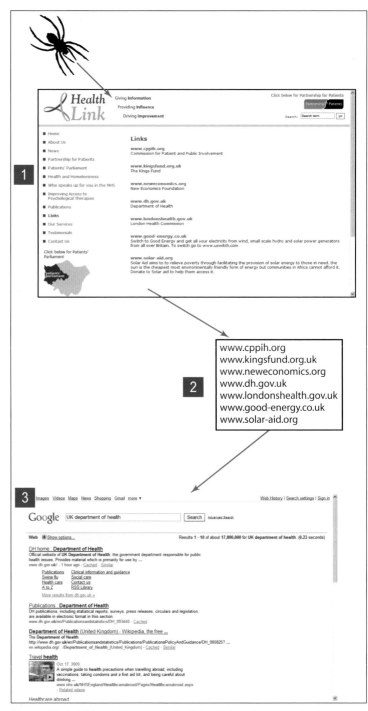

Figure 13-1 Web spiders search the internet for relevant content

When indexing and ranking sites, search engines give specific features of a site more weight than others. Features that are deemed more significant are shown below:

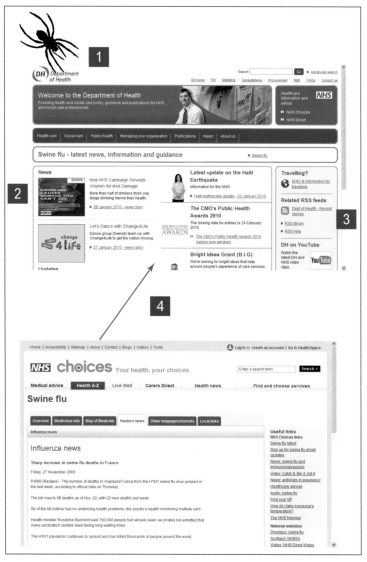

Figure 13-2 You can make your site more attractive to web spiders

Understanding how search engines work (cont.)

1 Web spider accessibility to pages – see Figure 13-2.

2 Relevant content, including titles, headings and keywords in the content.

3 Internal links.

4 Incoming links.

13

Did you know?

Features such as meta keywords, which web developers have often tried to use to trick search engines into raising a site's ranking, are deemed less important. Search engines may even penalise a site's ranking for attempting such tricks.

Using links strategically ▶

Because web spiders discover content through links, having an effective link strategy in place and executing it properly are key ingredients to search engine optimisation. See Figure 13-3 for an example.

1 Link through your site's main navigation bar or menu system to every page you want indexed.

2 Maintain a shallow folder structure. The deeper the spider must crawl, the less relevant it deems the content.

3 Use internal links generously to reinforce the importance of the pages you want search engines to focus on the most. For example, if you want your home page to have the highest ranking, make sure all pages contain one or more links back to the home page.

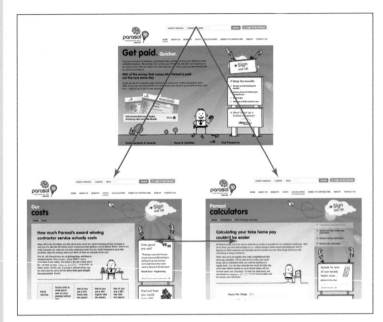

Figure 13-3 Internal links help search engines index your site more accurately

? Did you know?

Limit the number of links back to a certain page to no more than 100. Otherwise, search engines may penalise your site for trying to employ SEO tricks.

! Important

Avoid overusing JavaScript or Flash in a page's main site navigation. These technologies hinder search spiders' ability to locate and index content.

One of the biggest factors in SEO requires no tricks and no incredible amount of SEO expertise. You simply need to populate your website with relevant content that contains the keywords you want search engines to spot.

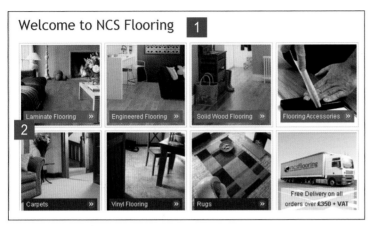

Figure 13-4 Keywords will attract search engine attention

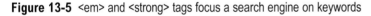

Figure 13-5 <em> and <strong> tags focus a search engine on keywords

SEO optimising content

1 Give pages descriptive titles. If possible, include keywords that you want search engines to focus on, such as in Figure 13-4.

2 Include keywords and phrases in the body of each page, especially in any headings.

3 Use HTML tags to emphasise keywords and phrases embedded in the content, as in Figure 13-5.

13

Timesaver tip

Many CMS platforms include tools for SEO optimisation or have plugins to add these features. The SEO All-in-One pack plugin for WordPress, for example, enables you to add a custom page title, meta description and meta keywords, without having to edit the page's HTML.

Adding a robots. txt file ▶

A robots.txt file works behind the scenes to provide search engines with the information they need to identify content they should not index, including directories with CSS files and support files.

1 Create a robots.txt file listing specific directories or files that should not be indexed. See Figure 13-6, for example.

2 Upload the robots.txt file to your site's root directory, as in Figure 13.7.

Timesaver tip

Several WordPress plugins are available for adding a robots.txt file to a site without having to create the text file and upload it.

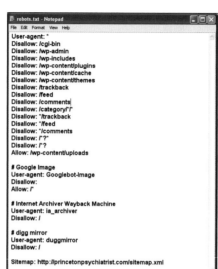

Figure 13-6 A robots.txt file tells search engines what not to index

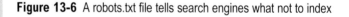

Figure 13-7 Upload the file to your site's root directory

A sitemap serves a purpose opposite to that of a robots.txt file. It tells search engines what to index and may even indicate the relative importance of each page. Use robots.txt and sitemap.txt or sitemap.xml in tandem to provide search engines with specific instructions on what to index.

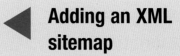

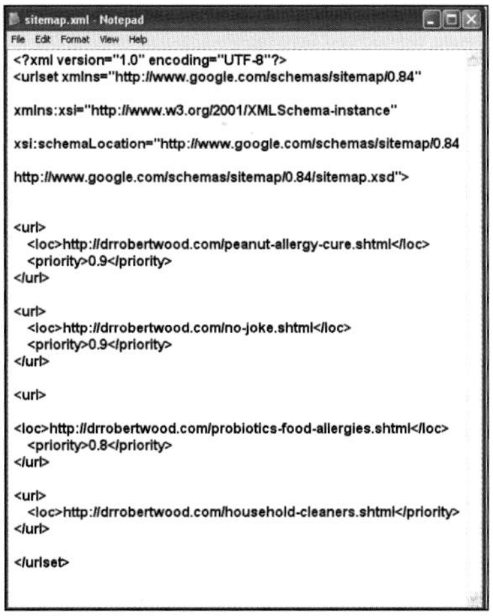

Adding an XML sitemap

1 Create a sitemap.txt or sitemap.xml file listing specific directories or files that should be indexed. See Figure 13-8.

2 Upload the sitemap.txt or sitemap.xml file to your site's root directory. See Figure 13-9.

Figure 13-8 A sitemap.xml file facilitates search engine indexing

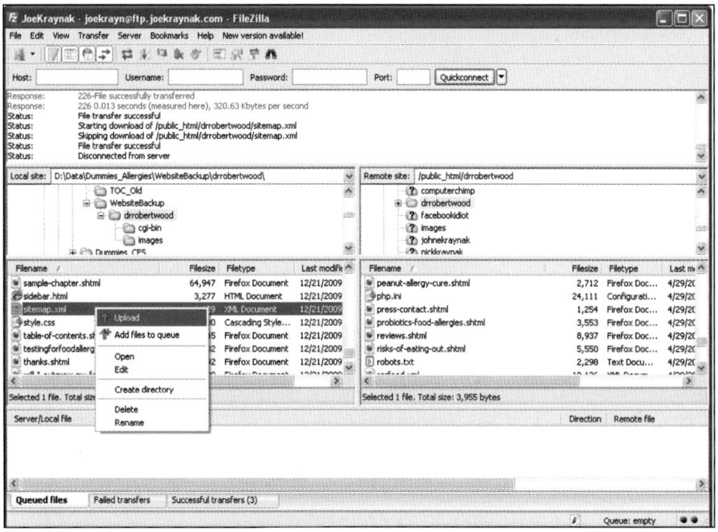

Timesaver tip

Although you can create your own sitemap.txt or sitemap.xml file using any text editor, consider using Google's Sitemap Generator at *www.google.com/webmasters/tools/home*. Better yet, if you are using a CMS platform, such as WordPress, look for a plugin that allows you to add a Google sitemap to your site so that you do not have to upload the file after creating it.

Figure 13-9 Upload the file to your site's root directory

13

Adding a meta description ▶

A meta description briefly describes the contents of a web page. It serves two purposes. First, it helps search engines properly index and rank the site. Second, search engines often display the meta description in the search results.

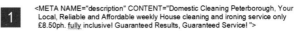

Figure 13-10 A meta description indicates what the page is about

Adding a page description

1 Insert the tag <META NAME="description" CONTENT="your description"> right after the closing </TITLE>, shown in Figure 13-10.

2 In CMS, you may be able to enter a description without having to edit HTML. See Figure 13-11, for example.

SEO Details and Additional Style

Custom Title Tag [+] more info

Art of Clean - Carpet Cleaning

custom `<title>` tag

Meta Description [+] more info   **2**

Art of Clean carpet cleaning serving Cambridge, Royston, Saffron, Walden, Ely, and Newmarket, UK.

`<meta>` description

Meta Keywords [+] more info

`<meta>` keywords

Noindex this Page [+] more info

☐ add a `noindex` robot meta tag to this page

"Read More" Text [+] more info

use custom "Read More" text for this entry

CSS Class [+] more info

CSS class name

Figure 13-11 A meta description in a content management system

---

For your information

To optimise your meta descriptions:

■ use a unique description for each page

■ limit the description to 150–200 words

■ include descriptive and precise keywords and phrases

■ write for users, not just for search engines.

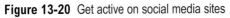

Figure 13-20 Get active on social media sites

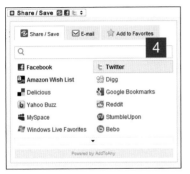

Figure 13-21 Add content-sharing links to your site

3 Become active on Facebook, Twitter, Digg, YouTube and other social media sites, so that you can link to your website from these accounts. See Figure 13-20.

4 Add content-sharing links to your site to enable users to easily share your content on Facebook, Twitter, Digg and other social media sites. See Figure 13-21.

13

Did you know?

Avoid cheap tricks, such as paying for incoming links. Designing a site with engaging, relevant content for the industry or community it serves and SEO optimising the content with search engines and users in mind is the best way to gain and maintain a high ranking.

Avoiding bad SEO practices ▶

Certain web design practices may reduce a spider's ability to find pages or access them, including the following bad practices:

- using frames to structure pages
- designing websites in Flash
- overusing Javascripts, which hinder search engine ability to index a site
- requiring mandatory user interaction to access content.

Avoiding frames

1 Avoid using HTML frames. See Figure 13-22.

2 Create columns using CSS. See Figure 13-23.

Did you know?

HTML frames were commonly used in the old days to structure a site's content. They made it easy, for example, to create a two- or three-column layout. Unfortunately, frame-based web pages negatively affect a search engine's ability to locate and index content.

Timesaver tip

Most CMS and blog platforms include CSS-based templates to manage the overall structure of a page on the site. Editing a template that is close to the desired design is usually easier than starting from scratch.

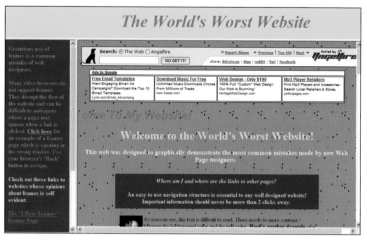

Figure 13-22 Avoid HTML frames

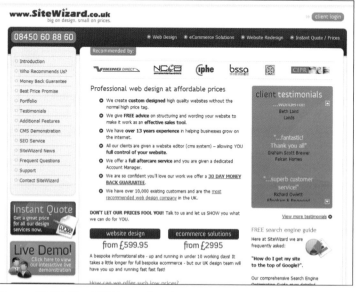

Figure 13-23 Use CSS to create columns

If a user is required to enter information to access your site or a specific page on the site, as illustrated in Figure 13-24, search engines are unable to gain access to the content and are unable to index it.

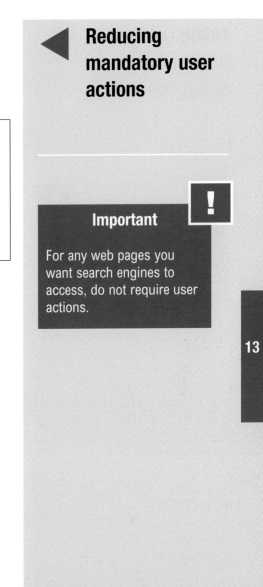

Please Verify Location and Age

Access to this website is prohibited to anyone under the age of 18 years old. To gain access to this site, please verify the country you are residing in currently along with the day, month, and year you were born.

Where are you?
United States of America ▾
When were you born?
Day ▾   Month   ▾   Year ▾

By entering this site you accept our terms and conditions and privacy policy.

Submit & Enter Site

Figure 13-24 Cut down on mandatory user actions

Reducing mandatory user actions

Important

!

For any web pages you want search engines to access, do not require user actions.

13

Using secure servers only when necessary

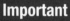

You may often be required to use a secure socket layer (SSL) technology to protect information users enter, but use it only when necessary. Search engines will not access any pages with a URL that begins with https:// (which indicates a secure server), such as the one shown in Figure 13-25, so they cannot index content on those pages.

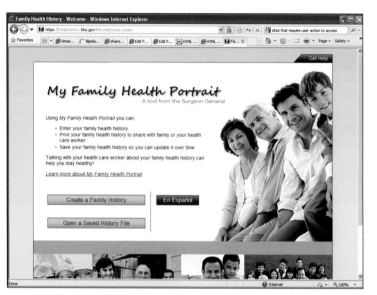

Figure 13-25 Place web pages on a secure server only when necessary

If you need to redirect browsers from one domain or URL to another, avoid using temporary redirects, which prevent any search engine momentum your site may have gained from transferring to the new domain or URL. This negatively affects a site's search engine ranking. Use a 301 permanent redirect instead.

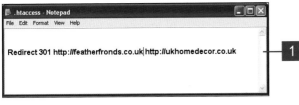

Figure 13-26 Use 301 redirect when moving pages permanently to a new address

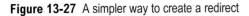

Figure 13-27 A simpler way to create a redirect

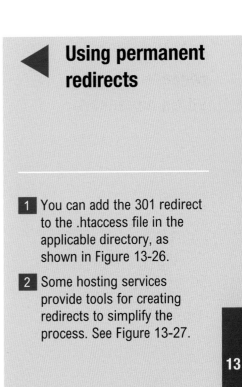

1 You can add the 301 redirect to the .htaccess file in the applicable directory, as shown in Figure 13-26.

2 Some hosting services provide tools for creating redirects to simplify the process. See Figure 13-27.

13

Avoiding Flash sites

Flash sites are multimedia-based, making it difficult for search engines to identify specific pages by unique URLs and properly index the content. The easiest solution is to stick with text-based sites that rely on HTML and CSS. But if you must include Flash, you have two options for optimising SEO on a Flash-based site:

1. Create an SEO-optimised text-based (HTML) site, using Flash movies as components of the pages rather than designing the entire site with Flash.

2. Create two sites with similar content (one HTML and one Flash) and employ user-agent detection to deliver the Flash site to people and the HTML site to search engines.

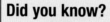

Did you know?

Flash sites are cool, but they may be difficult for search engines to index.

Cloaking is an underhand way of gaining a high search ranking for a site that does not deserve it.

With cloaking, a site contains separate content for users and search engines. The search engine indexes the content intended for it, but when users click the link in the search engine index, they receive content that does not match the site's description in the index.

- Serve the same content to search engines and users.

- Avoid any strategies designed to trick search engines into indexing your site.

◀ **Avoiding cloaking tricks**

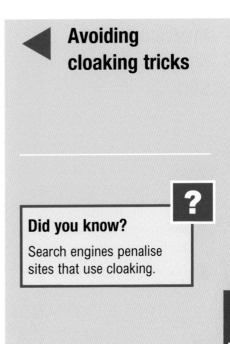

Did you know?
Search engines penalise sites that use cloaking.

13

Jargon buster

Cloaking: An SEO strategy in which a site delivers different content to search engines than it delivers to users, so the search engine will index pages it would normally reject.

Analysing and adjusting your SEO

After you optimise your site for search engines, analyse it to identify any problem areas. You can use any of the many free SEO analysers available on the web.

Follow the suggestions to further optimise your site for search engines.

1 Go to *www.rankingtoday.com*.

2 Click in the Insert key box and type the requested verification code.

3 Click in the URL to Check box (see Figure 13-28) and type the address of the page you want to analyse.

4 Make sure all the tasks to perform are ticked to ensure a thorough analysis.

5 Click Check.

Site CheckUp
Analyze and optimize your pages for a better search engine ranking now!

Google Analytics - Free
Gain traffic and optimize your site with Google Analytics. Free!
www.google.com/analytics

Ads by Google

Check your website and optimize your hidden and visible content to achieve the best search engine ranking for your targeted keywords!

Insert the domain name or the URL of the page you want to optimize and start the check-up of your website to find its eventual leaks or errors. Learn instantly how to improve your site's usability and positioning. To access the complete set of the available features sign up with no charge to our Member's Area.

Security key: 0962   Insert key » 0962   **2**

URL to Check: www.artofclean.co.uk   **3**

Results by E-mail: (Optional)

Choose the tasks to perform:

☑ Loading time and page structure ☐   ☑ Keyword density ☐
☑ Meta tags ☐   ☑ Link integrity ☐   **4**

Check   **5**

SEO Tools

Site Analysis
+ Site CheckUp
+ Meta Tag Analyzer
+ Link Check
+ Real PageRank
+ Alexa Rank

Site Optimization
+ Image Optimizer
+ Meta Tag Generator
+ Sitemap Generator
+ Google Sitemap Generator

Search Engine Ranking
+ Site Indexing
+ Site Popularity
+ Keyword Ranking

Competitor Analysis
+ Compare Site Indexing
+ Compare Site Popularity
+ Compare Keyword Ranking

Figure 13-28 Analyse a page on your site to identify any problems

238

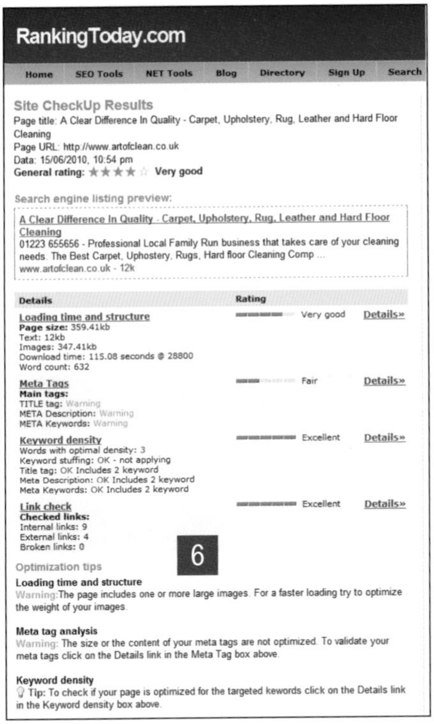

Figure 13-29 Optimisation tips can help you improve your site's search engine rank

For your information

Additional free SEO analysis sites include:

www.w3optimizer.com

http://spydermate.com

www.reactionengine.com

www.webseoanalytics.com/free/seo-tools/web-seo-analysis.php

Analysing and adjusting your SEO (cont.)

6 When the analysis is complete, RankingToday.com displays the results followed by additional optimisation tips – see Figure 13-29.

13

Securing your website

Introduction

Although the internet is generally a safe and friendly place to build a website, some people on the web have nothing better to do with their time and talent than break into sites to steal information, vandalise sites or hijack sites for other nefarious purposes.

Although you cannot possibly make your site completely secure, you can take steps to make it reasonably secure and to protect any data people enter on your site.

In this chapter, you will learn website security basics, identify the primary risks to your website and acquire strategies to help increase security on your site.

What you'll do

Grasp website security basics

Identify the primary security risks

Assess your need for increased security

Secure your computer

Choose a secure web hosting service

Update your blogging platform or CMS

Manage your site from a secure network

Choose and protect passwords

Lock down file permissions

Maintain a separate database for each site

Hide your site's login page

Implement SSL (secure socket layers)

Back up your site

Grasping website security basics ▶

Your website resides on a web server. Unless you have built an intranet that is completely self-contained on computers you control, the web server is connected to the internet, so anyone on the internet can access your site's resources and information. This is exactly why most people build websites.

However, you usually want to provide visitors with only *limited* access. In most cases, you want them to view the web pages you have created, but you do not want them to have the authority to edit or delete those pages. If your site is e-commerce enabled, you want people to be able to enter information to order and pay for products, but you must prevent other users from accessing your customers' information.

Website security simply ensures that users have only the level of access to your site's information and resources that you want them to have.

These are the goals of website security, as shown in Figure 14-1:

- Prohibit unauthorised access to the web server.
- Protect any sensitive information stored on the web server.
- Protect any sensitive information transferred between the web server and the end user.
- Prevent viruses, worms and other malware from infecting files on the web server.
- Prevent unauthorised users from logging on to the site as administrators and hijacking the site.

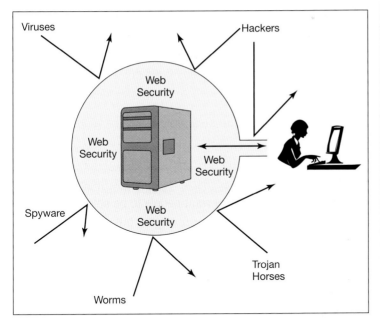

Figure 14-1 Website security blocks unauthorised access

14

Identifying the primary security risks ▶

Security risks include those illustrated in Figure 14-2:

1. Insiders, such as disgruntled workers or former employees, stealing information or damaging the site in some way.

2. Malicious hackers...

   ■ breaking into a site to steal information or vandalise the site

   ■ hijacking the site and possibly locking you out of it, or

   ■ obtaining access to the site's servers to use its resources, which could ultimately slow down your site.

3. Criminals intercepting sensitive information in transit between the site and end users.

4. Malware, including viruses and worms, that could infect files and possibly jeopardise security.

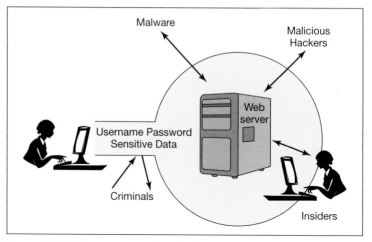

Figure 14-2 The primary security risks for a website

Some sites require stricter security than others. For example, a medical centre may store patient information that is highly sensitive. E-commerce sites, such as the one shown in Figure 14-3, require tighter security to protect customers. A website that functions simply as an information kiosk or business brochure, however, is probably not a very attractive target for hackers.

Tighter security may be required if your site meets any of the following criteria:

- collects or stores valuable information you want to remain private
- collects or stores sensitive information that must remain private
- may be an attractive target for someone to vandalise or hijack to seek revenge against you or your business, make a name for themselves or use as a way of collecting valuable information from users
- is critical for you or your business to operate. If you cannot operate without your site, you may need to tighten security to protect the site from the worst possible scenario, even if risks are relatively low.

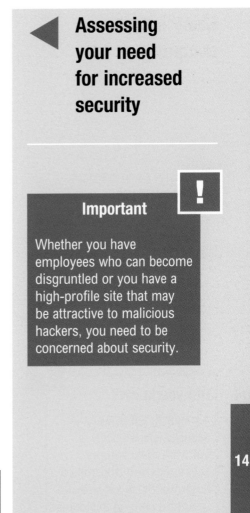

Assessing your need for increased security

!

Important

Whether you have employees who can become disgruntled or you have a high-profile site that may be attractive to malicious hackers, you need to be concerned about security.

14

Figure 14-3 Some sites needs to be more secure than others

Securing your computer ▶

1 Install a good antivirus program, such as avast (*www.avast.com*), shown in Figure 14-4.

2 Install all updates for your operating system and application software. Many updates contain security patches.

?

Did you know?

A major threat to website security is a *keylogger* – software that captures keystrokes and transmits a record of those keystrokes to a third party. A keylogger may be able to capture the login information you use to access your website for management purposes. Antivirus software can help protect your system from keyloggers.

Some of the most serious threats to website security may come from your own computer, so make sure it is free of spyware, adware, viruses and other malicious software, and is running the most up-to-date versions of all your applications.

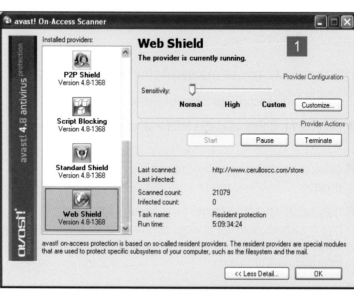

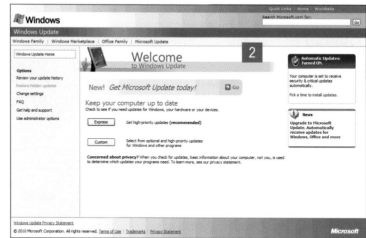

Figure 14-4 Protect your computer

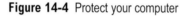

!

Important

Make sure all computers used to manage your site are secure.

The server on which your website resides is also vulnerable to attacks and malicious software. Choose a hosting service that has a good history for securing its web servers, such as the one shown in Figure 14-5.

A trusted web host performs the following tasks to maintain security for its web servers:

1. Ensures the web server software is secure and stable.

2. Installs any security patches required.

3. Carefully monitors its servers for any suspicious activity.

4. Stores backups of your files.

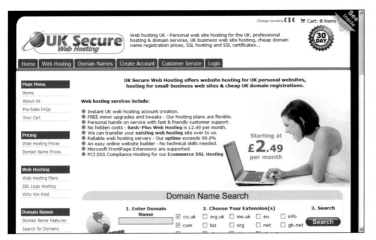

Figure 14-5 Choose a secure web hosting service

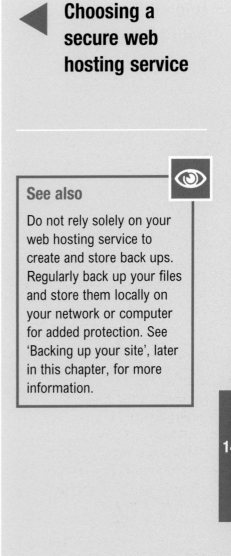

◀ Choosing a secure web hosting service

See also

Do not rely solely on your web hosting service to create and store back ups. Regularly back up your files and store them locally on your network or computer for added protection. See 'Backing up your site', later in this chapter, for more information.

14

Updating your blogging platform or CMS

If you manage your site with a blogging platform or CMS, keep your installation up to date. Upgrade to the most recent version of the blogging platform or CMS, as in Figure 14-6, for instance. Many updates include security patches to prevent unauthorised access.

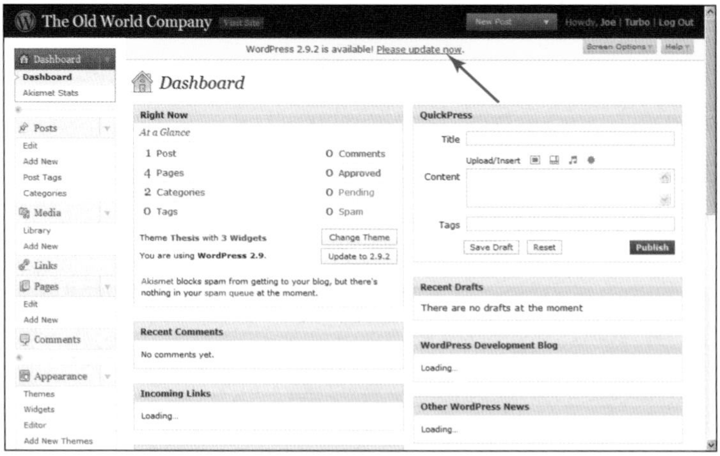

Figure 14-6 Upgrade your blogging platform or CMS

Whenever you connect to your site, make sure you are working behind a firewall (see Figure 14-7), which protects your system from unauthorised access and helps protect any login information you enter.

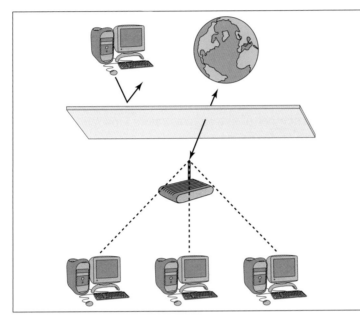

Figure 14-7 Work behind a firewall

Choosing and protecting passwords ▶

Jargon buster

Brute force attack: Typically a strategy of trying all possibilities to identify a decryption key. However, the term can also be applied to a strategy of trying different login names and passwords in order to guess the right ones.

Did you know?

Do not use your name as your user name or password.

Do not use any word from any dictionary as your password.

Do not use a string of four numbers (such as a PIN or personal identification number) as your password.

Hackers often launch a *brute force attack* to break into a site. To prevent unauthorised access, choose a user name and password that are difficult to guess.

- Choose a unique user name that does not reflect your real name, such as the one shown in Figure 14-8.

- Choose a password at least eight characters long that includes letters (a mix of upper- and lowercase), numbers and symbols (such as dashes or underline characters).

- Change your password every month or two.

- Limit the number of site administrators – people who can log in and configure the site.

- Instruct site administrators not to share their user names and passwords with anyone.

- Remove login access for anyone who is no longer an administrator or at least change the password.

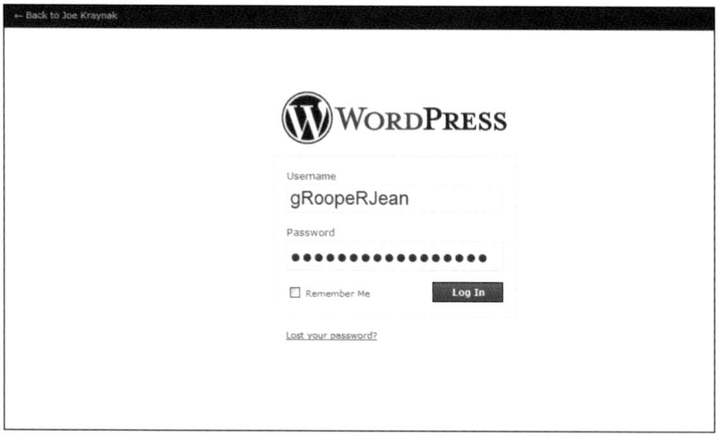

Figure 14-8 Use a user name and password that would be difficult to guess

You can use an FTP program or a utility provided by your web hosting service to adjust file permissions, restricting public write access to files and folders.

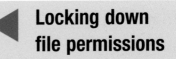

Figure 14-9 Keep a rein on file permissions

1 Retain owner rights to read, write and execute all files and directories. See Figure 14-9.

2 Assign group rights to read, write and execute only those files and directories that other authorised users must have to perform their assigned duties.

3 Provide public write access to only those files and directories that absolutely require it to function properly.

i

For your information

Test your site thoroughly after changing file permissions to ensure it functions properly. The public may need write access to some files and folders in order to enter information on your site – for example, if your site has a blog component where visitors can post comments.

14

Maintaining a separate database for each site

Many modern websites are built using blogging platforms or a CMS, which stores data for the site in a database. Keeping a separate database for each site provides added protection through containment – if database security is breached, it affects only one site.

1 When installing a CMS or blogging platform, create a separate installation for each site, as shown in Figure 14-10.

2 Each site has its own database, so if one database is broken into or damaged, other sites are not affected.

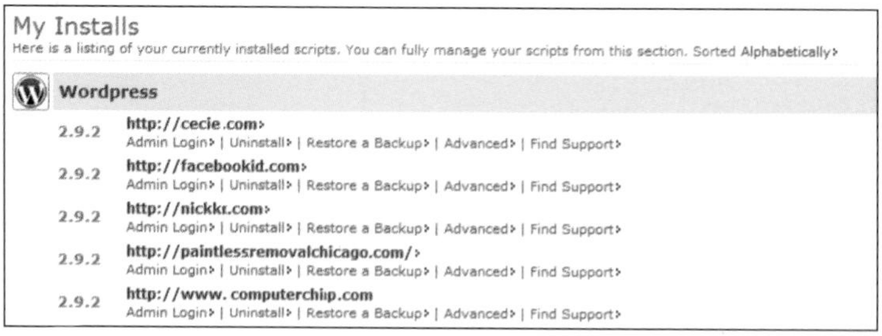

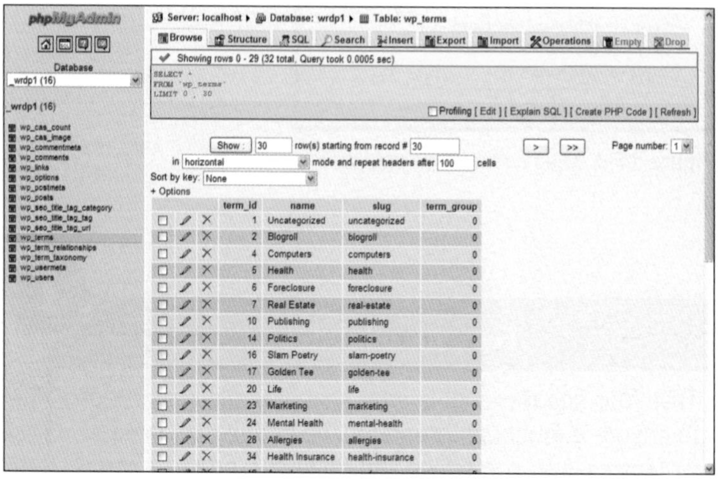

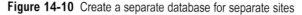

Figure 14-10 Create a separate database for separate sites

If your site is built on a blogging platform or CMS, you can usually pull up the site's administrative login page by going to a site address such as *www.mysite.com/wp-login.php* (Figure 14-11) or *www.mysite.com/joomla/administrator*. By installing to a less obvious folder or assigning a less obvious address to the login page, such as *www.mysite.com/w67X1-y62/wp-login.php*, you can make the page more difficult for novice hackers to locate.

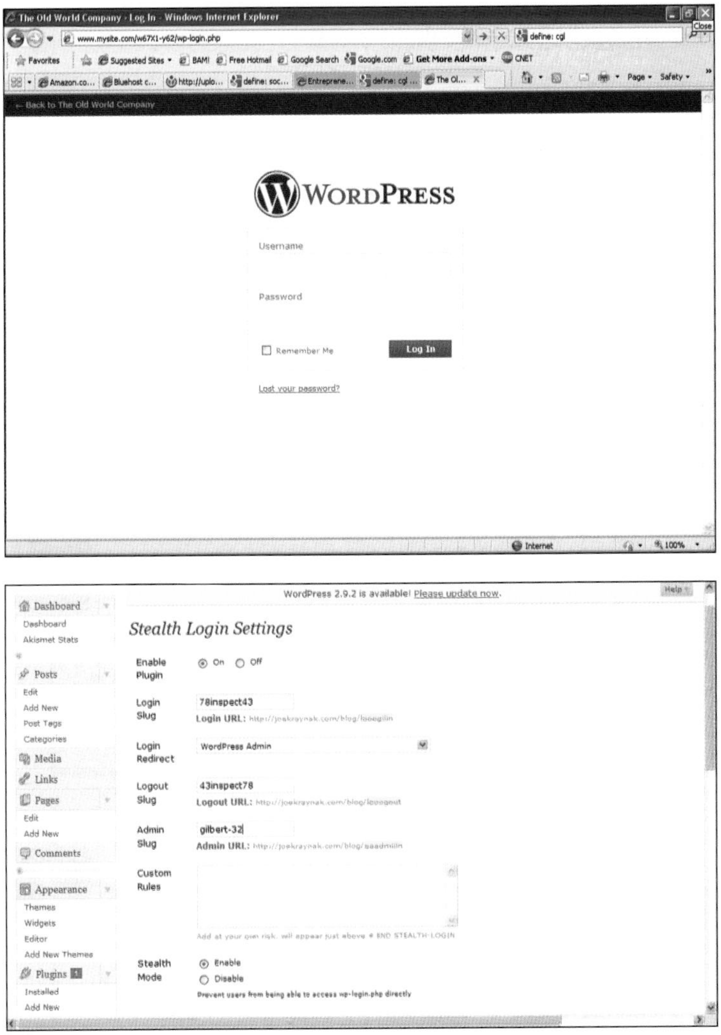

Figure 14-11 Make it difficult for hackers to find your login page

Hiding your site's login page

You can hide a site's login page using either of the following techniques:

1 If possible, install your CMS or blogging software in a separate directory within the site's root directory.

2 Install a plugin that enables you to change the address of the login page.

See also

For more about plugins, see Chapter 3, 'Assembling your tools'.

14

For your information

Additional security plugins may be available for your CMS or blogging platform. Look for plugins that can encrypt your login information, monitor your site for suspicious activity or scan for potential vulnerabilities.

Implementing SSL (secure socket layers)

When web users connect to a website secured with SSL, https:// appears in the address bar and the browser typically displays a lock icon in the status bar to indicate the site is secure, as illustrated in Figure 14-12.

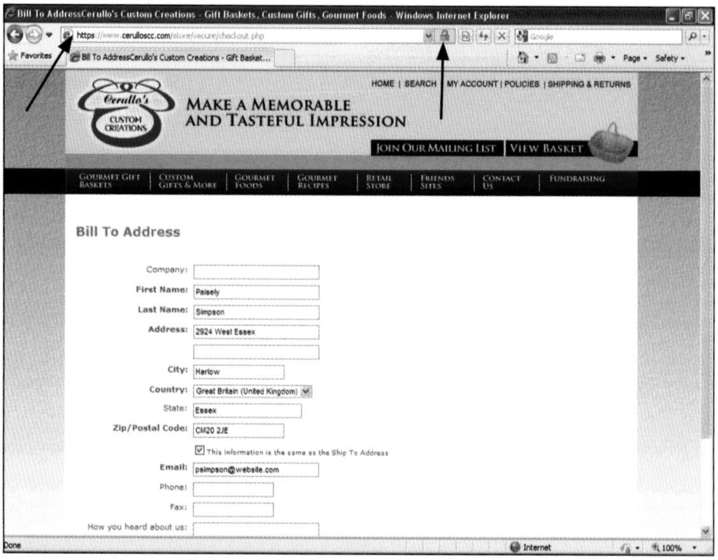

1 Obtain a dedicated IP address.

2 Obtain an SSL certificate.

3 Install the SSL certificate on your web server.

Timesaver tip

Your hosting service should be able to provide you with the dedicated IP address and SSL certificate, and install the SSL certificate on your web server.

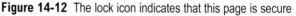

Figure 14-12 The lock icon indicates that this page is secure

For your information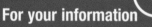

Certifying authorities (CAs) issue SSL certificates.

Jargon buster

Secure socket layers (SSL): A communications protocol that encrypts the channel between a browser and a website to ensure a secure exchange of data.

Did you know?

If your website is enabled for e-commerce, securing the site with SSL is essential to protect customer information, including credit card numbers.

To transmit form data securely, you must secure the connection between the end user and the form and between the form and the recipient. By placing the forms on an SSL server, you enable people to enter data securely into the form. You must then encrypt that data and send it via a secure email connection to the recipient or to a secure database.

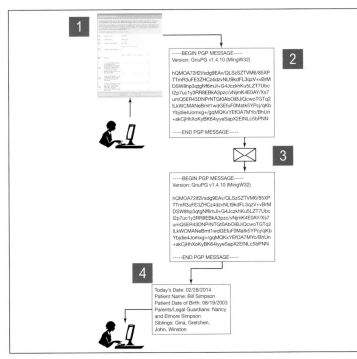

Figure 14-13 Steps for transmitting form data securely

◀ Transmitting form data securely

Steps for transmitting form data securely vary depending on your hosting service and the various tools and techniques available. The general procedure, as shown in Figure 14-13, is as follows:

1. Place the form on a secure (https://) server.
2. Encrypt the form data.
3. Email the encrypted form data over a secure email connection or store it in a secure database.
4. Decrypt the data upon receiving it.

See also

For more about secure servers, see the previous task, 'Implementing SSL (secure socket layers)'.

14

Timesaver tip

Your hosting provider may provide you with a secure email connection that prevents email messages from being intercepted and read in transit.

For your information

If your hosting service supports it, check out Gnu Privacy Guard (GnuPG) for encrypting and decrypting the form data: *www.gnupg.org*.

See also

Transmitting credit card information via email is typically prohibited by credit card companies. For more about processing credit card transactions, see Chapter 1, 'Getting started with web design'.

Backing up your site

For a less comprehensive backup, at least do the following:

1. If you built your site on a blogging platform or CMS, back up the database that contains the site's content.

2. Back up any themes or CSS files that control the appearance and layout of your site.

3. Back up all images and note the location of the folder in which they are stored.

4. Make a list of all plugins installed, so that you can easily reinstall them.

With a current backup of key website files, you can quickly recover your site if it is vandalised, damaged or hijacked.

Using an FTP program, you can copy your site's directory from the web server to your computer (Figure 14-14). Be sure to also create a separate backup of any databases your site uses. This gives you the most comprehensive backup but is the most time-consuming.

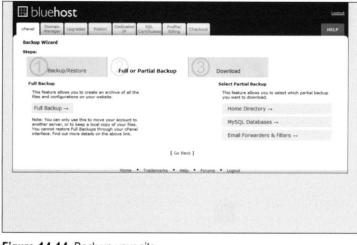

Figure 14-14 Back up your site

Timesaver tip

Your web hosting service may have utilities that can help with backups. Learn how to use these utilities and perform an actual backup and restore operation on a test site before trouble strikes, so you know exactly what your backups can help you recover and how to proceed in the event of catastrophe.

Developing an e-commerce site

Introduction

E-commerce is the term for the purchase of goods or services through a website. E-commerce sites follow certain procedures, such as the use of the 'basket' (or the 'cart') and 'checkout'. There can be bells and whistles, such as user accounts, having other goods suggested to you based on what you've picked out, or being able to later add reviews of purchased items.

Nearly all transactions involve credit card use. As such, security and privacy are big factors. Some websites will collect the sensitive information on the site, other configurations send the purchaser to another website to complete the purchase – and that is where the credit card info is entered.

Of course, any site that has items to purchase should clearly state a return policy, customer service availability and so forth. The reality is that the top-notch sites have everything in place and the small operators are unable to provide full support. So they may use a third-party service or website to provide what they cannot – at a piece of the profits, of course!

What you'll do

Understand the purchase cycle

Review how third-party services are involved

Review some common shopping basket applications

Consider what you need for an e-commerce site

The purchase cycle

▶

Buying on the web is very similar to buying in a store. You look at items for sale, perhaps read reviews, some items might be discounted, or there might be special deals going on. An additional part of purchasing on a website is shipping. Unlike a store, you are not walking out with your purchase – all web purchases are shipped.

The first step to online purchasing is browsing or searching for items. Consider this the 'store' part of the site. There can be any number of ways to present items – and this also depends on the items. For example, an article of clothing might be shown in a variety of colours. Figure 15-1 shows a shirt and allows you to see it in different colours by running the mouse over the colour swatch.

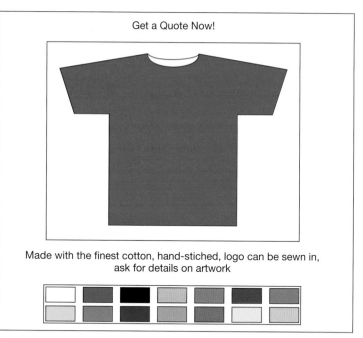

Figure 15-1 A colour swatch lets you see the shirt in different colours

When web shopping you fill up the basket and then either keep shopping or check out. This is shown in Figure 15-2.

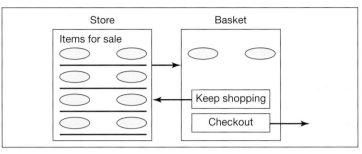

Figure 15-2 The store and the basket

A well-designed e-commerce site will let you get to the basket and see what is in it at any time – in other words, from any page. A 'View basket' link or button might therefore be included in the header. Certainly, a way to view the basket should be available from any product page. Figure 15-3 shows an example of a product page and towards the upper right is a 'basket' button.

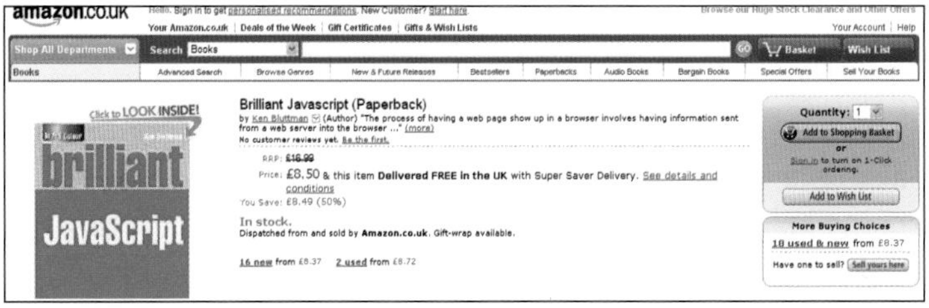

Figure 15-3 A product page has a button to view the basket (© 2010 Amazon.com, Inc. or its affiliates. All rights reserved.)

15

The purchase cycle (cont.)

The basket fills up with all your selections. On the basket page, for each item is the ability to change the quantity or delete the item from the basket. The price of the item is shown and the subtotal. Figure 15-4 shows a basket.

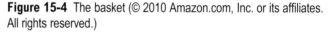

Figure 15-4 The basket (© 2010 Amazon.com, Inc. or its affiliates. All rights reserved.)

'Checkout' is where you pay, indicate shipping options and so forth. High-quality sites will usually have a membership-type system so that you do not have to enter all your information each time you shop. Once you've paid and checked out you should be led to a thank-you page and it will probably have suggestions for future purchases, perhaps a coupon for your next purchase or some other enticement.

Also within the ending process you should be able to print out a receipt and it is likely that one will be emailed to you as well.

One of the challenges in designing a site is to set up your own e-commerce system. You can have one custom developed from a web programmer or use a free open-source cart system, or one that you pay for.

Why pay for one when others are free? Well, there are factors such as:

- types of features
- vendor support
- whether the paid-for version includes payment processing.

Remember that taking sensitive input – credit card numbers, for example – might be something you wish to avoid doing on your site. Some cart systems are tied into payment gateways or at least ready for integration with one.

In a larger sense, consider your site as the store and the payment gateway (also known as the payment processor) as the equipment that you swipe a credit card through when in an actual store. Services such as PayPal and Authorize.net act as gateways for website purchases.

Many sites opt to use an open-source cart product such as OSCommerce (*www.oscommerce.com*) or Zen Cart (*www.zen-cart.com*). You will need technical know-how or assistance to install a cart product. Since these are open source they can be customised. Some carts, such as Magento (*www.magentocommerce.com*), provide both free and cost-based versions.

The available cart products are set to integrate with a variety of payment gateways. If you have a custom cart built, services such as PayPal provide snippets of programming code to put into your checkout page and then the purchaser is sent to the PayPal website to complete payment as the final action. This scenario is shown in Figure 15-5.

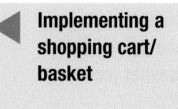

Implementing a shopping cart/ basket

Jargon buster

Payment gateway:
Service that handles the authorisation of credit card purchases.

15

Implementing a shopping cart/ basket (cont.)

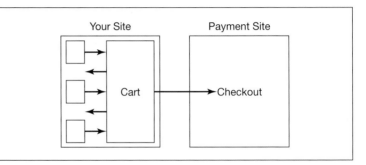

Figure 15-5 Only the final checkout process is on an external site

A number of services provide the payment gateway and keep the cart on their site while your customer is shopping. In this scenario, the product pages are on your site and the cart is on the other site. If multiple items are being ordered, the purchaser is sent back and forth between the sites until they check out. This is shown in Figure 15-6.

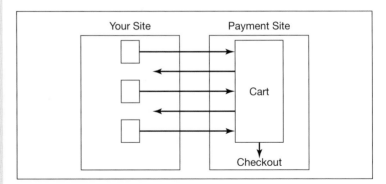

Figure 15-6 The cart is kept on the external site

Some companies make products that encompass the entire shopping process and the website itself. In other words, the product is installed and the site is built using utilities and features that come with the product. One such product is available from Interspire (*www.interspire.com*). Using a product like this can be costly but also alleviates much of the work of putting together an entire site. Typically, a comprehensive product like this will provide customisable templates from which to build the site.

Shopping online is a common activity and vendors are constantly coming up with ways to make the experience easy and exciting so that you will want to come back for future shopping. Here are some ideas that sites use and for you to consider including in yours:

User accounts: for the benefit of repeat business, having a login system for customers – that maintains shipping and other information – is quite useful. A buyer has to register once only (free, of course!) during their first purchase. In subsequent purchases they log in and therefore avoid having to enter their name, address and other typical information.

Recommendations: when an item is selected for purchase, other similar or complementary items are suggested. These should be easy to add to the cart.

Categorisation of products: make it easy for potential buyers to find an item – categorise your inventory and have category pages in addition to the individual product pages.

A search feature: when browsing through categories does not help a visitor find something, a search feature is great. A keyword, item name or model number is entered and the search feature returns a page of results.

A mailing list: keep in touch with your customers via a mailing list. You can send notices of new items, perhaps a newsletter, or just the occasional coupon or some other enticement to come to the site and shop.

View the cart/basket from anywhere: your site should be designed in such a way that a visitor can view what is in the cart from wherever they are with a single button click.

Gift certificates and coupons: a great item to offer is a gift certificate. This way a person can buy one and forward it to a friend. A numbering system keeps each gift certificate unique and it can be used only once. Coupons can be used in the same way, only in this case it is you – the website owner – sending coupons to your mailing list.

What to consider

15

What to consider (cont.)

Tell a friend: this feature is one in which a person can enter an email address and a message about your site and the message is then sent to that email address. It is similar to word-of-mouth advertising.

Product reviews: it can really help potential customers to make a decision to buy if they can read how other purchasers fared with the item. Have a way on your site for people to enter reviews of the products they have purchased. If you are running your site well, selling respectable items and keeping on top of shipping and customer service, you should end up with numerous favourable reviews.

Monitoring and improving your site

Introduction

Whew! Your website is live and people are visiting. However, there is a world of analytical feedback to implement and review that gives specific information about how visitors are interacting with your site. A website is like a living entity: it needs attention with regard to its strengths and weaknesses. Fortunately there are tools available to help get the full picture.

Even before analysing the traffic (aka the visitors to the site), it is helpful to make sure that all the pieces are in place. A broken link – a link that when clicked leads to a non-existent page – is a key thing to look for. Ease of use – for example how many clicks it takes to get to some vital information – is important.

And let's not forget marketing. Just because you have a live site does not mean the world is running to see it. You have to work at making it known. There are many ways to go about this and these will be explored in this chapter.

What you'll do

Test your website

Use available online tools to find problem areas

Learn the key points about web analytics

Review how Google Analytics is used on a site

Learn how to market your site

Testing your website

A well-designed site with a fair amount of content should naturally have many internal links. All of these should be tested to see that a click leads to where the navigation should go. There is presumably a menu or navigation system on the site, as well as links on individual pages that go to other pages.

Take some time and try clicking around. Test every link on every page. Some links could also be to external sites: these should be tested as well. Keep in mind that a link could be broken (leads to nowhere), but could also just lead to an existing though incorrect page. You need to watch out for this, too.

Timesaver tip

Not all of us tend to work in the same sequence. Therefore it's a good idea to ask a friend to check the links as well. They will probably click around in a different order from you.

A broken link will create a '404 error', which indicates a page cannot be found. Figure 16-1 shows just such an error.

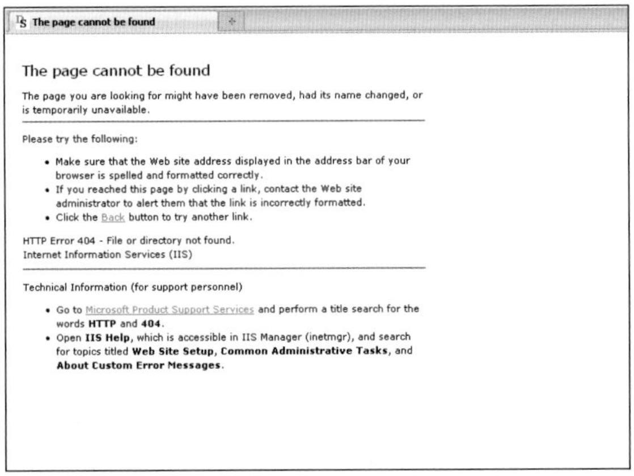

Figure 16-1 Navigating to a page that does not exist

The page shown in Figure 16-1 is not particularly enticing. It serves its purpose but does not look like much. Imagine that such a page could be shown in the style that the rest of your site is built around. Well, you probably can! Your ISP may provide options for how to handle a non-found page. For example, you could get the site to redirect visitors to the home page or a custom page, or perhaps make use of a default page the ISP provides.

Testing your website (cont.)

Many sites take advantage of providing a more appealing '404 error' page. Figure 16-2 shows the one that Facebook uses. Besides stating that the page cannot be found, it gives you options such as going to the home page.

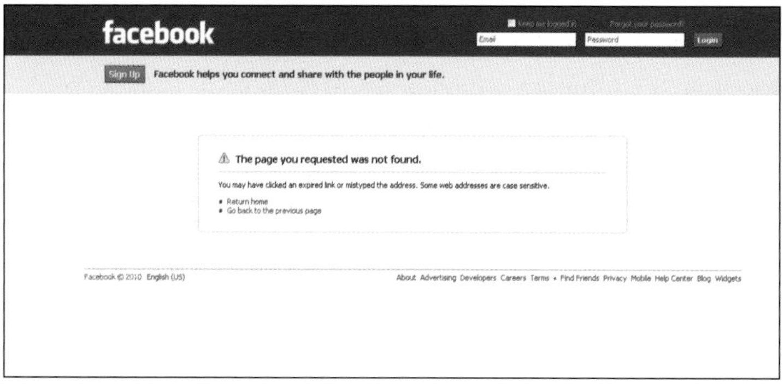

Figure 16-2 A page that cannot be found on Facebook

Besides links working correctly, you should look over your site to ascertain whether pictures are correct, make sure there are no typos in the content, see how functionality behaves in different browsers and so on.

Some webmasters like to validate their site with a tool provided by the World Wide Web Consortium (W3C). Navigate to *http://validator.w3.org* and enter the URL for a web page. Figure 16-3 shows the validator. It is not the only one to be found on the internet but it is the best known and most used.

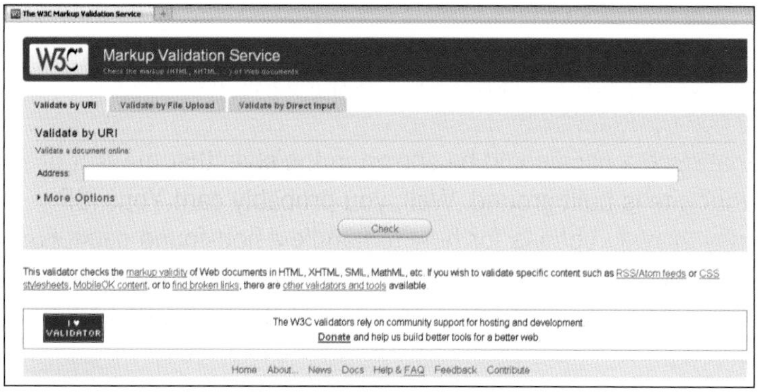

Figure 16-3 The W3C page validator

Did you know?

Clicking a broken link is not the only way to end up with a non-page issue. It could also be that a web address was incorrectly entered directly into the address bar.

Testing your website (cont.)

Jargon buster

World Wide Web Consortium: An organisation that sets many of the standards used on the web. Often referred to as the W3C (*www.w3.org*).

When you enter the address for one of your web pages you will get back a list of errors that were found. You then fix the errors and test again. You will probably need to do this a few times until all the errors have gone. Is this necessary? No, not really. However, it is considered good practice for a webmaster to follow.

Another great utility for finding issues with your website is Google Webmaster Tools. You need a Google account to use this, but don't worry, it is easy to join Google. Just go to *www.google.com*, click the Sign In link and then follow the link to create an account.

Google Webmaster Tools is one of many services Google provides. With this particular one, you add a site (or sites) to the tool and then can get a report about your site. Figure 16-4 shows such an overview. From this you can find information about links and more.

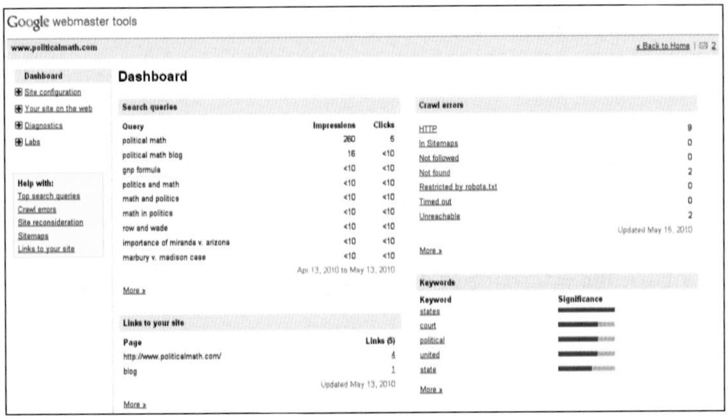

Figure 16-4 Google Webmaster Tools

Analytics tells you about visits, visitor behaviour and other important data about what is happening with your site. Picture this – you have a website with six pages and you find that most people never look at more than the first one they see (known as the bounce rate). Why? The reason clearly is that an immediate impression of any of the pages on your site is not a good one. This is a good example of what analytics is for.

Now turn this around a bit. People are visiting five of the pages regularly, but barely does that sixth page get seen. Why? Probably because it is not easy to find from the navigation or menu system on the site. You have to dig around and figure that one out.

Unless you have put a site on the internet just to show friends and family, then analytics is key to running your site. Traffic – how many people come to your site – is something you want to keep growing. Some of that traffic will be repeat visitors. In other words, they have come to your site more than once. Well, that's great. But you also want to have new people coming to your site too.

There are many analytic tools and utilities. Some are very simple, such as the logs that your ISP keeps about your site. At the other end of the scale are costly, high-level packages that provide a wealth of information. These are often used by busy, high-traffic sites that can justify the price for the analytical package.

And there is Google Analytics. This is a free utility provided by Google that shows you quite a bit about what people are doing on your site. When you have an account with Google, you can set up analytics. It works by putting some JavaScript near the bottom of each page on your site. Google provides the exact instructions and also generates the snippet of code that you need.

Analytics

16

Analytics (cont.)

Once you have put the JavaScript into the pages and uploaded them, analytical data will begin to appear within, typically, a few days – the site needs some visits to report on! Google Analytics provides reports on as many sites as you enter to have tracked. Each one will have a different bit of JavaScript code to keep the data unique to each site. Figure 16-5 shows the top-level view of Google Analytics. As you can see, a number of sites is included. Some have good numbers to report, some not so good – this is in regard to percentage change, green (up) or red (down).

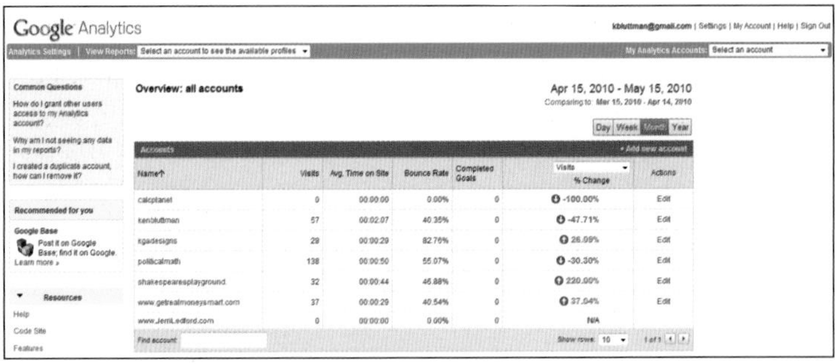

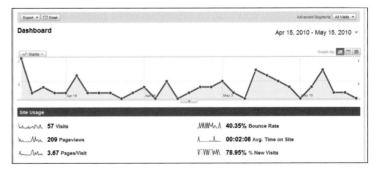

Figure 16-5 Overview page of Google Analytics

From the overview you can drill down to a single site and get further statistics. Figure 16-6 shows a drill-down into *www. kenbluttman.com*. In a period of one month there were 57 visitors. On average they viewed 3.67 pages and spent an average of 2 minutes and 8 seconds on the site. Of these visits, 78.95% were new – from visitors coming for the first time. The bounce rate was 40.35%.

Figure 16-6 Overview of website activity

What do these numbers mean? Although the number of visits was small, a visitor on average looked at three pages at least. That's not bad – their interest did not diminish upon entering the site. To back this up the bounce rate was around just 40%. Taken another way, more than half of visitors stuck around.

With the information here alone, goals could be set, such as attracting more traffic or getting people to spend more time on the site. Improving the numbers requires various approaches. For example, to encourage more visitors you could visit other sites with blogs where you can leave comments – and you can leave your URL. Or you could write articles and submit them to article directories such as Ezine Articles (*http://ezinearticles. com*). Article directories always let you have an 'author block' where you can give a quick blurb about yourself or product and have URLs that link back to your site. These 'backlinks' bring traffic and also help raise your positioning in search engine results.

Google Analytics breaks out the data into useful areas. Figure 16-7 shows four major areas – Visitors Overview, Map Overlay, Traffic Sources Overview and Content Overview. Drilling down into these areas provides more information. Note that each area has a view report link.

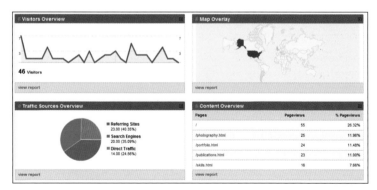

Figure 16-7 Different ways to use analytics

Analytics (cont.)

Drilling down into the Visitors Overview I can find out that of the 57 visits, 45 were new visitors and 12 were returning visitors. Of the 45 new visitors, further drilling down shows where they came from. Some were direct (the person typed in the URL in their address bar), 20 came as a result of Google searches and the rest came from a variety of other sites. This is all seen in Figure 16-8.

Visits		Pages/Visit		Avg. Time on Site	
45		**3.60**		**00:01:29**	
% of Site Total: 78.95%		Site Avg: 3.67 (-1.82%)		Site Avg: 00:02:08 (-30.57%)	

	Source ⌄	None ⌄	Visits ▾ ↓	Visits
1.	■ google		20	44.44%
2.	■ (direct)		12	26.67%
3.	■ headfirstlabs.com		4	8.89%
4.	▫ guru.com		2	4.44%
5.	■ homeschoolphonebook.com		2	4.44%
6.	■ images.google.com		2	4.44%
7.	▫ kgadesigns.com		2	4.44%
8.	▫ monstersearchengine.com		1	2.22%

Figure 16-8 Sources of new visitors

From the Traffic Sources Overview I can drill down to see what keywords were used in search engines that led to visits. Not surprisingly, several were variations of my name, but other search phrases such as 'funny food photography' brought traffic to the site. See Figure 16-9.

	Keyword ⌄	None ⌄	Visits ↓
1.	ken bluttman		5
2.	"first day of sixth grade"		1
3.	bluttman		1
4.	bluttman ken		1
5.	bluttman, ken		1
6.	food photography		1
7.	funny food photography		1
8.	ironies of world		1
9.	ken bluttman.com		1
10.	kenbluttman		1

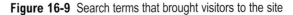

Figure 16-9 Search terms that brought visitors to the site

The Content Overview is useful to see the popularity of the various site pages, shown in Figure 16-10. Usually the page with the highest view is the home page, which is indicated simply with a slash (/). The next most popular page is photography.html.

Page	None ⌄	Pageviews ↓	Unique Pageviews
1.	/	55	43
2.	/photography.html	25	13
3.	/portfolio.html	24	15
4.	/publications.html	23	13
5.	/skills.html	16	13
6.	/blog/	12	10
7.	/contact.html	12	8
8.	/index.html	10	8
9.	/foodfun.html	5	5
10.	/nature.html	4	4

Figure 16-10 Pages ranked by view popularity

Google Analytics can do much more than is shown here. You can tie it in with goal setting, with AdWords campaigns and more. For example, of the 53 visits, I could see that three came from visitors viewing the site on their iPhone.

Marketing your site

A site on the net is a site unseen by many unless you take the steps to promote it. This is not simplistic work and takes dedication. Always be on the lookout for opportunities to get your site known. The activities involved do not even have to be done on the internet. If you are running a business, all your letterheads, business cards and other office items that end up in the hands of clients should carry your web address.

Your email signature block is a great place to put your website name, web address and a blurb about your site. Talk to people about your site. Let the entrepreneur in you do its thing and keep the focus on increasing traffic.

On the internet, these activities are all helpful in increasing traffic, keeping people coming back and increasing knowledge of who you are and what you do:

- Keep a constant stream of new content added to your site. This is typically in the form of a blog, but it can also be updates of pages, colour schemes or any other techniques that make people take notice. But do keep content as the leading factor in all this. You may find that constant new content is difficult to come up with. In this case outsource to writers. There is a world of freelance writers itching for the chance to make some money to provide you with quality content. Visit the various freelance sites and explore how this all works. Some top sites are Guru (*www.guru.com*), Scriptlance (*www.scriptlance.com*) and Get A Coder (*www.getacoder.com*)

- Submit articles to article directories. You (or someone you hire) writes an article that is of the same interest that your site is about. You submit it to the directory and it has the possibility of being seen and used (read the terms of service) by many people. An article always carries a link back to the URL that you designate so the thought of someone stealing your work should not be of great concern. In this arena are many sites, including Ezine Articles (*http://ezinearticles.com*), isnare (*www.isnare.com*), and Article Dashboard (*www.articledashboard.com*).

- Follow blogs and add comments to relevant postings. When you do so, include a link back to your site.

- Build a mailing list. You can have this feature on your site – where people click to be added to your list. You can maintain the list yourself but should consider using a service such as Constant Contact (*www.constantcontact.com*). The laws are testy with what is considered spam, whether a person 'opted in' to receive emails and so on. By using a service this burden is removed from your plate. Of course, don't ignore your list. Prepare a monthly newsletter, offer a coupon for shopping on the site, or whatever makes sense. Think this all through before collecting names. You may have heard that it is important to have a list, but this is different from a typical client list that a salesperson might keep. People enter their information and expect something in return. Don't disappoint them or you will lose them.

- Make use of an AdWords campaign (*https://adwords.google. co.uk*). AdWords is another Google goodie. It is advertising, but certainly not the traditional type. With AdWords you bid on certain keywords or phrases that match the content you have on your site. You may or may not win a bid as others could be bidding on the same keywords. What you are bidding on is the cost per click of an advertisement. AdWords are shown as ads all over the internet. When someone clicks on one of yours, it costs you the bid amount (for example, you might have bid €1 to have the phrase 'dog collar'). This means when someone clicks on your ad it costs you €1. Luckily you can control how much you want to spend each day. The person clicks the ad, is brought to your site and hopefully your site is compelling enough to make a sale. You can tie in your AdWords campaigns into Google Analytics and see how your pay per click (PPC) effort is succeeding.

- Prepare a YouTube video. This is very effective as visitors get to see something that is more than just a static picture and text. Videos are great for displaying your products, your company, yourself or whatever it is that your site is about.

Marketing your site (cont.)

- Use SEO (search engine marketing). This is making the best match of your content to what people are searching for. A goal is to rank high in SERPs (search engine result pages). The higher your listing, the more likely it is that people will click to go to your site. SEO is an art unto itself and beyond the scope here. In essence, there is organic SEO – the concept that your content is exactly what it should be without the need to play games with it. The other side of SEO is to explore keywords, with regard to what people enter when searching and adjusting your content to match. There are sites and tools that analyse keywords. A popular site for this is Wordtracker (*www.wordtracker.com*).

- Create interfaces between your site and popular social networking sites such as Facebook and Twitter.

- Lastly, stay on top of internet trends. The internet is a dynamic arena and the rules and best practices change constantly. Social networking is a perfect example. A few years ago it had little meaning. Now it is paramount. Don't get left behind. Update your site to keep up with what is popular.

Jargon buster

ASP/ASPX – Active Server Pages (Classic version and .Net version) – a server side programming language.

Body – a HTML tag. Visible parts of a web page are in between the opening and closing Body tags.

CSS – Cascading Style Sheets. This is the browser side programming language that provides styling to web page elements.

CYMK – a subtractive colouring system used more for print than web pages. Stands for Cyan, Yellow, Magenta and Black. Mixing varying amounts of these colours provides the full colour spectrum.

DTD – Document Type Declaration. The top line in the source code of a HTML page. Defines certain behaviour of the page, and defines the variant of HTML to be used on the page. There are many DTDs. The two most common are Strict and Transitional. See *www.w3c.org* for more information.

Encryption – a method of taking understandable text and making it garbled and unreadable. It becomes readable again when a key and algorithm are applied. The purpose for the most part is to have sensitive data be unreadable during transmission (such as from your web browser to a web server).

FTP – File Transfer Protocol. The standard method for transferring files to and from a web server and another computer.

Golden Ratio – a number, approximately 1.618, that is applied to measuring out elements of a design. It is often associated with geometric shapes such as a pentagon. The Golden Ratio has been known for thousands of years and is represented by the Greek letter phi. Research the Golden Ratio and you can find examples of how it has been used in construction and even appears in nature.

Head – The top part of a HTML page. It comes after the DTD and before the Body.

HTML – Hypertext Markup Language. The programming language used to make web pages. Some do not consider it a programming language because it does not have the ability to do many of the sophisticated functions a full programming language can. HTML consists of tags – which the web browser reads and then displays the appropriate visual elements.

HTTP – Hypertext Transfer Protocol. The method for which data moves between a web server and a web browser.

HTTPS – Hypertext Transfer Protocol Secure. This is a method for moving data between a web server and a web browser, but encrypts the data for the transfer. It is a secure method used on the web for when sensitive information is needed, such as a credit card number to make an online purchase.

Inline – often termed with regard to CSS. CSS (for styling web page elements) is often used by a web page by linking to an external CSS file. However CSS can be put directly into a web page, either between a set of style tags (`<style></style>`) or directly within a HTML tag; for example `<input type="text" style="color: red;" />`. The indication of the colour being red is the inline CSS.

JavaScript – a web programming language that works in the web browser instead of the web server. It is a powerful language that is used subjectively for three purposes – animation, calculations and form input validation.

PHP – a server side programming language, possibly the most popular one in use. The acronym originally was for Personal Home Page, but has long since instead been for Hypertext Preprocessor.

Pixel – a single addressable point on a computer monitor. Pixels are so small they blend together to create one continuous image. The resolution of a computer screen is expressed in pixels. For example a screen resolution of 1,366 × 768 means there are 1,366 pixels horizontally on the screen (the width), and 768 pixels in the vertical direction (the height). Each pixel displays a colour.

RGB – Red, Green, Blue. An additive colour model used for rendering colours on computer screens (such as in a web browser). Each of the three colours can have a value between 0 and 255. This allows for over 16 million colour combinations.

Rule of Thirds – a design principle that states a visual image is best composed by dividing the image space into evenly spaced horizontal and vertical thirds, and having key elements of the image be placed along a border or at the intersection of a horizontal and vertical border. The immediate effect of this is that the key element of an image does not appear in the centre.

Tag – A HTML element. HTML is composed of tags, such as `<body>`, `<div>`, `<form>`, and `<img>`. There are dozens of tags. Getting familiar with them is a good objective for a web designer. Even though designers often use a graphics program that shields them from the HTML, being aware of it is often helpful.

Title – a HTML tag that appears inside the Head tag. The value of the Title tag determines what is seen in the head of the browser or tab of the browser. For example, a construct such as `<title>My Web Page</title>` will cause the browser to show My Web Page in the header area of the browser (each browser does this a bit differently).

Validator – an online utility that reviews the structure of a web page and reports back errors about the HTML or other parts of the page. A popular one is at *http://validator.w3.org*. You enter the web page to be validated and results are returned about errors (or hopefully that no errors were found). When errors are found, you can then fix the web page to correct the errors and try the validator again – do this repeatedly until all errors are gone.

W3C – an international community that works to set standards for the web. It is found at *http://www.w3.org*.

Wireframe – a simplified representation of a web page used during the design process. In essence, it resembles the web page but with areas marked off where text and graphics will eventually go.

Troubleshooting guide

Full colour, step-by-step guides to get you working more efficiently and creatively on your computer

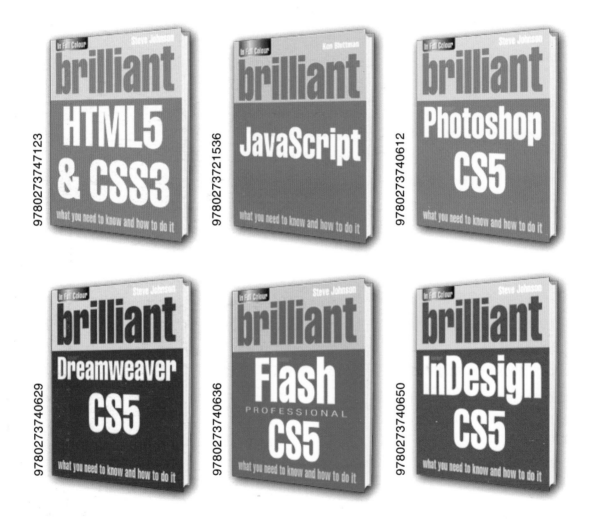

Explore exciting new design possibilities, achieve superior results and produce exactly the images you want

Prentice Hall
is an imprint of

PEARSON